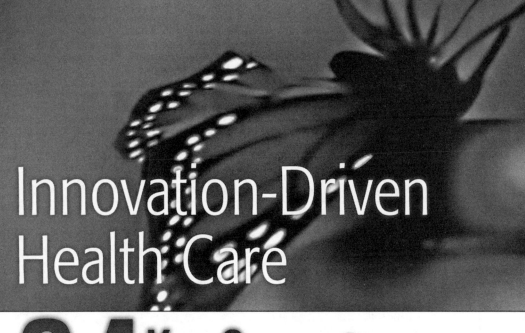

Innovation-Driven Health Care

34 Key Concepts for Transformation

Richard L. Reece, MD
Editor-in-Chief, *Physician Practice Options*
Medical Advisory Board, *America's Top Doctors*
Historian, Center for Practical Health Reform

JONES AND BARTLETT PUBLISHERS
Sudbury, Massachusetts
BOSTON   TORONTO   LONDON   SINGAPORE

World Headquarters

Jones and Bartlett Publishers	Jones and Bartlett Publishers	Jones and Bartlett Publishers
40 Tall Pine Drive	Canada	International
Sudbury, MA 01776	6339 Ormindale Way	Barb House, Barb Mews
978-443-5000	Mississauga, Ontario	London W6 7PA
info@jbpub.com	L5V 1J2	UK
www.jbpub.com	CANADA	

Jones and Bartlett's books and products are available through most bookstores and online booksellers. To contact Jones and Bartlett Publishers directly, call 800-832-0034, fax 978-443-8000, or visit our website www.jbpub.com.

Substantial discounts on bulk quantities of Jones and Bartlett's publications are available to corporations, professional associations, and other qualified organizations. For details and specific discount information, contact the special sales department at Jones and Bartlett via the above contact information or send an email to specialsales@jbpub.com.

Production Credits
Executive Editor: David Cella
Production Editor: Renée Sekerak
Editorial Assistant: Lisa Gordon
Production Assistant: Mike Boblitt
Associate Marketing Manager: Jennifer Bengtson
Composition: Auburn Associates, Inc.
Manufacturing Buyer: Amy Bacus
Cover Design: Anne Spencer
Senior Photo Researcher and Photographer: Kimberly Potvin
Cover Image: © Tracy Siermachesky/ShutterStock, Inc.
Printing and Binding: Malloy, Inc.
Cover Printing: Malloy, Inc.

Library of Congress Cataloging-in-Publication Data
Reece, Richard L.
  Innovation-driven health care : 34 key concepts for transformation / Richard L. Reece.
    p. ; cm.
  Includes bibliographical references.
  ISBN-13: 978-0-7637-4681-0
  ISBN-10: 0-7637-4681-9
  1. Health care reform—United States. 2. Medical innovations. 3. Diffusion of innovations. I. Title.
  [DNLM: 1. Health Care Reform—United States. 2. Diffusion of Innovation—United States.
  3. Entrepreneurship—United States. WA 540 AA1 281i 2007]
  RA395.A3R374 2007
  362.10973—dc22

                      2006100263

6048

Printed in the United States of America
11 10 09 08 07 10 9 8 7 6 5 4 3 2 1

To Loretta for everything

Richard (Dick) Reece is that rare breed of physician commentator who admires his colleagues. How long has it been since you read an article in a medical or health policy journal that applauded the skill and compassion of doctors, scientists, and administrators and/or bemoaned their increasing loss of autonomy to health insurers and governments? Well, you won't read about how greedy and incompetent they are in *Innovation-Driven Health Care: 34 Key Concepts for Transformation.*

What you will read is an intelligent, knowledgeable analysis of the impact of innovations on the future of U.S. health care; and it's supportive, too. As Dick says, God love him, "being a physician is being part of a brotherhood or sisterhood."

But why should you read yet another health care future book? Because Dick Reece has nailed it: His view of the future is exactly right. If you want to continue doing what you are doing, this book will enable you to assess how you fit into this new world and to adapt yourself if needed.

I had the good fortune to meet Dick Reece some 30 years ago at the Harvard Business School's Program for Health Systems Management. Then, as now, Dick was a big man with a gruff affect, piercing intellect, heart of gold, and a sunny, bemused view of life.

I learned of the qualities because I taught Dick accounting in the program, a course that quickly separates the intellectual and emotional wheat from the chaff—the analysts from the analyzed; the "let's-cut-costs" types from the "let's–increase-productivity" ones; and those with a sense of humor (believe me, you need this quality in an accounting course) from the deadly serious.

These qualities inform *Innovation-Driven Health Care.*

However, Dick is not merely a cheerleader. He believes that innovations will increase the productivity of the U.S. health care system so that it can provide better services, at a better price, to more people. What a contrast to the usual dour prescribers who contend that innovation is impossible and improved productivity a myth. Their cure? Uncle Sam rations health care. Hello, Canada!

To make the importance of this point of view concrete, consider the following excerpt:

Almost immediately (after the introduction of CAT scanning), political objections arose to widespread use of this new imaging technology. HEW Secretary Joseph Califano rose on his political haunches and declared, "There are enough CAT Scanners in Southern California for the entire western United States." (Califano, 1977)

Not to be outdone, Dr. Howard Hiatt, dean for the Harvard School of Public Health, compared the use of CT scanners to overgrazed medical commons in which too many were foraging for too little. He said a national center for technology assessment and suppression of new technologies should be established and argued:

There is no doubt that the scanners provide additional diagnostic information, and frequently with less discomfort and hazard to the patient, however, it is not clear that the diagnostic information very often leads to a better outcome for the patient. Until this important information is available from careful studies, would we not be better served limiting the use of such expensive technology. (1976)

Califano and Hiatt overestimated the power of federal regulations and underestimated the thirst of doctors and the public for this clearly superior technology. Neurosurgeons immediately embraced CT scans. Their enthusiasm soon spread to orthopedic surgeons, who saw the potential of MRIs for joint, bone, and soft-tissue imaging. Most recently, oncologists have welcomed PET scans to check for subtle cancer spread. CT and MRI scanning has become the modus operandi for evaluating all manner of physiological anomalies.

In 2001, 225 internists, when asked to evaluate the relative importance of 30 medical technologies, rated CT and MRI scans as the "number one innovation" (Fuchs & Sox, 2001).

However, Reece is no ideologue. He is a pragmatist. With illuminating case studies, he provides news you can use, as illustrated by the following examples:

- How stand-alone, onesie-twosie physician practices can thrive.
- How to make your intellect, training, and experience work for you, if you want to leave medicine.
- How to empower consumers and embrace new high-deductible health plans without disemboweling yourself.
- How large groups—Mayo, Kaiser—have avoided "mid-life" crises.
- How to flourish in insurer–physician and hospital–physician relationships, which are typically more akin to the relationship between a salmon and a bear.

I have merely mentioned only five of the 34 topics in this book. If you want to know more, read on!

Why am I so sure that Dick Reece's views of the future are right? It's not only that he agrees with my own views, but also, and, more importantly, because he has been right so often before. For example, a dozen years ago, as chairman of a physician hospital organization, Dick created the case-based pricing that payers are finally coming to some 20 years later. And while living in the midst of managed care-loving Minnesota, Dick predicted the threat HMOs posed to physicians. The observation, which now seems obvious, was radical when he made it—a quarter century ago.

Best of all, Dick's sunny belief in the transformative powers of innovation are mirrored by his bright, witty writing style. Here are some samples:

> Question: What do you call farmers who convert fallow into fertile ground?
>
> Answer: Farmers with a sense of humus.

And on pay for performance: "An ounce of performance is worth a pound of lucre." It's great to laugh, especially when the laughter is accompanied by such useful advice.

Regina E. Herzlinger
Harvard Business School

Endnotes

Califano, Joseph. (1977). "Remarks Before the American Medical Association." *Minnesota Medicine 60:* 601–605.

Fuchs, V., & Sox, H. (2001). Physicians' views of the relative importance of thirty medical innovations. *Health Affairs, 20,* 30–42.

Hiatt, Howard. "Too Much Medical Technology?" *Wall Street Journal* (1976, June 24), p. 1.

This book contains six parts:

1. **SMALL-PRACTICE INNOVATIONS:** Seventy to 80 percent of American doctors practice solo or in groups of 10 or less. Health industry changes threaten these physicians. These changes may even make primary care doctors obsolete. Health care innovations favor larger groups. In these chapters, new practice models and innovations within existing practices that tell of innovations allowing small practices to survive and thrive are described.

2. **LARGE-GROUP INNOVATIONS:** Twelve percent of physicians practice in groups of 50 or more. Most often these doctors are in multispecialty groups, academic faculty practices, and, to a lesser extent, single specialty groups. Because of greater capital, technological expertise, and other resources, these groups often create major innovations. Experienced practice managers, economies of scale, and physician teamwork make innovations work well.

3. **HOSPITAL–PHYSICIAN JOINT VENTURE INNOVATIONS:** Hospital–doctor joint ventures may be the largest enterprise in any given town or region. These ventures may be detached walk-in units offering surgical, diagnostic, and imaging services. This part relates stories of why hospitals and doctors seek higher ground and market leverage, often against one other. One development that may bring hospitals and physicians closer together is regional health information organizations (RHIOs).

4. **EMPLOYER AND HEALTH PLAN INNOVATIONS:** Employers pay 54 percent of total health costs. Business owners and health plans innovate to save money, raise quality, and please employees and provider clients. This is perhaps the newest and most fertile ground for innovations, as owners and health plans struggle to cut costs. They are now focusing on using technologies to manage consumers who are buying and using health care on retail, rather than entitlement, basis.

5. **CONSTRAINING COSTS AND EXPANDING MARKETS:** These sometimes contradictory twin issues are central to health reform. Innovations to reduce costs have been sparse. Innovations will multiply as costs escalate, information

technologies grow, and data mining matures. The health industry will have no other choice but to reduce costs. At the same time, companies want to expand market share. As a rule of thumb, if no growth occurs, margins shrink, and stockholders and stakeholders become unhappy. This combination may cause the firing of executives and will not be tolerated for long.

6. **CONSUMER INNOVATIONS:** The consumer movement is young, but it is rocketing to the ascendancy. It drives many innovations as physicians, hospitals, and health plans strive to lure consumers and make them the health system centerpiece.

How Each Chapter Is Organized

Each chapter kicks off with a brief prelude and quote or quotes. The prelude sums up the essence of what follows. Sometimes a quote comes from an historical figure. More often the source is a recent newspaper account. Most quotes are contemporaneous. Following the quote is a discussion of the innovation involved: its background, relevance, and impact.

On occasion, I describe a commercial company's innovation. In medical journalism, it is a "no-no" to highlight a single company—but truly innovative ideas may start with entrepreneurs who launch small companies. They sense a niche, they want to make a difference, and they go for broke—often the consequence of risk-taking ventures.

A tongue-in-cheek entrepreneur once said, "There is nothing mysterious about innovation. It's about niches—and sons of niches."

- Consider the entrepreneurial spin-offs from Healthcare Corporation of America (HCA) in Nashville. Nashville now has over 300 for-profit innovative health care-related enterprises.
- Think of Boston's Medical Industrial Complex with its nexus of academic medical centers and health care firms sprouting around Route 128.
- Look at Minnesota's Medical Alley stretching from Rochester to the Twin Cities, with the Mayo Clinic, Medtronic, St. Jude Medical Inc., UnitedHealth Group, MinuteClinic, and the 800 registered medical device manufacturers. Innovation breeds replication and transformation.

A section entitled "Innovation Talking and Action Points" highlights what has been said, what lies ahead, and what type of innovation was discussed.

Most chapters end with one or more case studies. I have written a few of these case studies; mostly, however, I call upon others more informed of the topic. Case studies vary in style and format. Some are more classic case studies while others are commentaries and company profiles. In soliciting case studies, I did not seek sameness; I simply asked case-study authors to "tell your story in your own words."

The Glue

As you read through these six parts, information technologies' central role in innovation takes shape. These technologies glue together health care innovations, reduce costs, ease use, and improve care and outcomes. For example, today's doctors submit 75 percent of claims online, thereby improving payment rates, turnaround time, and accuracy. Four years ago, that figure was 44 percent. This rapid rise in e-claims submission—that is, the rate at which doctors submit claims online—shows how fast IT catches fire in health care when it fills a needed niche; in this case, the need is prompt payment for doctors whose accounts receivables are spinning out of control.

The Book

This is not a health policy, health reform, or politically correct book. It is the view of one man who sees U.S. health care as it is, not the way it ought to be; who has been there, done that—and seen that; and who has talked, listened, and observed those who have seen it—and done it.

This book does not defend U.S. health care. It explains it. It is pragmatic, not phlegmatic. It preaches action, not reaction. It is more about technology than ideology. It espouses energy—and synergy. It speaks of proinnovation need, rather than preaching any antigovernment screed. It is more contextual than intellectual. It seeks clarity, verity, and parity between market and government sectors, rather than ideological purity. It is about restructuring the health care infrastructure. It is about how the here and now may lead to the then and there.

Consider:

- If you think of yourself as a humanitarian, remember that through innovations, one can always better the health of the well and the care of the sick.
- If you regard yourself as a cultural anthropologist, keep in mind the U.S. culture and its never-ending search for innovations shape our values and our health care.
- If you are an innovator and entrepreneur, think of this book as a string of nuggets waiting to be mined and refined.

Please enjoy this book; I certainly enjoyed writing it.

Richard L. Reece, MD
Old Saybrook, Connecticut
August 1, 2006

Acknowledgments

To "acknowledge," Webster's New World Dictionary, Second College Edition, says is "to confess, avow, or admit the existence, reality, or truth of."

I confess writing this book has been a labor of love. I love being a doctor, a student of care delivery, an admirer of those who work within health care's boundaries, and a servant for patients, who have been patient long enough and who should welcome the new patient-centric system.

I confess this book has too few profundities (wisdom is not my strong suit) and too many redundancies (these are inevitable when one writes of health care's overlapping sectors, functions, and vectors). I avow, and openly admit, the truth of the reality that I could not have done it alone.

I thank:

My wife, Loretta, who supported me every step of the way. She thought I had something fresh, immediate, even historic to say. I have tried to justify her faith.

My editor, Dave Cella, and his editorial assistant at Jones and Bartlett, Lisa Gordon, who have gently led me down the winding path of producing a good book, pointing out bear traps, pratfalls, potholes, boulders, and sharp turns along the way.

My computer, a Dell, that held up throughout the writing of the book. It allowed me to till more easily the literary ground. When I sat before the blank screen, I was reminded of the nursery rhyme: "The farmer in the dell, the farmer in the dell, Heigho! the derry, oh, the farmer in the dell." This reminder prompted me to start plowing new ground.

Finally, I thank those whom I quoted or who wrote the case studies that follow each of the 34 chapters. In my opinion, the case studies make the book, by taking it out of the abstract and setting it in the concrete. For Chapter 22, about runaway imaging costs, I had a coauthor, Brian Baker. I was out of my depth technologically, and I needed his knowledge.

Contents

About the Author

Richard L. Reece, MD, is a pathologist, writer, editor, consultant, and speaker. This is his eighth book. He was educated at Duke University and the Duke University School of Medicine and did his postgraduate training at Hartford Hospital and an 8-week stint at Harvard Business School.

He resides in Old Saybrook, Connecticut, with his wife, Loretta, a former nurse, and Paris, a male French bulldog of impeccable heritage. Dr. Reece and his wife have two sons: Spencer, who lives in Juno Beach, Florida, and Carter, a resident of New York City. Dr. Reece can be reached at rreece1500@aol.com. To read more of Dr. Reece's writings on health care innovation, visit his blog: http://www.medinnovationblog.blogspot.com

Other Books by Richard L. Reece, MD

A Collection of Editorials from Minnesota Medicine, 1975–1982. (1982).

And Who Shall Care for the Sick? The Corporate Transformation of Medicine in Minnesota. (1988)

A Managed Care Memoir: A Physician's Whistle-Stop Journey, 1988–2003. (2003)

Hello Health Care Consumer: The Transformation of the Patient-Doctor-Hospital-Health Plan Relationships in America. (2004)

Paris, the Blue French Bulldog. (2004)

Voices of Practical Health Reform: Interviews with Health Care Stakeholders at Work Options for Repackaging American Health Care. (2005)

Sailing the Seven "Cs" of Hospital–Physician Relationships: Competence, Convenience, Clarity, Continuity, Control, Cash, and Competition with James A. Hawkins. (2006)

Past Innovations

During the past thirty years, an unprecedented number of innovations have had great clinical and economic importance for U.S. medicine. New medications, new diagnostic techniques, and new surgical procedures have helped millions of patients to live longer, better-quality lives.

At the same time, leading health economists believe technological advance is the major cause of rising expenditures. The need to compare the value to patients of new technologies with their effect on spending is a major source of tension among physicians, hospitals, patients, insurance companies, and government policymakers.

Victor Fuchs and Harold Sox, Jr., 2001

Present and Future Innovations

I see five huge innovations going forward:

1. *Consumer-driven health care*

2. *Chronic care management*

3. *Health care IT (particularly tools for consumers to better manage and pay for their health care)*

4. *Public–private partnerships to manage care for seniors (Medicare) and the disadvantaged (Medicaid)*

5. *Customized care centers (chains to deliver high quality, cost-effective patient services locally, regionally, and nationally)*

The regulatory environment has got to change to allow these innovations to occur. We've got to open up Stark, eliminate corporate practice laws, eliminate Certificate of Need, and eliminate a few other things, too.

Brooks O'Neil, senior analyst, Avondale Partners, 2006

Part One

Small-Practice Innovations

The elephant in the living room in what we're trying to do is the small physician practices. That's the hardest problem, and it will bring this effort to its knees if we fail.

**David Brailer, then national coordinator
of Health Information Technology, 2005**

Chapter 1

American Health Care Innovates

The entrepreneurial disciplines are not just desirable; they are conditions for survival.

Peter F. Drucker, 2004

It's never too late to innovate. You can always do better.

Anonymous

In this book, I lay bare the ins and outs of innovative processes. I tell why innovation is important; I explain why innovation contributes so much to American health care's vitality and viability.

"Innovations" differ from "issues." *Issues* tend to be political, divisive, insoluble, and despairing. Where you stand, in other words, depends on where you sit. *Innovations*, on the other hand, may transcend politics, heal old wounds, inspire hope, and even solve vexing problems in a practical and impersonal fashion. Where you stand depends on who benefits—and how much. It boils down to win-win, win-loss, and loss-loss situations. A win-win is another word for innovation.

Policymakers say health reform is at worst in gridlock; at best in a state of quivering Brownian movement. I do not believe it. Many things, good things, are going on. They are just beneath the surface, often beyond the reach of those who make and preach policy changes to conform to their philosophies.

Bottom-Up Innovations, Not Top-Down Impramateurs

While the nation debates a single-payer versus a market-based health system, significant, underreported innovations are blossoming under the radar. These innovations mostly bubble up from the marketplace, rather than filtering down from government. Whether by marketplace innovation or government action, Americans are seeking a system offering prompt access to affordable, compassionate, and effective care.

Voices of Health Reform

In *Voices of Health Reform* (2005), I interviewed 41 national health care stakeholders, concluding that superimposing a government system upon existing health care infrastructures was unlikely to happen soon.

Three political realities support that conclusion:

1. Congress has been debating universal coverage off and on since 1912 without resolution.
2. Medicare and Medicaid are the two fastest growing federal entitlements, and Congress will blink before extending either to cover everybody unless the country has a deep depression, a worldwide war, or an overwhelming national disaster.
3. A "universal" program requiring tax increases will be a hard sell to Americans. (Reece, 2005c)

Here is what E. J. Dionne, a *Washington Post* columnist, said about selling universality, after a universal child preschool care program went down to a resounding 61–39 defeat in California.

> *Hardest of all is the issue of "universality." In principle, programs that cover everyone—Social Security and Medicare are prime examples—are usually better programs and commend broad political support. But universal programs carry large price tags. In retrospect, is there a lesson here on how to expand health insurance coverage? Realism is not the enemy of idealism, and taxpayers aren't selfish just because they place a heavy burden on those who would ask them to part with some of their money. Advocates of public action need to meet that test. (Dionne, 2006)*

Innovations tend to be realistic; reformations idealistic. Pragmatic Americans lean toward the real rather than the ideal.

Innovation alone will not lift U.S. health care to where it ought to be. As Dr. George Lundberg, editor of *Medscape General Journal,* observed:

> *Yes, there are lots of innovations, and a lot of them might be very helpful, but we're talking about 293 million people, and innovations tend to be limited and localized. For the masses, innovation would have to propagate like crazy.* (Reece, 2005c)

The government must pitch in to improve health care—but government by itself, however well intentioned, cannot improve care. It may impose equity. Equity does not ensure quality or access. Instead it may induce stagnation. Government is a muscle-bound giant. It cannot flexibly adapt or completely control health care marketplace events in a vast decentralized continental nation. It can, however, lead by inspiring public-private partnerships.

New Directions, "But..."

Innovations are pushing health care in new directions. These innovations may be more powerful than rules being imposed from Washington, D.C., and state capitals. "But," as Dr. Regina Herzlinger (2006b), the nation's leading consumer-driven care advocate, says in a *Harvard Business School* article, "strong forces undermine health care innovations." To understand why, she says one must examine forces constraining innovations. Here are some innovations Dr. Herzlinger says are now making health care better and cheaper:

1. those involving how consumers buy and use health care
2. those that are technology enabled or technology driven
3. those producing new business models

Unfortunately, the health care system often blocks these innovations. Sometimes, organizations can overcome barriers by managing six forces affecting health care players.

Six Forces Shaping Health Care Innovation

1. *friends and foes* helping or destroying innovations
2. *funding* differing from funding in other industries
3. *policies and regulations* handicapping innovations
4. *technologies* making health care delivery more efficient and convenient
5. *consumers* of health care
6. *safe, cost-effective, and accountable innovations* demanded by health plans, consumers, and government

Add to these six forces the belief among some that the United States has a cruel health system. It is a system, they believe, driving people into bankruptcy while letting them bleed, even die in the streets. They believe all people everywhere are morally entitled to government-sponsored universal care. These beliefs pose political and psychological barriers to market-based entrepreneurship and innovation because there are only so many resources to go around for both public and private sectors.

Market-based care, as with all things human, may fail to protect all, will let a few people fall through cracks, and may partially shred the safety net. So, too, do government systems, a seldom-mentioned truth. It would be great, of course, for all health care stakeholders and government technocrats to act for the common good, not their own self-interests, but that would require repealing the laws of human nature and of Adam Smith.

It may be the public, business, and government will unite to build momentum for universal, or at least mandatory, coverage as a moral imperative. However, many do not see a big move toward universal coverage taking place soon.

Infant Mortalities, Life Expectancies, Uninsured, and Costs

U.S. health care critics and universal coverage advocates routinely trot out four statistics:

1. The United States ranks 17th in infant mortality.
2. The country is rated 22nd in life expectancy.
3. Forty-five million people are uninsured in the United States.
4. The country spends 50 percent more than any other nation. (WorldHealth Organization, 1997)

Critics argue these numbers flow from lack of universal coverage, limited government regulation, "fragmentation" of the system, and racial biases. It follows no amount of innovation, short of sweeping federal health policy changes and the remaking of American cultural values, will right these wrongs. There is some truth to these arguments, but governments cannot and will not solve all health problems.

- First, national health systems, despite their social justice virtues, marginally affect life expectancies. Better health habits often lead to longer lives than broader health coverage does.

  Consider centenarians living in remote villages in Ecuador, Hunza in Kashmir, Abkazian in Georgia, or in Okinawa. In a closely reasoned book, *The Health of Nations: True Causes of Sickness and Well-Being* (1987), Dr. Leonard Sagan, a Stanford-based epidemiologist, observed health care systems have *little to do* with reducing death rates or extending average life expectancy. Sagan says social, family, and personal factors loom larger than health coverage.

"Technical fixes," he says, "only marginally affect longevity." (See Table 1–1.) Medical care accounts for about 15 percent of the health status of any given population, life style for 20 percent to 30 percent, and other factors—poverty, inferior education, income differences, and lack of social cohesion—for the other 55 percent (Satcher and Pamies, 2006).

- Americans may spend more on health because of the vibrant U.S. economy, higher discretionary incomes, and strong belief in powers of medical technologies to "fix" anything that goes wrong. As Dr. Iona Heath, a general practitioner in London, shrewdly observed, "I have heard it said that the U.S. believes more in the perfectibility of humanity and the role of science than Europeans" (Kolota, 2006a).
- The uninsured are a mixed lot. Some choose to be uninsured. Some choose to pay out of pocket. A Colorado study (Fletcher, 2006) showed three-quarters of Colorado's total uninsured adult population had jobs. Many were uninsured by choice, preferring to spend their money on other lifestyle choices. Nevertheless, the uninsured pose a serious cost problem for hospitals obligated to treat them.

From 1993 to 2003, the U.S. population grew by 12 percent, but emergency room (ER) visits grew 27 percent, from 90 million to 114 million. Meanwhile, 425 emergency departments, 700 hospitals, and 200,000 beds closed. About 14 percent of ER patients are uninsured, and 16 percent are covered by Medicaid, and 21 percent by Medicare (MSNBC, 2005). More than half of hospitals lose money in ERs.

How one thinks about universal coverage depends on one's point of view. Dr. Brian Gould, a former UnitedHealth executive and now a consultant, who has organized health companies around the world, says the case for U.S. universal coverage is overstated.

Table 1–1

Ethnic Origin	Total Population	Percentage of Population	Growth Rate, 2000–2004 (%)	Average Life Expectancy (years)
White	197,525,000	68	1.2	81.0
Black	35,577,000	12.3	4.8	73.6
Hispanic	39, 340,000	13.6	17	74.0
American Indian	2,181,000	0.8	5.2	75.5
Asian	11,667,000	4.0	16.5	75.2
Hawaiian or Islander	381,000	0.13	8.5	75.0
Interracial marriage	3,747,000	1.3	13.5	No Answer

Source: Abstract of the United States, 2000–2004.

Gould says:

> *What happens if an uninsured person in the U.S. is hit crossing the street. They are taken by ambulance to a tax-supported hospital where they get the highest quality care. In France or Italy, that's called "universal coverage." In the United States, we call that being "uninsured." (Reece, 2005c)*

In 1960, 56 percent of 200 million Americans' personal medical spending was out of pocket. This meant some 112 million Americans were uninsured, although that was not the term used then. Then it was called being personally responsible. The significance of being uninsured varies with the beholder. Paying out of pocket is not automatically or axiomatically a bad thing. Others persuasively argue there ought to be at least a "floor" for "essential care" in a humane nation. Many concur, but defining what is essential is as slippery as catching an oiled eel.

- Life expectancy may have more to do with ethnicity, family structure, and culture than health systems. The United States receives 85 percent of the world's immigrants. Its diverse population is now nearly one third African American, Hispanic, or of other ethnic origins. American minorities' life expectancies profoundly affect overall U.S. longevity statistics.

Most Americans consider racial diversity a good thing. Regrettably, interacting variables—insufficient education, lower socioeconomic status, fear of being exposed as an illegal immigrant, violence, language barriers, racial biases, and lack of health care access—converge to cause whites to exceed nonwhites in life expectancies.

Immigration and cultural circumstances skew health statistics. Except perhaps for Canada, the United States has proportionally more immigrants than countries with "pure" populations. Japan, for example, whose citizens lead the world in life expectancy at 81.2 years, is 99 percent ethnically Japanese. Scandinavian countries have homogeneous populations with average life expectancies over 80.

Overall, U.S. life expectancy differences are not great. Britons, who spend half as much as Americans do for health care, live 77.6 years. In the United States, life expectancy is 77.1 (though latest figures put that number at 77.6). Social justice aside, and that is a huge "aside" for progressives, in a conservative nation like the United States, these differences may not justify completely overhauling the health system.

Health care policy innovations are to be desired and pursued. There is always room—and gloom—for improvement. Massachusetts has shown government can politically innovate around barriers to universal coverage, Florida is innovating to make health care pricing more transparent, and a handful of other states—Oklahoma, South Carolina, and Massachusetts—are introducing health savings accounts to control Medicaid expenses (Herzlinger, 2006a). These political innovations' consequences are not yet evident. They may fail, but they are worth trying.

The General Proposition of This Book

What differentiates the U.S. health system from single-payer counterparts in other Western nations? This book puts forth this general proposition: What separates the United States from other countries are its dynamic market economy, its continuous innovation, its remarkable entrepreneurship, its robust infrastructure, its experiments with new ideas, and its proximity to buyers. These cultural characteristics spill over into health care.

The government supports but slows innovation, yet government–private sector partnerships are essential. After all, according to the Congressional Budget Office, the Centers for Medicare and Medicaid and other federal programs pay 46 percent of total U.S. health costs, and they depend on the private sector for delivering health services.

The private sector, in turn, depends on government. As Joseph Antos, an American Enterprise Institute economist and an inside-the-Beltway health care expert, asserts, "Medicare is the Sheriff of the System. You better heed the Man with the Badge" (Reece, 2005c). Improving health care will come through incremental enlightened interactions and a cooperative consensus between government and the private sector rather than through sweeping government-imposed reforms.

Innovation and Entrepreneurship Do Not Occur in a Vacuum

Innovation requires large organizations' support and resources, yet many often look down at the fragmentation of U.S. health care. However, large organizations—representing government, managed care, integrated hospital systems, community hospitals, drug companies, and supply chain manufacturers—dominate U.S. health care.

This dominance is seldom mentioned in assessing U.S. health care—yet it may take government and corporate management and monitoring systems to control costs, judge quality of vendors, and make sense of U.S. health care.

Rarely does innovation stem from a single entrepreneur's bright idea. Innovations are like frog eggs; only a few make it to maturity. Nine of 10 bright ideas fail from lack of capital and team support (Drucker, 1985). It takes an organization to sustain innovations, and large health care organizations have resources to be innovative. A good example is Kaiser Permanente. It has invested $3.2 billion into its information technology system. Its goal is a computer at the fingertip of every physician (Halvorson and Isham, 2004). Another example is the Mayo Clinic. It thinks of itself as a "learning organization" committed to learning from its successes and failure (Cortese and Smodt, 2006).

Innovation lunges forward in fits and starts. Successes and failures dot the process. Change-adverse physicians, pining for the "good old days," may block change. That may be why electronic medical records have been slow to enter the small-practice physician market. In a group of 10 doctors, two will refuse to use the computer (Wenner, 2006).

Indeed, their resistance may be an unspoken but central reason only 15 to 25 percent of medical practices have installed electronic medical records systems (Cortese and Smodt, 2006). This percentage may be climbing. As of 2006, the American Academy of Family Practice reports 20,000 of 59,000, or 34 percent, of its actively practicing members use electronic records (Freudenheim, 2006d).

Another example is e-prescribing's (electronic prescribing) tardiness in catching on among physicians. E-prescribing failed and died a quick death at Cedar-Sinai in Los Angeles. The medical staff revolted because it slowed them up (Berger and Kichak, 2004).

This revolt reminds one of Harrison Salisbury, a *New York Times* reporter, who, after visiting Los Angeles, remarked, "I have seen the future, and it doesn't work" (Salisbury, 1959). Salisbury was talking of the gasoline engine, but the analogy may hold because computer data entry is considered fuel for health care efficiency.

Computer pharmaceutical data entry is not yet widespread. Tethering doctors to keyboards and forcing them to follow computer protocols rather than facilitating or speeding their practicing patterns is not a winning strategy.

Physicians' resistance to e-prescribing will fade as young doctors armed with PDAs (personal digital assistants) and laptops enter practice. As EHR (electronic health record) systems with embedded e-prescribing functions, such as the Allscripts EHR, become more common and convenient, e-prescribing may flourish.

Dr. David Brailer who resigned as President George W. Bush's health care information czar on April 24, 2006, maintained a "seamless inoperable national health information system" will not work unless small practices adopt electronic health records. Indeed, he said lack of electronic adoption by small practices is "elephants in the room," the key thing blocking a successful national system (Lohr, 2005).

Seven Lodestones for Systematic Innovation

According to Jane C. Linder, research director at the Accenture Institute for High Performance Business in Wellesley, Massachusetts, innovation is incremental. She says, "Companies don't have to wait for the stars to be aligned before they innovate. They can start with incremental improvements right now" (Salz, 2006).

Linder gives seven points for overcoming innovation constraints:

1. **Top management support.** Speed to market and business effectiveness improve when senior executives lead innovation.
2. **Internal networking.** Innovation flourishes when teams across organizations combine talent.
3. **Pushing innovations downward.** Innovation opportunities grow when responsibility for innovation flows down to individual workers.

4. **Supply-driven partnerships.** Suppliers are an important and untapped source of rapid innovation. It is in the best interests of suppliers for their clients to succeed.

5. **External partner–intensive.** Innovation yields better results when it leverages ideas and expertise and talent and resources of external organizations to coinnovate and collaborate.

6. **Competitor driven.** Enviable business returns can be achieved by innovating to be first-to-market; in other words, taking the lead.

7. **Customer driven.** Innovators must be closely connected to customers, deeply understanding their true wants and needs. (Salz, 2006)

Why U.S. Health Care Differs

Why does U.S. health care differ from other countries?

- Is it because other nations have homogeneous populations supporting, depending upon, and trusting single-payer systems?
- Is it because Americans distrust government-run systems? Perhaps this distrust exists for good reasons. According to John Goodman and associates (2004), government systems ration high technology and stint on care for the sick.

  These systems often feature waiting lines and rationing of expensive technologies. Americans might not tolerate rationing, waiting times, and limited access to high technologies—inherent features of universal systems. The Canadian Supreme Court in Ottawa ruled in June of 2005 that "access to a waiting list is not the same as access to health care." The Court found parts of the single-payer Canadian system (exclusion of private care) unconstitutional (Knauss, 2005). In England, citizens are so weary of waiting, they have given up getting dental care and are pulling their own teeth (Lyall, 2006).
- Is it simply because Americans lack a unified national vision of how things ought to be? Scott Serota, chief executive officer (CEO) of the Blue Cross Blue Shield Association, says, "The phrase 'U.S. Health System' is a misnomer. The first thing we need to create is a unified U.S. health system. We have a terribly fragmented approach to serving the needs of the American population" (Reece, 2005c).

The U.S. system has roots in the country's unique national culture. Since its founding more than 225 years ago, Americans have:

- distrusted centralized federal power
- reveled in virtues of self-improvement
- sought freedom of choice
- believed in equality of opportunity, not results, for all citizens

Flawed though the system may be, it fosters an innovative market-driven approach to health care, as opposed to government coverage for all. As Winston Churchill observed, "The inherent vice of capitalism is the unequal sharing of blessings; the inherent virtue of socialism is the equal sharing of miseries" (Bartlett, 1992).

These characteristics may explain why Americans:

- Prefer a multiplayer to a single-payer system.
- Reject federally mandated universal coverage.
- Want to make their own health care decisions.
- Seek immediate access to new medical technologies.
- Allow market- and public-based institutions to coexist and compete.
- Permit doctors to practice where they want.
- Let private health care organizations innovate, sometimes even self-destruct.

This contrasts to government-sponsored health agencies. They never go out of business.

The Role of Innovation and Entrepreneurship

Given these American cultural traits, innovation and entrepreneurship, as defined by management theorist Peter F. Drucker, may offer the country's best hopes for reforming health care (Drucker, 1986). Drucker makes the following key points:

1. **In the United States, decisions are based on proximity to performance.**

   The American entrepreneurial economy distinctly differs from socialistic European economies. American organizations must be able to make decisions based on proximity to performance, the market, technology, society, environment, and demographics. In Europe, on the other hand, distance from the market of centralized systems makes innovation and responsiveness difficult.

2. **The United States has shifted from a managerial to an entrepreneurial economy.**

   Thirty years ago, the American economy shifted from a managerial to an entrepreneurial economy. It has generated millions of American jobs in its wake and outpaced Europe in growth and employment by roughly two to one. The American economy is now growing at 3 to 5 percent a year, while Europe's growth rate remains stagnant at about 1 percent. Certainly the American health industry's growth rate is robust. The industry now consumes one of every seven dollars of the U.S. economy and generates one of every 11 jobs.

3. **U.S. innovation adjusts quickly to change.**

   Entrepreneurship and innovation thrive when there are demands for change, structural industry adjustments, demographic shifts, and changes in perception. With consumer-directed care, the market is shifting from:

- *HMOs and PPOs to HDCDHPs (high-deductible consumer-directed health plans)*
- *doctors being paid by third parties to doctors being paid by patients*
- *a young country to an aging and more affluent nation*
- *passive patients to assertive consumers*

For excellent background reading materials for health care professionals to promote the ideas of innovation and entrepreneurship, read two of Peter Drucker's books:

- *Innovation and Entrepreneurship* (1986)
- *The Daily Drucker* (2004)

The latter book is a daily diary consisting of Drucker quotes with lessons for the day. For health care teams, it might be useful to take the diary entries under innovation and entrepreneurship and review one entry each week at a staff meeting to see if the health care company, the hospital, or the medical practice is on course or is sufficiently innovative.

The following is an example of what might be used as a daily reading for a team of innovators.

BOX 1.1

Sample for Daily Drucker Reading
2 March

• •

Test of Innovation
Measure innovations by what they contribute to market and customer

The test of an innovation is whether it creates value. Innovation means the creation of new value and new satisfaction for the customer. A novelty only creates amusement. Yet, again and again, managements decide to innovate for no other reason than they are bored with doing the same thing with the same product day in and day out. The test of an innovation, as well as the test of quality, is not, as Drucker states, "Do we like it?" but rather it is, "[Will it do] what the customers want and will they pay for it?"

Organizations measure innovations not by their scientific or technological importance but by what they contribute to market and customer. They consider social innovation to be as important as technological innovation. Installment selling may have had a greater impact on economics than most of the great scientific advances of this century.

ActionPoint   Identify innovations in your organization that are novelties versus those that are creating value. Did you launch the novelties because you were bored with doing the same thing? If so, make sure your next new product or service meets your customers' needs.

"Under the Radar" Innovations

This book describes 36 U.S. health care innovations. Most of these innovations, but not all, are infrastructure adjustments from the bottom up, rather than government mandates from the top down. Some are responses to these mandates.

The Centers for Medicare and Medicaid (CMS) is the engine driving the reimbursement train. Indeed, the Bush administration in 2006 announced Medicare plans to make a 25 percent to 30 percent cut in fees for complex procedures like cardiac stents, defibrillator implants, and hip and knee replacements (Pear, 2006a).

However, government is not a fertile source of innovations. Government mandates command the most attention, but fundamental changes on the ground—in the clinical trenches, hospital corridors, health plan boardrooms, and supply-chain company headquarters—may be more important.

The idea of these 35 innovations was borrowed from a 2001 *Health Affairs* article by Victor R. Fuchs and Harold Sox, Jr. Fuchs is a Henry J. Kaiser Jr. Professor Emeritus at Stanford University and a health care economist. Dr. Harold Sox, Jr., is the former chair of the department of medicine at Dartmouth and the editor of *Annals of Internal Medicine.*

The Fuchs and Sox study revealed a strong consensus among 225 general internists on the relative importance of 30 major medical innovations. General internists were given a list of 30 innovations. They were asked to select five to seven that would have the most adverse effect on their patients if the innovations did not exist, as well as the five to seven that would have the least adverse effect. The result was a top-10 ranking of innovations of the 30 innovations based on the physicians' ratings.

Here, in alphabetical order, were the 30 medical innovations from which 225 primary care physicians chose the top 10:

1. ACE inhibitors and angiotensin II antagonists (for treatment of high blood pressure)
2. Balloon angioplasty with stents (a procedure to open blocked blood vessels of the heart)
3. Bone densitometry
4. Bone marrow transplant
5. CABG (cardio-arterial bypass grafts)
6. Calcium channel blockers
7. Cardiac enzymes, for example, CPK, troponin
8. Cataract extraction and lens implant
9. Fluoroquinolones
10. Gastrointestinal endoscopy
11. *H. pylori* testing and treatment
12. Hip and knee replacements

13. HIV testing and treatment
14. Inhaled steroids for asthma
15. IV-conscious sedation
16. Laparoscopic surgery
17. Long-acting and parenteral uploads
18. Mammography
19. MRI and CT scanning (magnetic resonance imaging and computed tomography)
20. Nonsedating antihistamines
21. NSAIDs (Non Steroidal Anti-Inflamatory Drugs) and Cox-2 inhibitors
22. Proton pump inhibitors and H2 blockers (used to treat gastroesophageal reflux disease)
23. PSA (Prostatic Specific Antigen) testing
24. SSRIs (selective serotonin reuptake inhibitors) and recent non-SSRI antidepressants
25. Recent hypoglycemic agents, for example, metformin
26. Sildenafil
27. Statins (drugs used to improve lipid metabolism and reduce risk for coronary heart disease and other vascular diseases)
28. Tamoxifen
29. Third-generation cephalosporins
30. Ultrasonography, including echocardiography (Fuchs and Sox, 2001)

Physician Choices for Top 10 Innovations

Here, in order of importance, are the internists' rankings of the top 10 medical innovations:

1. MRI and CT scanning (magnetic resonance imaging and computed tomography)
2. ACE inhibitors and angiotensin II antagonists (for treatment of high blood pressure
3. Balloon angioplasty with stents (a procedure to open blocked blood vessels of the heart)
4. Statins (drugs used to improve lipid metabolism and reduce risk for coronary heart disease and other vascular diseases)
5. Mammography
6. CABG (cardio-arterial bypass grafts)
7. Proton pump inhibitors and H2 blockers (used to treat gastroesophageal reflux disease)

8. SSRIs (selective serotonin reuptake inhibitors) and recent non-SSRI antidepressants

9. Cataract extraction and lens implant

10. Hip and knee replacements (Fuchs and Sox, 2001)

These are, of course, technological medical innovations, rather than social or organizational innovations. Most innovations (except for MRI and CT, originally developed in England), originate in the United States (Hounsfield, Ambrose, Perry, and Bridges, 1973).

This country is a nation of innovators. Over the last 30 years, the United States has produced more medical Nobel Prize winners than all other nations combined; drug companies headquartered here have created 8 of the 10 top selling drugs; and, in the 30 innovations listed by Fuchs and Sox, 8 of 10 came from the United States (Cogan, Hubbard, and Kessler, 2005). These technological innovations' downsides are high costs and, in some instances, unregulated entrepreneurialism (the operative words criticizing those who profit are *greed,* and for those favoring profit *opportunities*) on the part of manufacturers and physician users of these wonderful innovations. American patients are often willing accomplices to overuse, for they, like their doctors, have insatiable appetites for medical technologies as a quick fix for their ailments.

What Follows Are 34 Operational Innovations for 2006

This book features the top 34 operational innovations picks for the United States. Some of these "innovations" may strike the reader as nothing more than a response to major government decisions. However, remember it takes innovations and ingenuity to deal with sweeping government programs, like the Medicare Part D benefit for 42 million beneficiaries or the 53 million Medicaid recipients.

To give you, the reader, a sense of the relative importance of innovations discussed in this book, 100 health care stakeholders—hospital executives, physicians, consultants, editors, and contributors to this book and previous books—were polled. They were asked to rank the 10 innovations out of 34 innovations presented in this book in order of importance. Here is their consensus.

Top 10 Innovations

1. **Pay-for-performance (P-4-P) programs**
2. **Introductions of electronic health records (EHRs) into medical practices**
3. **Add-ons to EHRs; instant medical histories, coding devices, prescription-enabling modules, or Web sites that permit registration, virtual visits, prescription refills, and open-access scheduling**

4. Software that facilitates office dispensing and prescription writing
5. Self-care, self-service, and self-empowerment of consumers
6. New practice business models (concierge, cash, or other new types of innovative practices, such as retail clinics or home-disease management)
7. High-tech/high-touch remote patient monitoring with patient interactive capacity
8. Personal health records with and without EHRs
9. Disease-management programs
10. The transparency movement as part of consumer-driven care movement

This survey revealed this consensus among health care stakeholders:

- They foresee pay-for-data-driven quality care (pay-for-performance) as a new reality.
- They think the most fruitful site of innovations resides in physicians' offices, retail outlets, and patients' homes.
- They have a deep faith in information technologies' capacities to transform the system by making transparent cost data widely available.
- They believe the combination of EHRs in medical offices and PHRs (personal health records) will be a watershed event.
- They project consumer-driven care, fueled by health savings accounts (HSAs), will be powerful.
- They think technology-aided disease-management programs will be big.
- They believe new physicians business models will be necessary to deal with change.

As with any list, some suggested important innovations were left out. Here are two examples of omissions:

- Regina Herzlinger, Harvard Business School professor and consumer visionary, mentioned "focused factories," specialized clinics to treat certain chronic diseases. These focused factories, she noted, may evolve into a new practice model, namely, hospital–doctor partnerships for treating such costly diseases as diabetes and HIV/AIDS, with hospitals and doctors sharing in the savings made possible by these specialized models.
- Larry McGovern, a Montana-based practice management consultant, commented, "What about malpractice innovations?" It was mentioned that high malpractice rates are driving specialists into the arms of hospitals as employers. Certain innovations, other than legislative reform, or other innovations are under way to minimize risks—hospital/physician offshore insurance entities with strict protocols to avoid suits and realistic video presented to patients before surgery to ensure realistic expectations as to what will take place. In any event, Larry's reminder led to Chapter 34, "Pragmatic Malpractice Innovations."

Policy Issues and Innovations Deserve Equal Places at the Reform Table

Health reform usually focuses on policy issues: mandated employer coverage, tax credit subsidies, Medicare and Medicaid, health savings accounts, managed competition, quality incentives, personal mandates, single-payer proposals, and universal vouchers (Reece, 1988a). Innovations deserve an equal place at the reform table.

In a 1963 address in Frankfurt, Germany, President John Kennedy declared, "As they say on my own Cape Cod, a rising tide lifts all the boats." Similarly, the rising tide of innovations lifts American health care to new heights. Critics of the health system often quote Pogo, "We have met the enemy, and he is us." The U.S. system is undoubtedly uneven, and Americans are often their own worst enemies, but one could counter, "We have met our friends, and they are us—American health care innovators."

Chapter 2

The Search for New Careers and New Primary Care Business Models

Prelude: A hard but fresh look at practice downsides and upsides and realistic nonclinical career options escapes for doctors.

When I read about new types of innovative practices they all write about same day access, better communication with patients, computerized medical records, 'medical homes,' 'team practices,' use of non-physicians for routine care, but none write about the need to strengthen the doctor-patient relationship.

There is no other profession as personal as the medical profession. If physicians continue to allow non-physicians and businesses such as hospitals and insurance companies to control them, they will lose their patients and will be nothing more than over-educated hired technicians.

Donald Copeland, 2006

March 28, 2006
To my patients:

I am saddened to inform you all that as of June 1, 2006, I will resign from my position with Old Saybrook family practice.

My reasons for leaving are a combination of personal and professional. The action I have chosen to take, for better or worse, is to leave the practice of medicine entirely. I will be joining a company called Executive Health Resources (EHR), whose function is to help doctors and hospitals claim the money they have earned from insurance companies. They will require me to move from the region into the suburbs southwest of Philadelphia.

Steven Regatti, 2006

Health Care Is Personal for Doctors Too

Medical practice is a personal thing. Opening this chapter with a letter from a physician to his patients highlights the personal aspect of medical practice.

Being a physician is part of being a member of a brotherhood and sisterhood. Physicians pass through similar rites of passage, and they tend to cluster together and take each other's problems personally.

In the mid-1980s, HMOs were growing explosively. Many physicians, mostly internists and hospital-based specialists, were hurt financially as HMOs ratcheted down on reimbursement, excluded doctors from networks, and narrowed the number of hospitals where doctors could admit. One frustrated internist, Dr. Richard Frey, said, "You know, it doesn't pay to be a good doctor anymore" (Reece, 1988a).

Hospitals were shutting down or closing. HMOs preferred to say euphemistically that hospitals were "consolidating." Meanwhile, some doctors, particularly internists, were taking their children out of private schools and universities, moving out of high-priced suburbs to more modest quarters, or shutting down practices.

Doctors were learning what downward mobility meant. In heavily penetrated managed-care markets, this is a still a largely untold story. Health system restructuring with downsizing of hospital and physician capacities and discounting their pay has economic consequences for physicians.

Dr. Regatti's letter strikes at the core for two reasons:

1. Dr. Regatti practiced for 7 years.
2. His departure symbolizes many young primary care doctors' frustrations.

According to Dr. Regatti, in 2007, Executive Health Resources will recruit a dozen more primary care physicians. Executive Health Resources, a physician-advisory company, provides medical management services to improve hospital revenues and maintain physician compliance.

A company such as Executive Health Resources gives insight into why companies recruit physicians for alternative careers. According to their Web site, the company provides specialized solutions for:

- concurrent clinical denial reduction
- retrospective clinical denial management
- Centers for Medicare and Medicaid compliance
- managing length of stay/coordinating patient care
- screening of transfers from one center to another
- screening emergency department admissions
- improving physician documentation and compliance
- impacting quality and pay-for-performance metrics
- changing physician behavior

These functions show how complex medical practice has grown, how closely payers monitor physician behavior, how outside entities influence practice, and why physician knowledge of other physicians is important in tracking and controlling activities of other doctors. Experienced physicians' skills are in demand outside of their practices. Doctor Regatti's decision may have been based on this reality. Companies offer more security, less hassle, and more personal and family time than current medical practices.

PRIMARY CARE ON THE EDGE OF COLLAPSE

Primary care may be collapsing. Fewer younger doctors are entering primary care residencies. More older doctors are leaving primary care practices. Multiple reasons exist for this decline: fragmentation from too many scattered small practices, inadequate reimbursement, insufficient capital, operational inefficiencies, poor business practices, too little prestige, low morale, too few doctors entering primary care specialties, competition from nurse practitioners and retail clinics, patients choosing alternative practitioners, and too many doctors leaving with resulting stresses on those who remain. Suggestions abound on how to salvage primary care: more teamwork, a single-payer system, income narrowing between primary care practitioners and specialists, better business practices, more focus on consumers (Lawrence, 2002; Halvorson and Isham, 2004).

Other business models have been tried. Most of these models have failed to change the fundamentals of primary care office practice—small practices with too little mobility, inadequate resources, and too much to know.

Pay of Nurses and Doctors

In a 2006 summary report of physician recruiting incentives, Merritt, Hawkins, and Associates, a physician recruiting firm, noted the average starting salaries of certified nurse anesthetists ($155,000) now exceeds the starting salaries of family physicians ($145,000) and approaches that of internists ($161,000).

This may be a bad time to be a family physician, who may feel 10 to 12 years of post high school education is not a good return on investment for years of training and money for education expended. The typical medical school graduate carries a debt burden of about $150,000. Internists were once considered American medicine's intelligentsia. Apparently cerebral differential diagnosis skills of general internists are no longer highly regarded enough to be sufficiently rewarded.

In his book, Dr. David Lawrence, chairman emeritus of Kaiser Permanente, describes the dilemma of Adam Landers, a fictitious solo practitioner:

> *In spite of his motivation to be a high quality physician, Dr. Landers can't deliver on the promise of modern medical care. He lacks the time, the money, and the organization to do so. And he will fall further and further behind if he continues to practice as he does today.*

Unfortunately, his patients and their families are the ones who pay the price. For the simple and routine illnesses, he provides a valuable service. But for more complex illnesses and chronic conditions, neither he nor his colleagues in other solo or small group practices are prepared for what medicine now requires and patients demand.

The forces are too strong and the changes too profound. Physicians like Dr. Landers and his colleagues—independent, autonomous professionals who practice as craftsman, along or in small, single-specialty groups—are already being overwhelmed by those forces; as a consequence, the dangerous and expensive gulf between what patients need and expect and what they get grows wider every day. (Lawrence, 2002)

Failed Physician Business Models

Carcasses of independent practice associations (IPAs), group practices without walls, physician–hospital organizations, hospital-based employment, and absorption into larger multispecialty groups litter the health care landscape.

Many practice management methods have been tried, but few have been found to correct most small practices' problems. Proposed solutions include:

- consistent coding for all work done
- collecting at the point of care after visits and before procedures
- open-access scheduling
- installing electronic medical records
- triaging by nurse practitioners and physician assistants
- extending hours
- following evidence-based clinical protocols

Breaking loose from the old business model—a stationary, immovable, small, office-based practice with overheads of 50 percent to 70 percent—is hard. Doctors often enter practice with idealistic hopes of being their own boss and of being a servant to no one but their patients. Instead, they find themselves subservient to government and private insurers, and, to a lesser extent, to malpractice lawyers lurking in the wings.

The plight of primary care cries for innovation. Primary care physicians need a model to provide enough income to pay off medical school and postgraduate training debts, afford a home, finance their children through college, and offer a decent retirement income (Reed, 2006). These economic benefits or assurances are more common with employment by large organizations or new business models.

One model that has impressed physicians is ProHealth Physicians, Inc., headquartered in Farmington, Connecticut. The 200 members of this primary care group practice in multiple locations, mostly original practice sites, throughout central Connecticut.

Venture capital money originally financed the group, but it has stood on its own financial feet for 10 years. It is a patient-focused, physician-owned, and physician-directed group. Although most doctors remain at their original practice sites, a few solo and two practices have consolidated into larger groups.

The group innovative activities include uniform coding, stringent quality standards, establishing diagnostic centers (laboratories, X-ray, imaging centers, and physical therapy, sleep apnea, and attention-deficit clinics), and in 2006, the opening of clinics in retail pharmacies and grocery chains.

By merging and owning their own organization, ProHealth Physicians organization has more power to influence legislation and hospitals and to negotiate better contracts with insurers and HMOs by offering a greater number of value-added propositions. Each of the 200 doctors owns shares in the organization and controls decision making through committees and frequent group-wide meetings. The group concentrates on setting and monitoring quality control standards. The executive director of the group, Jack Reed, says, "Our basic attitude is to first establish uniform standards and then to go with the flow of market-based changes rather than resisting them."

New business models restoring autonomy, vitality, and profitability of primary care interest many. Physicians working together in decentralized practices under a centralized administrative structure can effectively compete and thrive in the medical marketplace. At the end of this chapter is a case study written by Dr. Charles Staub, an internist in ProHealth Physicians. He believes the ProHealth practice model can lift primary care physicians out of their economic doldrums and give renewed hope.

Exit Strategies from Medicine: The Other Side of the Coin

The other side of this chapter is helping physicians who are dissatisfied with their current practice of medicine; in fact, so dissatisfied, they choose to leave the profession. A number of companies have sprung up to help place these disgruntled physicians in nonclinical careers.

One of these is CareerLab, Inc., in Denver, Colorado. In 1978, William S. Frank, who may be the country's leading authority on nonclinical careers for physicians, founded CareerLab, a consulting firm specializing in career management, executive coaching, leadership development, and outplacement. Frank has sold more than 300 consulting contracts to brand-name corporations, including the American Cancer Society, Blue Cross Blue Shield, CIBA Vision, Columbia/HCA, GAMBRO Health Care, Kaiser Permanente, LifeCare, Medtronic HemoTec, the College of Medicine at the Pennsylvania State University, and Sunrise Health Care.

In 1998, he cofounded a subspecialty practice called the Physician Career Network (PCN). This became the authoritative source for doctors wanting to improve their careers. PCN has physician clients from all 50 states.

After psychological testing and interviews, Frank and his associates help doctors find their career footing, inside and outside of medicine. In some cases, doctors can restructure their existing practices and find more satisfaction than in switching careers. Others find happiness in nonclinical work.

SEAK, Inc., a company in Falmouth, Massachusetts, also helps physicians find nonclinical careers by sponsoring national conferences, in concert with CareerLab, for physicians seeking nonclinical employment opportunities.

Yet another company is Creative Strategies in Physician Leadership in Bellevue, WA, an executive coaching, leadership development, career counseling resource for physicians, physician executives, health care leaders, and entrepreneurs. It was founded by physician leader and health care consultant Francine R. Gaillour. She and her coaching associates provide executive coaching and leadership consulting to high-potential and high-performing physicians, health care business leaders, and clinical teams.

Their goal is to help doctors succeed as a new breed of health care executives who take personal responsibility for leading health care—whether as a clinical practice leader, a medical management executive, an entrepreneur, or a business innovator.

Case Studies 1 and 2

Two Case Studies of Doctors Who Choose to Leave Clinical Practice
Dr. William S. Frank

William S. Frank, CEO of CareerLab, wrote these case studies. He started CareerLab 27 years ago. Initially the company focused on industries outside of medicine. But in 1998, Frank co-founded the Physician Career Network, which is devoted to helping physicians seek new careers inside and outside of medicine. The following case studies were written with permission of the physicians involved in making career transitions.

● ●

Case Study 1: Middle-Aged Woman Internist Finds Career Outside of Practice

A middle-aged woman internist, married, and the mother of three children, sought an alternative career outside of private practice. She did so even though she said she was happy and successful in a three-person group. She got along well with her two colleagues. She was the busiest of the three and earned $100,000 to $150,000 a year.

Her problems were threefold: demanding work and home schedules that frequently conflicted, a sick child, and unhappiness with the way medicine was evolving. "I decided that I thought the health system was really broken. I became very interested in looking at the big picture, and I was interested in the ways I could change what 100 doctors did in a good way. I was interested in systems. I was interested in how care actually could be changed."

Although her family supported her when she decided to leave practice, she had an identity crisis with herself and her colleagues. Her partners said she would merely become "one of the suits." She thought that was short-sighted. So she persisted, she said, "Because physicians need to get management training, and they need to communicate on an equal level with CEOs, and they need to take a leadership role in medical affairs. I wanted change, to learn new things. I wanted to avoid getting stale."

She committed to leaving the practice. She went to work in an academic setting, teaching other internists. She took on administrative responsibilities, worked as a medical director for an insurance company, earned an MBA, worked full time as the vice president of a community hospital, and finally became vice president of medical affairs of a large hospital, where she earned $250,000 a year.

She was happy in her new situation. She liked the money—but she left that job to start her own consulting business. She had other priorities. Her family had grown up, and her husband made plenty of money. In her consulting business, she could do things she wanted to do and to work with people with whom she wanted to be associated.

Not everything was perfect. She disliked the "sales component" of her work, and her duties and income were "much less predictable" than with practice or her previous positions. However, the new work fit her priorities. It was realistic financially.

Case Study 2: General Surgeon Finds New Career Outside of Operating Room

He is a 55-year-old male surgeon, married with children, who made about $200,000 a year as a busy practicing surgeon at a Denver hospital.

"The biggest challenge I had was balancing my professional and my personal life. There was always a tension between the two. If I was busy, I would worry I was forgetting things. After a while, I got used to that. I took advantage of the opportunities for time as they came," he said.

"My greatest satisfaction was in treating patients and the relationships with them. I became more aware of this as I was leaving. My least satisfaction was in performing administrative duties. I hadn't planned on leaving. I went on disability because I developed arthritis. I was a part-time consultant for about 2 years before I went full time into a new field. My family was 'very positive' about my change in career, but my colleagues were jealous," he stated.

"I am now in medical risk management for an insurance company. I analyze claims and occurrences to help physicians lower their risk of making errors and being sued. My job title is physician risk manager and I make about $240,000 a year. I am satisfied with the income and the new position. My options were not to do this job and just take the disability."

Although there is some travel, he is no longer on call and rarely works weekends. He is satisfied that he is "continuing to work in medicine and feeling I could make an impact in medical claims and patient safety." He also gets to spend more time with his family. He has no regrets about how things have turned out and said he would do it again.

"I was enjoying what I was doing and I planned to do it until I retired. What I miss from my old job is the relationships with the patients, and the satisfaction of being in the operating room, just doing surgery with other professionals, and working in a highly skilled environment where you are, quote, the captain of the ship. But the tradeoff is that this job has a lot less stress, obviously," he said.

"I think the key for my ability to make the transition is that, when I was in practice, I got involved in a number of leadership areas that were training grounds for what I am doing now. I think physicians tend to get very isolated and they tend stay in their silos. But I was a chief of staff, chief of surgery. I was and remain involved in medical missions (including an annual, regional health fair), and I was involved in building a clinic in Juarez, Mexico. I was also involved with a couple of HMOs in their infancy, and I learned a lot about managed care. I got involved in peer review of physicians. All this helps in my current job of helping physicians in a nonclinical way. And that's been a source of fulfillment. I guess my message is that you can find fulfillment in whatever you're doing. You can bloom where you're planted."

Case Study 3

The ProHealth Physicians Practice Business Model

By Dr. Charles Staub

Here Charles Staub, MD, FACP, Chairman of ProHealth Physicians, Inc., tells why he believes the ProHealth group practice model may prove to be the salvation for other primary care practices across the country. Dr. Staub practices family medicine.

Despite the atmosphere of crisis today, primary care doctors already possess the potential to shape the future of health care in this country. The challenge is whether we can realize how to harness this inherent power and restore primary care to its rightful place in our health care system.

Our success in ProHealth Physicians, a primary care group practice, has been based on three basic forces that underlie this power: alignment with the goals of people, a practice model that delivers care reliably, and the market presence to be paid fairly for our work.

• •

My Practice Experience

It's 2006: I am 53 years old and will attend my 25th medical school reunion in a few days. My practice experience as a general internist has ranged from a Laotian refugee camp, to a neighborhood clinic in an inner city, to solo and small-group practice and now to serving as chairman of the largest primary care group in the region.

While helping to lead this organization, I see patients every day in my practice site in Litchfield, Connecticut, a town of 9,000 where I live with my family. I am surrounded by family, friends, and patients. I am a small-town doctor. As chair of our group, I am also fully engaged in the challenge of breaking new ground to develop a practice model that strengthens primary care.

Melding Together ProHealth Physicians

Ten years ago in the ProHealth Physicians organization, 120 primary care doctors took their 80 independent practices and melded them together into a jointly owned group practice. Over the ensuing decade, this entity has evolved from a loose federation of practice sites into a truly unified group practice, designed and led by primary care physicians.

The Essence of New England Medicine

The group practice that we have formed is one that preserves the essence of New England medicine: individual doctors and providers connecting with patients in a personal relationship founded on trust, respect, and accountability. Understanding people and what they want is one of the central forces of health care; one that uniquely empowers primary care providers.

Providing What People Want from Their Health System

Simply put, people want to maintain their health and live their own lives. They would like to have minimal contact with the health care system; just enough to maintain wellness, find illness early, and manage chronic conditions as efficiently as possible.

Primary care stands in a singular position to fulfill this promise of living a longer and better life. Through alignment with the goals of the people we serve, primary care doctors can reassert their influence on a health care system preoccupied with treating end-stage disease through high-tech specialty care.

Choosing the Right Practice Model

However, just engaging this basic force is not enough. We must choose the right practice model that can deliver reliably on the clinical agenda for prevention, wellness, and disease management.

The cottage-industry model of small-group practice with one to four physicians still accounts for 75 percent of the practice settings in our country. This venerable structure has served us well for over two centuries, but now struggles to meet the requirements of health care delivery in the modern era.

The Group Practice Model

In ProHealth Physicians, we have adopted a group practice model that has enabled us to upgrade our ability to deliver better care to people; the right care to the right person at the right time.

With this enhanced level of organization, we can more easily implement basic management principles to improve the human and technological systems that underlie the effective delivery of primary care. We have built and are continuing to expand a lab, practice facilities, ancillaries, and information systems that support us in the care we provide every day, both to individuals and to our entire population of patients.

The Importance of Market Presence

The final element in this triad of forces is market presence. Our health care system operates on the interplay of negotiations between powerful entities: hospital systems, insurers, the pharmaceutical industry, and government. Ever since the antitrust decisions of the 1970s, physicians have been divided and conquered by these other entities.

Without legal practice organizations that could negotiate directly for us, physicians have been relegated to the marginal role of a commodity in the health care arena. The alternative strategy of unionization concedes ownership of the means of production to others, ownership that should be held in the hands of physicians in trust with their patients. It is only through building our own practice entities with significant presence in a given market that we can begin to garner our fair share of health care resources to do our job properly.

ProHealth Physicians Today

In ProHealth Physicians, we have 350,000 patients today; about 10 percent of our state's population. Our 200 providers in pediatrics, family practice, and internal medicine are represented by a skilled management team who can negotiate contracts that improve the fee schedule and also access additional revenues derived from the value created by the efficient delivery of high-quality primary care. These contracting tactics will change over time, transitioning from pay for performance to other formats that have yet to be developed. We feel confident in our ability to move with the market on these developments, as long as we maintain alignment with the needs of people and provide effective medical care.

Replicable in Other Parts of the Country

The model that we have developed here in ProHealth Physicians can be replicated in other areas of the country. A number of similar primary care groups have been established in the last 10 to 15 years. Different paths to the same end could be pursued; perhaps three modest practices could join together in a local area with a plan to double their size in 5 years.

Vision and Stamina Required

Building a group practice takes vision and stamina. Successful group practices mark their lifespan in quartiles of 25 years, and our most prominent medical groups are over a century old. I believe that our own professional organizations could assist us in founding these new entities through education, mentoring, and encouragement. Small-group practice will not disappear, but we cannot rely on it to serve as the sole vessel to bear our futures as physicians.

Putting Primary Care Back at Center Stage of the Health System

Primary care is in crisis today because we lack leadership, organizational structure, and resources. As primary care doctors, we must look to ourselves and not rely passively on government, hospitals, or academic centers to solve our problems. We possess the ability to create practice organizations that can bring primary care back onto center stage in the medical arena through helping people achieve what they truly desire: reaching their own goals through longer and better lives. In ProHealth Physicians, we are living proof that primary care can flourish as an equal partner in a health care system that works better for people.

Chapter 3

New Practice Paradigm for Preventing Vascular Deaths

Prelude: A fundamental mind-set shift is occurring among physicians across the Southeast, namely, their role is preventing, monitoring, and minimizing metabolic risk factors producing the vascular death epidemic and restoring health rather than merely treating causative diseases.

The Consortium for Southeastern Hypertension Control (COSEHC) is a professional organization of physicians, scientists, and health care providers working together to reduce the incidence of high blood pressure and hypertension-related cardiovascular disease outcomes (heart attacks, strokes, renal disease and heart failure) in the southeastern region of the United States.

COSEHC home page, 2006

Why COSEHC Is Innovative

- Would you consider it innovative if a widely dispersed group of community physicians worked together to prevent significant numbers of vascular deaths across a wide geographic region?
- Would you consider it innovative if this group of physicians located in 16 separate community practices collaborated with 23 cardiovascular centers of excellence and seven medical schools to coordinate care of patients located throughout a wide geographic region of the United States?

This is exactly what the Consortium for Southeastern Hypertension Control (COSEHC) has done.

COSEHC is an organization of physicians, scientists, and health care providers working together to reduce high blood pressure and hypertension-related cardiovascular deaths (heart attacks, strokes, renal disease, and heart failure) in the southeastern region of the United States.

The Founding of COSEHC

Carlos Ferrario, a professor from Wake Forest University, and Michael Moore, a community doctor on the Wake Forest Medical School clinical faculty, founded COSEHC. Others who led hailed from both academic institutions and community practices. Twenty-three centers of excellence, a subsidiary of COSEHC, came from adding together 16 community practices and 7 medical schools. The community practices range from 10 providers at the smallest to the Holston medical group with 115 providers. The organization touches hundreds of doctors and many thousands of patients.

Dr. Ferrario is the president of COSEHC, a more traditional Continuing Medical Education (CME) organization like the American Society of Hypertension.

The COSEHC Cardiovascular Centers of Excellence is a subsidiary function, and Dr. Bestermann, an internist in Beaufort, SC, is president of that function.

COSEHC Goals

COSEHC's goals are to:

- Improve knowledge of hypertension and its related risks
- Improve medical care of cardiovascular disease in the Southeast
- Promote research in hypertension and cardiovascular disease

Throughout the southeast and in collaboration with its centers of excellence network, COSEHC provides Category I Continuing Medical Education professional education, public education, cardiovascular benchmarking, and trending of risk factors and evidence-based management interventions.

Comments from Bestermann

Dr. William Bestermann, an internist, shared his insights into the centers component of COSEHC. A self-confessed data addict, he began by citing overwhelming evidence that type 2 diabetes, hypertension, and dyslipidemias considered as a group of diseases culminates too often in vascular deaths.

According to Bestermann, these diseases represent a global metabolic disorder. In diabetics, vascular events account for 65 percent of deaths. As a private physician in his multispecialty group, Bestermann and a large number of other physicians have compiled evidence that a systematic protocol best practice approach can prevent significant numbers of vascular deaths.

Bestermann also noted in the world at large among diabetic adults only 7.3 percent achieved the recommended goals of an HbA1c of less than 7 percent, blood pressure of less than 130/80, and total cholesterols of 200 or less.

The following figures compare data from the Hypertension Initiative of South Carolina and Bestermann's care of diabetics. The first figure represents the South Carolina figures; the second, those achieved by Bestermann:

- Hemoglobin A1c of less than 7: 52 percent, 59 percent
- Blood pressure under 130/80: 22 percent, 48 percent
- LDL under 100: 74 percent, 86 percent
- LDL less than 70: 27 percent, 45 percent

To achieve these results across a wide swath of practices, Bestermann says physicians must organize around best practice guidelines, launch a major program to target bad-risk behaviors, develop information technology infrastructures to support care protocols and measurements, and be paid for achieving these results. In other words, doctors must be reimbursed for their performance.

Bestermann commented on the current practice of medicine, "Our profession is organized in top-down single risk silos that ensure a fragmented approach to a global condition. Furthermore, professional and advocacy societies are based on a single risk factor. This structure cannot work." He continued, "Progress toward integrated, coordinated management of global risks will require totally new organizations. What we need is connection and coordination of goals." Bestermann's work is insight translated into innovation. What is impressive is that he, COSEHC, and their cardiovascular centers of excellence have done this without a pooling of money. They have done it with like-minded physicians paying attention, sharing evidence, and learning together how to defuse the explosion of chronic disease.

Innovation Talking and Action Points

In this chapter, a new practice business model that focuses on systematically monitoring and altering risk factors in related diseases (hypertension, diabetes, and dyslipidemias) that lead to vascular deaths is described. Some experts have said that as many as 30 percent of American adults suffer from the "metabolic syndrome," an expanded version of what Bestermann mentioned. The components of the metabolic syndrome include:

- Abdominal obesity (excessive fat tissue in and around the abdomen)
- Atherogenic dyslipidemias (blood fat disorders—high triglycerides, low HDL cholesterol and high LDL cholesterol—that foster plaque buildups in artery walls)
- Elevated blood pressure
- Insulin resistance or glucose intolerance (the body can't properly use insulin or blood sugar)

- Prothrombotic state (e.g., high fibrinogen or plasminogen activator inhibitor–1 in the blood)
- Proinflammatory state (e.g., elevated C-reactive protein in the blood)

Tracking all of these components is impractical because of expense. What Dr. Bestermann and his COSEHC colleagues have achieved has been done by using existing tools within the constraints of their existing practices, and without funding or financial rewards. They have nothing to sustain them but a passion for continuous learning. Yet they have:

- shown that vascular deaths can be reduced across a broad spectrum of cardiovascular-producing diseases
- applied evidence-based practices to induce death risk reductions
- persuaded academic medical centers to engage in the process
- stuck with their plans without an increase in reimbursement
- done all of these within the context of a loose confederation of private practitioners

The Opportunity

Based on these five achievements, an opportunity exists to:

1. extend this new model to markets outside the Southeast
2. persuade payers that a procedure-based model is too expensive and doomed to fail
3. introduce a new paradigm of addressing risks across the entire spectrum of atherosclerotic-producing diseases (diabetes, hypertension, hyperlipidemias)
4. create enormous cost-saving and life-saving benefits
5. build a new model for care given the pay-for-performance movement

This new model might be a shot in the arm for primary care physicians, provided, of course, they are paid more for achieving superior outcomes.

What Is Needed to Support a New Model

According to Brian Klepper, president of the Center for Practical Health Reform, a former practice consultant, and a fan of Bestermann and his colleagues, what is needed to support the spread of this effective model for preventing vascular diseases, the biggest killer of Americans, is strong physician leadership, a well-conceived and detailed business plan, technical skills, early relations with key payer and technology firms, and a transition plan to a new business model.

A Suggested Role for the Pharmaceutical Industry

The pharmaceutical industry now sells $17 billion worth of drugs to control hypertension (Saul, 2006). A controversy is brewing because many of the nation's leading hypertension experts are functioning as consultants for the industry. These experts are advocating the criterion for hypertension be lowered from 120/80 to 110/70. This would raise the number of Americans labeled as having hypertension. Controlling blood pressure is a mainstay of the pharmaceutical industry. About 65 million Americans have high blood pressure under the current definition; another 59 million people are borderline.

If doctors were to treat these borderline hypertensive patients, money expended on controlling hypertension could expand to $25 to $30 billion. Rather than redefining hypertension, why doesn't the pharmaceutical industry, now spending millions sponsoring lectures on drugs, spend more of their monies on broad-scale preventive measures such as those advocated by COSEHC and Dr. Bestermann's centers of cardiovascular excellence? Why not take a broader and more cost-effective approach to a national health problem affecting nearly one third of American adults?

Case Study 1

The COSEHC Story
By Dr. Bill Bestermann

Dr. Bestermann is an internist in the 18-person Lowcountry Medical Group in Beaufort, South Carolina. He serves as president of COSEHC's Cardiovascular Centers of Excellence Program. He has joined Holston Medical Group, a 115 provider group in Kingsport, Tennessee. His job will be to develop a cardiovascular and diabetic center of excellence. The Holston Medical Group has 24,000 diabetics in their practice, which is paperless and uses the AllScripts electronic health record system. In addition to developing the center, Dr. Bestermann will conduct clinical trials and will manage diabetic patients and others with cardiovascular disease.

William H. Bestermann, Jr., was born in Brooklyn, New York, and grew up in Myrtle Beach, South Carolina. He did his undergraduate work at Furman University and attended Wake Forest Medical School. Dr. Bestermann went onto internship and residency training at Portsmouth Naval Hospital and completed 7 years of naval service before beginning private practice in Beaufort, South Carolina, as the first full-time internist.

He became president of the South Carolina Affiliate of the American Heart Association in 1993 and was the test practice for the Hypertension Initiative of South Carolina. He began to practice vascular medicine in 1998 and in 2006 served as president of the Cardiovascular Center of Excellence program under the auspices of the Consortium of Southeast Hypertension Control.

• •

The *Annals of Internal Medicine* published a review article in 1998 on managing stable angina. That single article changed my professional life. The piece offered a revolutionary view of coronary artery disease; namely, medical treatment effectively prevented myocardial infarction. On the other hand, percutaneous and surgical revascularization did nothing to reduce the incidence of heart attacks in stable angina patients and in reality only relieved symptoms.

That article almost knocked me out of my chair. Until then I had thought of myocardial infarction as a result of a fixed atherosclerotic blockage in an artery, the block finally reached a critical point and revascularization was the ultimate preventive measure.

I began right away to look for confirmation of this concept. I was quickly able to find the 1995 article in *Circulation* by Peter Libby, the noted cardiologist from the Harvard system.

Libby said, "It is of interest in this regard that despite the well-accepted benefit of coronary artery bypass surgery on anginal symptoms, this treatment aimed at severe stenoses does not prevent myocardial infarction. To reduce the risk of acute myocardial infarction, one must stabilize lesions . . . particularly the less stenotic plaque."

Even in the Deep South

The medical prevention and treatment of atherosclerotic vascular disease could be done anywhere, even in a small town in the Deep South. I had come to Beaufort, South Carolina, in 1976 as the first full-time internist. By 1995, I was feeling a bit overwhelmed by the avalanche of new information in the broad field of general internal medicine.

I had always really enjoyed work in cardiovascular disease and I decided to devote my full-time practice to the medical prevention and treatment of atherosclerotic vascular illness. I first thought I would emphasize and manage high blood pressure and cholesterol. I learned very quickly the highest risk patients are adult-onset diabetics. I understood I was going to have to dramatically improve my management of those vulnerable individuals.

Not long after I made this decision, I ran into Dr. Brent Egan from the Medical University of South Carolina. Dr. Egan told me he was about to initiate a program to improve blood pressure treatment in our state. The Hypertension Initiative of South Carolina would track core measures in the prevention of vascular disease—BP, HbA1c, and LDL—using 3×5 cards which treating physicians would fill in by hand and send to the medical school periodically for manual entry into a computer database. The program would improve results by tracking data and improving knowledge with continuing medical education lectures. I agreed to be the test practice and began to produce encouraging results.

Improving the Process of Measuring Quality Improvement

Very early in this effort, it became apparent this was essentially a quality-improvement effort. Now with a means to measure performance, it seemed to me the critical second step would be to work on the process of care. I became more and more convinced vascular risk factors were interrelated. The key next step would be to develop an evidence-based protocol addressing them in a coordinated and integrated fashion.

Unraveling a Complicated Metabolic Web

All of these risk factors were associated with insulin resistance and impaired endothelial function. The protocol should identify treatments improving endothelial function and insulin resistance while not causing weight gain. Medications should have beneficial effects on more than one risk factor if possible. Dr. Ralph DeFronzo described the metabolic syndrome as a 'complex metabolic web. The best protocol should unravel that complicated web.'

Not long after I met Dr. Egan, he introduced me to the COSEHC Cardiovascular Centers of Excellence program. I finally felt that I had found a home. The type of practice I had been drawn to was so new I did not even know what to call it or where to find other physicians with the same interests. The COSEHC Cardiovascular Centers of Excellence implied a focused effort to integrate the care of all cardiometabolic risk factors. It was just the right answer. The longer I have worked in this kind of practice and the Centers of Excellence, the more convinced I have become of the validity of the concept.

Crossing the Quality Chasm Strikes a Chord

That way of thinking received further affirmation when the Institute of Medicine published *Crossing the Quality Chasm* in 2001. The authors said that improvement in the care of chronic conditions would require a substantial reworking of the system of care. They said the current care model could not accomplish this vital function. They recommended focused efforts to address 15 priority conditions and the cardiovascular center of excellence addresses nearly half of those identified in a single clinic.

The IOM recommendations are extensive, but the core of simple quality improvement can be done in most communities.

1. Set up evidence-based protocols consistent with best practices.
2. Develop the information infrastructure to support care and measurement of care processes and outcomes.

COSEHC Centers of Excellence Evolves

That is exactly what the COSEHC Centers of Excellence program has been developing since then. We have formed a writing committee capable of updating protocols rapidly. We also have a database committee actively engaged in refining the information infrastructure to support and measure care processes. Our stated purpose is to provide an instrument to facilitate implementing *Crossing the Quality Chasm* concepts in communities across our region.

A Practical Real-World Innovation for Any Community

This is a practical, real-world innovation. It can be implemented in any community with physicians willing to adjust their practices to focus on certain priority conditions. Any well-qualified primary care person could become very effective within 6 months' time.

This is not "cookbook" medicine but rather a willingness to implement a proven strategy to improve care. As with most quality-improvement efforts, it will only cover about 80 percent of encounters. Our professional expertise will be tested as usual to address exceptions. This is the best example I know of that improves care and reduces cost in the fairly short term.

Case Study 2

Health Care's Season of Discontent and the Devil's Staircase: Recast the Debate

By Stephen Barchet, MD, FACOG, CPE, FACPE, Rear Admiral, MC, USN, Retired

Dr. Stephen Barchet is the managing partner of Benefit Payment Solutions, a limited liability company that consults on matters of electronic financial message interchange. In addition, he is the coordinator of Health Plan for Life (HP4Life), a model and concept developed and placed in the public domain for implementation and test in both public and private sectors.

Serving in the Navy first as an obstetrician-gynecologist and later in various executive positions, he completed over 27 years active military service. His final assignment was Deputy Surgeon General and Deputy Director of Naval Medicine.

After retiring from active naval service in 1983, he provided consulting services in the private sector initially emphasizing needed efficiencies in military health benefits and related programs. A past member of the editorial board of Managed Care Outlook, Barchet participates in numerous professional and civic organizations. He was principal investigator of the 1995 study of Medical Savings Account Programs funded by the J. W. Murdock Charitable Foundation. As project manager, he oversaw the Defined Health Contribution Project (DHC). Barchet coedited and coauthored the project members' deliberations in an April 2001 publication—a how-to/what-to primer for small employers who want to understand and offer defined contribution health benefits for their employees.

Barchet currently coordinates efforts to facilitate, enhance, and expand understanding of the economic and health effects in both public and private sectors under various methods of financing health benefits and purchase of health services. He is the coordinator of the Health Plan for Life (HP4Life), a strategy and method for improving the health of people and stabilizing the inevitable growth in health care spending. A draft form of the HP4Life model and concept was reviewed, modified, and refined at a 2-day workshop convened September 2003 at South Seattle Community College. The HP4Life workshop proceedings are Internet accessible at www.effwa.org/hp. In 2004, Barchet joined the board of directors of the Seattle-based Hope Heart Institute and chairs the education committee. He advocates patient responsibility, informed consumers, and individual empowerment.

••

In this season of discontent with an endless conundrum of our nation's health care crisis, the resolute but fruitless search continues for the "Killer App" of remedial innovations. Would that the omnipresent print and electronic proposals by pundits, experts, policy mavens, and others harboring opinions assure antidotes for every problem of access, quality, and cost of health benefits and health care services.

It is not for lack of published research; demonstrations large and small, newly minted and refined laws advocate, promote, or throttle various innovations. Despite all the noise, fury, and frustration, our discontent and the conundrum coexist as both descend the "devil's staircase"(the devil's staircase is a mathematical term meaning that with each step taken downward one descends into the abyss of infinity as explained in Munnecke, Tom, "Health and the Devil's Staircase," Business Enterprise Solutions and Technologies, "Veteran's Hospital Administration," January 31, 2001, Munnecke, 2000).

I'll not belabor familiar reports, studies, essays, opinions, and media interpretations of unending proposals but will instead share some examples.

- First, is the congressional-directed *Citizen's Health Care Working Group's June 2006 Preliminary Report,* directed in the 2004 Medicare Modernization Act. This report describes the results of multiple public community meetings held in many U.S. cities. The report summarizes the "values, principles, and recommendations" presumed to reflect the collective wants and preferences of the participants. This compilation synthesizes discussions and electronic collected answers to structured questions about health care, coverage, and financing. Predictably, citizen wants exceed by far capacities, capabilities, and resources but ignore constraints. Few, if any, will feign surprise at the conclusions.
- Second, that same month there appeared an immediately lauded book, *Redefining Health Care: Creating Value-Based Competition on Results.* Expanding on his popular essay in the *Harvard Business Review*, Michael Porter and coauthor Elizabeth Olmsted Teisberg diagnose the fatal flaw underpinning our national health care crisis. They offer a strategic prescription for what ails health care financing, access, and quality. This too should not surprise critical readers. Diagnosing the problems as the product of failed interventions these past years, the authors prescribe provider competition based upon measured value of their products.

  What an amazing innovation to lie upon a $2 trillion economy. Is value-based competition the long-sought after "Killer Application"? Amid well-outlined generalities, this innovation joins the overly crowded complex of supply-side cost management interventions.
- Third, in Washington State another study generated local and national headlines (Fox, Will, and Pickerington, 2006). Once more it was touted an important discovery. Blue Cross Premera/ Milliman found that public funded programs cost shifted health care services onto the private sector, mostly employers' purchased benefits and services. Surely no health expert would be surprised.

From each main-stage policy think tank, a plethora of proposals, small and large, focused and comprehensive, grabs daily media attention, but then both proposal and the latest headline disappear in the fog of relentless pursuit of increasing health care spending, its attendant revenues happily deposited nightly.

Finally, there are countless reports of health care services grossly misused, overused, and underused. Advocates abound with all manner of provider-focused interventions too numerous to list but widely known and practiced. Each counts upon heavily weighted supply-side interventions. Exhortations and demands for every kind of new reform, legislation, and mandates old and new occupy conferences, meetings, study groups, commissions, and sundry other congregations. As thinking and parlaying wears on and on, the spending continues unabated, unbridled. The discontent widens and deepens as does spending and its rewards.

- Is there an identifiable solution to widespread discontent; a truly effective remedy?
- Is there a results-based prescription groomed for prime time?
- Is there one acceptable to public and private sectors, academicians, philosophers, public policy decision makers, and everyday people?

Probably not! Our wants according to most Citizens' Health Care Working Groups are infinite no matter constraints, obvious or not. Is there an exit from the health care "devil's staircase" and its awaiting abyss? I think so: "Recast the health care debate!" Frame and adopt an individual, local, regional, and national policy focused not on health care first and its myriad services but instead on health itself—the health of individuals and the people.

Recast the Health Care Debate for Progress: Set a Prime Directive

The age-old, lifelong, unending debate over the health care conundrum rages with innumerable resolutions and tactics for relief proposed and promised but unrealized.

Though some people contend the United States offers the best health care in the world, numerous critics and studies assert the opposite, citing unacceptable problems of access, coverage, quality, and costs.

Complaints include patient safety, quality, outcome, provider and facility adequacy, generational, and income disparity. Increases in health benefits widely surpass wage increases. Health spending in 2006 exceeded $2 trillion. Medicare outlays in less than 35 years will exceed 8 percent of Gross National Product (U.S. Budget and Economic Data).

Call to Action: Gotta, Gotta, Gotta

With the focus on three principal issues (access, cost, quality and innumerable subordinate concerns), the mantra and calls to action are: " . . . gotta reform the health care system"; or ". . . gotta make health care a right for all"; and ". . . gotta provide universal coverage, insurance."

These goals and objectives are well intentioned. However, all actions beget little but more discontent. Neither outcomes nor the debate change for what I contend are likely but unstated reasons. The stakeholders, health care communities, and industry forces will tweak things for show only—notwithstanding public avowals and declarations of needed reforms.

Spending Pain, but No Health Gain

However, the spending continues with little if any gain in the health of the people. Hence, my assertion to recast the debate: absent real progress and absent an established national policy set upon the health of the people, it is time to reorder the approach to the principal issues that confound much needed real innovation with change and results. The framework upon which to make progress requires abandoning fixing the health care system and seeking universal coverage as the dominant goal and outcomes. Change the ground rules and the debate itself.

New Policy Objectives

In order to focus the issues and redirect the debate over reform, above all else is the need to adopt an overall national policy objective—as follows:

- **The sole overall national policy objective is:** Universal optimal attainable health of the people.
- **The prime directive becomes:** Permit a flourish of universal health system(s)—*emphasis plural*—that foremost improve, enhance, and maintain optimal attainable health of individuals, communities, and the general population.

- **The means to optimal health for all:** Systems of universal health will make clear precisely the purpose of health benefits, health services, and health care.
- **The purpose of health benefits, health services, and health care is:** To continuously lessen the burden, impact, and likelihood of human disease, illness, disability, and injury, thereby improving, enhancing, and maintaining to the extent possible the health, longevity, and quality of life of all.

Next Steps

Upon acceptance, agreement, and adoption of the previous points, it then follows to ask and to answer the following:

- What is the framework for universal health systems?
- What would these universal health systems look like?
- Who pays for—and how—for what services?
- How are health care outcomes, health status, and economic results compared, evaluated, and measured?
- What changes in behaviors, nutrition, and health patterns would people adopt to achieve optimal attainable health?
- What roles would exist for individual, community, and industry responsibility?
- How would universal health systems effect changes that are desirable, preferred, and measurable?

With the debate over reforms suitably recast, the old devil's staircase can be replaced for one upon which to descend anew.

Chapter 4

The KISS Trifecta, from Complexity to Simplicity

Prelude: Simple changes may pay off big in practice productivity, quality, and satisfaction.

Products based on disruptive technologies are typically cheaper, simpler, and, frequently, more convenient to use.

Clayton M. Christensen, Harvard Business School professor, 1997

Belief in Economies of Scale

Among many observers, this belief persists: Only large practices with system changes will solve small-practice problems. This belief is prominent among leaders of large multispecialty clinics and organizations like the RAND Corporation and the Institute of Health Care Improvement in Boston.

System Doctors and Simple Doctoring of the System

Many physician leaders regard large integrated multispecialty clinics as the most rational solution for solving small-practice woes; in other words, work together as teams in large systems or die. Dr. Fitzhugh Mullan, author of *Big Doctoring in America: Profiles of Primary Care* (2002) and a family physician on the board of editors of *Health Affairs,* describes these physician leaders as "system doctors," because many are medical directors of large health systems.

Disruptive (and Simplifying) Innovations

However, in *The Innovator's Dilemma* (2000), Clayton M. Christenson, a professor at Harvard Business School, says that "disruptive innovations" can undermine even the best managed large organizations. A disruptive innovation is a new technological invention, product, or service that eventually overturns the existing dominant technology or product in the market

Simple, convenient, and powerful innovations aimed at the low end of the market disrupt large organizations. In health care, the market's low end is primary care physician practices, and the high end is large multispecialty organizations. Like all large organizations, they may be mismanaged, develop bloated overheads, become overly bureaucratic, and suffer losses of physicians who seek more autonomy and incomes on the outside. In short, large organizations are complicated bureaucracies, and many physicians do not feel comfortable in complicated working environments.

Disruptive Innovations in Electronic Health Records Market

A good example of disruptive innovations (also called disruptive technologies) is EClinicalWorks, a small electronic health records (EHR) company in Massachusetts. In head-to-head competition with three larger EHR companies—GE Health, Allscripts, and NextGen—for small-group practices in three Massachusetts communities, 170 of 180 physician practices picked EClinicalWorks as their vendor of choice (Rowland, 2006b).

The reason was quite clear. The three larger companies developed their products for larger groups. They perceived these to be more profitable, while EClinicalWorks targeted the low end of the market, small-group practices. The EClinicalWorks system was simply easier for physicians in small practices to use, learn, and implement than other systems. This ease was partly because its users were constantly ironing out its bugs in a transparent Web site, www.ecwuser.com, where users could suggest how to continually improve the EHR.

Three Disruptive Add-On Technologies

The following are three disruptive add-on technologies that can be implemented in smaller practices. An "add-on technology" is a piece of software that can be added to an existing electronic record.

The First Three Options

In a *Minnesota Medicine* article, Rich Kirkpatrick (2006), a general internist in a nine-person primary care group in Longview, Washington, suggests three ways for primary care physicians to improve their economic lot.

1. "Skim the cream" of the patient pool by eliminating Medicare and welfare patients and collecting $40 to $50 more per visit. Kirkpatrick regards this as unethical.
2. Go to work for a health care company and shift your allegiance from patients to business interests. Kirkpatrick finds this distasteful; in effect, selling out to the enemy.
3. Get into the ancillaries—X-rays, lab work, ultrasounds, and MRI and CT ownership. Kirkpatrick says this is the acceptable alternative, though critics may condemn it as self-referral.

A Fourth Option: The "KISS Trifecta"

A fourth option might be the "KISS Trifecta." The KISS (keep it simple, stupid) method is a computing term that recognizes two things:

1. People want things simple and easy to use.
2. Use of simple services or products shortens time and reduces costs for customers.

In horse racing, the trifecta is a system of betting. Bettors who pick the first three winners in the correct sequence win. It is possible the following KISS Trifecta will work for practitioners with too little time to see patients at too high a cost.

First Leg of the Trifecta: Instant Medical History

The Instant Medical History is software that has been developed over the last 15 years and that is available at www.instantmedicalhistory.com.

This software saves time and answers several fundamental questions. What eats up time when you see a patient? Taking and documenting the history with a review of systems—correct? Moreover, third parties won't pay unless you extensively document what took place. Why not let patients document why they are seeing the doctor by entering their own histories and system reviews using simple software, either from their home or in the reception room? Why not permit patients to tell their story on their time, not yours? Why not place a desktop computer in your reception room to serve this ATM-like function; in other words, having customers enter the own data?

Why Not Let the Patient Enter Historical Data?

Why not let the computer take the history and record the review of systems? All of this can be done using a simple "yes" or "no" algorithm based on the patient's chief complaint, gender, and age. For the last decade, family physician Allen Wenner of Columbia, South Carolina, and John Bachman, head of primary care at the Mayo

Clinic in Rochester, Minnesota, has done precisely this, with mutual satisfaction for themselves and patients (Bachman, 2004). What's wrong with having patients enter the exam room with their story spelled out in a computer interview? Nothing. Once you know the patient history, you can enter your findings with a few computer key strokes based on their complaint and their story. If you wish, call this a focused physical. Further, using this approach, patients can leave the office with their electronic medical record with history, findings, and treatment plan in hand.

Costs and Gains of Patient-Generated Histories

What is the cost to you of patient-generated histories? Probably around $50 per month for software you can connect to any current EMR system. The gain? Four to 8 minutes time saved per patient and a documented electronic record. In addition, patient creation of this history and computer entry of your findings make most dictation unnecessary and it serves as a basis for claims initiation and enhanced coding—even a referral letter. Furthermore, the patient immediately has a clear record of what transpired, thereby eliminating confusion that may lead to malpractice suits. Finally, because of the impressive documentation made possible through patient input, you can often move the code up one level; in other words, from a 99214 to a 99215, a gain of over $37.00 (see the following).

Second Leg of the Trifecta: Electronic Coding within the Doctor's Control (www.dpnx.com)

Think again. How are you paid? Like most doctors, you are paid primarily through five ICD-9 codes: 99211 through 99215. For these payment codes, in the Longview, Washington, zip code, for instance, Medicare pays $21.20, $38, $51.90, $81.41, and $118.49, respectively. Medicare payments vary by zip code and are continually changing; Dr. Kirkpatrick and his colleagues are paid an average of $53 per patient because Medicare pays only 80 percent. To cover overhead, Dr. Kirkpatrick says the doctor must see 27 patients a day. Many doctors can't do this.

Addressing the Underpayment Issue with Self-Coding

What does an online coding system, listing Medicare fees for your zip code, offer doctors to address this underpayment issue?

- Doctors can quickly audit their current fees and upgrade them to make sure they exceed Medicare (third parties allow 125 to 150 percent of Medicare in most regions). Many practices haven't changed fees for years and are below current Medicare fees for their zip code.

- Doctors can use the DPNX.com translator function to find fees for things they don't usually charge for; for example, consultation fees. Different doctors use different language for the same procedure or service and often have a hard time locating the precise code. The particular doctor's language, in other words, needs to be translated to find the right code. This translator function is enormously helpful because many doctors have a hard time locating the precise code for seldom coded visits or procedures.

- Doctors can look up Medicare procedure fees for their zip code and charge accordingly. This last point brings up the third part of the Trifecta: Doing simple procedures in your office.

Third Leg of the Trifecta: Performing Simple Procedures in Your Office

In 1989, John Pfenninger, a family physician, founded the National Procedures Institute in Midland, Michigan (www.NPInstitute.com). Since then, he and his staff have taught procedure skills to thousands of physicians in Michigan and in regional conferences across the United States for CME (Continuing Medical Education) credits. Pfenninger's reasoning is straightforward: It can be spelled out as follows. Properly trained primary care physicians are perfectly capable of performing simple procedures (skin biopsies, skin repairs, incision and drainage, joint injections, colposcopic biopsies, colonoscopies, and so forth) in their offices—safely, effectively, conveniently, and for lower costs than can be done in specialists' offices.

Toward these ends, he and his staff have organized courses for CME credits, developed a reimbursement manual for office procedures, and written a textbook, *Procedures for Primary Care,* 2nd edition (1994). Codes for these procedures may be obtained at www.dpnx.com for your particular zip code. The procedure manual contains several reimbursement examples. These examples are procedures primary care physicians did routinely in the recent past and, with proper preparation, can be done in the future.

Three Simple Steps

Primary care physicians can afford to remain in practice if they do three simple things, all available thorough current software online:

1. Let their patients create their own medical histories (www.medicalhistory .com).
2. Use an online coding system to access up-to-date ICD-9, CP4, and Evaluation and Management (E&M) codes and to audit and upgrade their current fees (www.dpnx.com).
3. Perform simple office procedures (www.NPInstitute.com).

These three simple things, the KISS Trifecta, can be carried out without radically restructuring or altering current office practice patterns.

Innovation Talking and Action Points

As just noted, using small add-on information technologies and procedural innovations within the context of the existing practice model fosters efficiency, productivity, and revenues. Add-on technologies, however, feature *chunking*, the building of a better model from simple incremental changes. It benefits consumers by offering timesaving techniques that facilitate diagnosis, minimize the need for referral, and generate an electronic record people can take with them.

These three applications reduce the complex to the simple and follow Drucker's innovation principle of "if it isn't simple, it isn't right" (Drucker, 1986). This brings to mind two other principles, borrowed from complexity science:

1. Go for multiple actions at the fringes, let the direction arise rather than be sure before you do anything.

2. Grow complex systems by chunking by allowing complex systems to emerge out of links among simple systems that work well and are capable of operating independently. (Zimmerman, Lindberg, and Pisket, 1998)

One final word of wisdom from Alfred North Whitehead, the English philosopher, "Seek simplicity, but distrust it." We live in a complex world. Complexity is not going away, but sometimes it can be circumvented.

Shadow-Based Medicine

Ask any seasoned primary care practitioner what he or she honestly thinks of evidence-based medicine and pay-for-performance, and the person will likely express skepticism. Why?

- He or she knows that the value of physicians' services does not rest solely on hard evidence or diagnosing and treating specific diseases.

- He or she knows medicine is often practiced in the shadows; in other words, the diagnosis is not evident early and the visit may stem from loneliness or the need for psychological reinforcement.

- He or she knows that perhaps 70 percent of patients present with vague symptoms, fatigue, malaise, emotional problems, depression, Alzheimer's, driving difficulties, prediagnostic chronic diseases, hard-to-pin-down disorders that don't come bearing a label or carrying a code. (Wenner, 2006)

Practice is not black or white; it is gray and full of shadows. Those who pay only for concrete evidence do not understand it takes time to flush out what lurks in the shadows. As the old radio character Lamont Cranston said, "Only the Shadow knows." Similarly, the patient, given time and the right questions, knows something is wrong, and in time evidence will reveal what is wrong. That is why a computer-based interview like the instant medical history is a valuable innovation.

- It pushes aside or penetrates the shadows.
- It asks those questions that take time to ask and time to answer.
- It permits patients to "tell" the computer what they might be ashamed to tell a doctor or nurse.
- It allows the physician to categorize and code such diseases as alcoholism, depression, and obsessive-compulsive disorders by using the official scales for judging those disorders.

Paying for simple needed procedures is something evidence-based and performance advocates can understand. There is nothing shadowy about removing a basal cell, lancing a boil, or injecting a painful joint. It takes less time, pays more, and leaves time for exploring the shadows.

Doctors Not Paid for Work Done, but Work Documented

Doctors are not paid for work done, but rather for work documented—and rightly so. To document what is done, one can use checklists (payers tend to look at these skeptically), handwritten notes (one can write 30 words/minute), dictation (one can dictate at 150 words/minute), or patient-generated histories (patient entry rate as high as 3,000 words a minute using protocols with minimal time for doctors except for reading patient-generated narrative).

Codes are written in the abstract by committees and lawyers and paid by payers for concrete, documented action. Fair enough. However, none of those who wrote these codes or pay for them are present at the doctor–patient interaction. If the encounter is documented extensively through the innovative use of technology, it cannot be denied in retrospect.

Case Study 1

Workflow Using Instant Medical History with an Electronic Medical Record

By Dr. John Dugaw and Dr. Allen R. Wenner

Drs. John Dugaw and Allen Wenner are family physicians in Columbia, South Carolina. Over the last 15 years, they have developed, modified, and perfected the clinical algorithms that make up the Instant Medical History (www.instantmedicahistory.com)

. . . .

When it comes to innovation, technology is a two-edged sword. Technology may simplify complexity (as Drs. Dugaw and Wenner show in diagnosing and evaluating depressed patients) or it may complicate simplicity (many regard human-to-human interviewing as simplicity itself). Unfortunately, to complicate matters, as this case study shows, describing technological simplicity can be complicated.

The use of an electronic medical record changes workflow in the outpatient office. By adding Instant Medical History software to an electronic medical record, workflow can be faster, cheaper, and better for patients and providers. Here three simulations of the workflow by inexperienced and experienced providers are contrasted with any provider using Instant Medical History. The improvement in time, efficiency, diagnostic accuracy, coding, and patient satisfaction justifies inclusion of Instant Medical History in any computer-based medical record used in an outpatient setting.

Results

Instant Medical History can make health care faster, cheaper, and better for patients because by using the program, both patients and providers save time. As demonstrated in these clinical examples, the workflow with Instant Medical History saves the physician 21 minutes for three patient visits. How?

- By reducing paperwork
- By permitting the nurse to spend twice as long with the patient doing clinical duties including in-office patient education and providing advice not previously possible

The new patient in for a complete examination spends one third less time in the encounter. The patient spends less time waiting and is occupied with productive activity throughout the visit. The overall costs of the care are lower and the reimbursement is higher.

The provider would be able to see additional patients with the time saved as well as generate additional revenue because documentation becomes more accurate as it becomes a side effect of the visit rather than a primary focus of the encounter.

The physician is able to bill a higher code for the office visit because the computerized history alerts him or her to the proper diagnosis and automatically identifies appropriate computerized screening tests that are billable as CPT Code 96103.

He or she is able to bill substantially more for what is fully documented as a complex therapeutic intervention with interlinked problems. He or she is able to bill for the additional indicated testing and preventive health services. Using Instant Medical History, the patient often meets criteria for a comprehensive evaluation and management code because of the multiple diagnoses previously addressed but not documented.

Improving quality is economically justified in both capitated and fee-for-service environments. Capitation payment is based on a fixed monthly payment for patients in a defined population; fee-for-service is payment for an individual service at the time the service is delivered. In a capitated environment, early recognition of disease can lower costs substantially as evidenced by the inexperienced physician scenario if the depression is not recognized. If the provider does not prospectively diagnose depression (Reece, 2005), then the cost of this missed diagnosis is reflected in an emergency room visit after office hours for pain control. The following example contrasts three simultaneous patient visits with an experienced physician and a less-experienced physician using the same patient both with and without patient-entered data using Instant Medical History.

The cases are based on clinical experience of the users of this software to demonstrate the differences in outcome as revealed in the medical literature. The cases are not based on a specific patient.

Routine Office Visit

A. Inexperienced Physician B. Experienced Physician*	Cost/Time CPT/RVU	Using Instant Medical History (Any provider)	Cost/Time CPT/RVU
A new patient comes to the office with a bad headache. Immediately the patient completes a new patient business form that is entered into the billing system by the receptionist.	Patient waits 5 minutes.	Idem	Patient waits 5 minutes.
The receptionist gives the patient a paper medical history on a clipboard. The office has used this questionnaire for years. It is commercially produced, but must be stored, re-ordered, handled, and restocked. Patient completes it and returns it to the front desk. The receptionist is too busy to notice or let the nurse know that the patient has completed the paperwork and	$1.50 for forms. Patient waits 30 minutes	Patient is instructed by the receptionist to go to the computer kiosk in the corner of the waiting room and follow the on-screen instructions. The patient operates the software, gaining a sense of control of the medical process. New patients receive a review of systems and provide family and social history according to HCFA level 5 documentation guide-	Patient works on computer for 10 minutes.

(continued)

Routine Office Visit

A. Inexperienced Physician B. Experienced Physician	Cost/Time CPT/RVU	Using Instant Medical History (Any provider)	Cost/Time CPT/RVU
is ready to be seen by the doctor. This possible loss of satisfaction also impacts patient flow negatively.		lines. Preventive measures as recommended by U.S. Preventive Services Task Force are elucidated for provider and explained to patient.	
Nurse comes to get patient, takes vital signs, records them in the computer, and completes other required data. Nurse chats with patient about presenting problem and gives the patient a second paper form for completion about headaches. Patient completes the form and waits for the doctor or nurse. Nurse returns and looks at the initial patient history form and begins to enter pertinent clinical data into the computerized chart. Nurse stops after the Review of Systems. Nurse looks at the headache form and explains to the patient that the doctor will review it with him.	$1.50 for forms. Nurse time 12 minutes. Patient waits 10 minutes.	Nurse calls patient to the sub-waiting area and edits the data in the electronic medical record that the patient has entered using Instant Medical History. Nurse reviews the initial screening and mentally triages the patient. Quality assurance occurs as nurse makes certain that the patient is being seen 1) by the right provider; 2) for the proper complaint; and 3) in a time appropriate fashion. Nurse takes the patient's vital signs and records them in the electronic chart. Nurse initiates the second computer screening of the present illness section of Instant Medical History.	$0 paper materials. Nurse time 12 minutes.

Experienced Physician has at least 15 years of clinical experience.

Step 1—Waiting Room and Nurse Triage of Patient #1: The early use of the computer by the patient changes the workflow for the nurse and receptionist. The patient is entering the information that would normally be required of them.

The patient is occupied doing productive work. Preventive guidelines and patient education is occurring even before the interaction showing a remarkably different approach to the new patient. The nurse and receptionist can each perform more productive tasks like patient care. Using Instant Medical History the workflow allows for real-time quality assurance measurement at the start of the visit.

Case Study continues

Routine Office Visit

A. Inexperienced Physician B. Experienced Physician	Cost/Time CPT/RVU	Using Instant Medical History (Any provider)	Cost/Time CPT/RVU
Patient waits		The software program, Instant Medical History, interviews the patient with the interactive branching logic. She tells the patient to indicate the head and neck section to give details of her headache. Because of the patient's responses, the software automatically branches into a Zung Depression survey, a Hamilton Anxiety scale, and a Holmes Stress scale. The patient finishes the questioning, indicates that there are not further problems for today's visit, and notifies the nurse.	Patient works on computer for 20 minutes; 5 minutes Nurse time
Patient continues to wait. (Waiting time is the number one complaint by patients about medical care.)		Nurse administers a tetanus/diphtheria immunization and schedules the patient for a mammogram. These are examples of indicated preventive measure revealed by waiting room screening to comply with U.S. Preventive Services Task Force Guidelines. Nurse improves quality of care by meeting these HEDIS and NCQA standards. The nurse takes the patient to the examination room.	10 min nurse and patient time. Revenue increase is $19.00
Doctor comes in to see patient. Patient confirms history given on paper forms. Data flows from form to doctor to patient confirmation back to doctor to computer. **A.** The *inexperienced provider* would likely concentrate on the physical symptoms of the	**A.** $24.00. 20 min physician and patient time.	The physician sees the patient. He reviews the data entered by the patient indicating a history compatible with common migraine syndrome, a positive depression survey and a high Holmes Stress scale. Most of the template for depression has been completed by Instant	$12.00. 10 min physician and patient time.

(continued)

Routine Office Visit

A. Inexperienced Physician B. Experienced Physician	Cost/Time CPT/RVU	Using Instant Medical History (Any provider)	Cost/Time CPT/RVU
headache. The clinician might not recognize the underlying masked depression as a cause of the headache since it is missed in more than 50 percent of new cases.		Medical History. The physician verifies the DSM4 interview for depression. The physician asks open-ended questions about the patient's life and family. He discovers very quickly that the patient's clinical depression is aggravated in part by the recent death of the patient's father and loss of a pet. The physician documents quickly that the patient meets criteria for a Major Depressive Disorder, moderate severity without dysthymia. The physician then gives the patient a handout on depressive disorders. Physician instructs the patient to get undressed and he will return for the clinical examination.	

Step 2—Patient #1—HPI by provider: The patient waiting time is replaced by preventive interventions and data input into the electronic medical record by the patient, not the nurse.

Routine Office Visit

A. Inexperienced Physician B. Experienced Physician	Cost/Time CPT/RVU	Using Instant Medical History (Any provider)	Cost/Time CPT/RVU
Going to a second examination room, the provider treats a child with an ear infection and completes that visit.	$7.20. 6 min. physician and patient time. CPT 99212 RVU .72	Going to a second examination room, the provider treats a child with an ear infection and completes that visit. Instant Medical History documents the history of this child as well as parental feelings about the illness.	$7.20. 6 min. physician and patient time. CPT 99212 RVU .72
Physician returns to the other patient. He performs a detailed physical examination of the patient, discovering no significant diagnostic findings. He directs the patient to dress and leaves to see another patient.	$12.00. 10 min physician and 16 minutes patient time.	Idem	$12.00. 10 min physician and 16 minutes patient time.

(continued)

Routine Office Visit

A. Inexperienced Physician B. Experienced Physician	Cost/Time CPT/RVU	Using Instant Medical History (Any provider)	Cost/Time CPT/RVU
Patient is satisfied that his symptoms are heard and that he has been examined. His underlying condition is unknown to him. Physician gives the patient a pamphlet to read about depression until he returns.	$2.00	Nurse begins an interactive patient education program on the computer in the exam room. The patient completes it unassisted before the physician returns.	5 minutes nurse time
In a third examination room, provider treats a patient in follow-up with diabetes and completes that visit.	$14.40. 12 min physician and patient time. CPT 99213 RVU 1.0	In a third examination room, provider treats a patient in follow-up with diabetes. Instant Medical History documents the history of the present illness, including new symptoms, and reminds the clinician about diabetic eye and foot care.	$14.40. 12 min physician. CPT 99213 RVU 1.0

Step 3—Patient #2—HPI, Assessment, and Plan + Patient #1—Examination + Patient #3—HPI, Assessment, and Plan: The workflow diverges early with the nurse taking on new duties, instituting preventive interventions, and reviewing the patient information.

The clinician has more information before the visit. Computer interviewing aids both the experienced and inexperienced provider, providing them with the data about the patient's psychological condition causing the headache.

Unless automated by Instant Medical History, the clinician must go to a file cabinet and find the medical reference or paper version of the scale that he wants to administer. He must give it to the patient to complete on a clipboard and return to score it himself or use valuable personnel time for processing the test. Alternatively, he can guess what the results of psychological screening might be by entering them into a template in the medical record if he picks the correct template.

Otherwise, he will have no objective evidence of the underlying cause of the headache. If he feels uncomfortable because this is a new patient, the clinician might order a CT scan of the brain to reassure himself that no pathology exists. The nurse practitioner without the Instant Medical History data might refer this patient for a second opinion.

Case Study continues

Routine Office Visit

A. Inexperienced Physician B. Experienced Physician	Cost/Time CPT/RVU	Using Instant Medical History (Any provider)	Cost/Time CPT/RVU
Physician returns. **A.** *Inexperienced physician* explains to patient that he has common migraine headache syndrome. **B.** Reviewing the paper based depression screening, the *experienced physician* explains to the patient that he has depression in addition to common migraine headache. The recent death of the patient's father and loss of a pet aggravate the depression. The depression is documented with DSM4 criteria as moderate. The physician uses additional time counseling the patient regarding the diagnoses of common migraine headaches as a sign of underlying depression. The symptoms are entered manually by the physician on a template in the electronic medical record.	**A.** $14.40. 12 min physician and 24 minutes patient time. CPT 99203. RVU 1.4. **B.** $33.60. 28 min. physician and 40 minutes patient time. CPT 99204. RVU 2.59.	The self-assessment scales completed by the patient using Instant Medical History already provide full medical record documentation of the depression according to DSM4 criteria. The physician uses additional time counseling and educating the patient regarding the diagnoses of common migraine headaches as a sign of underlying depression. The treatment plan is determined by the patient and physician rather than the provider hurrying to document a template in the electronic medical record. During explanation of the treatment plan, the medication is given along with a drug side effect profile.	$12.00. 10 min physician. CPT 99205. RVU 3.22.
Counseling regarding the diagnoses is easily documented in the electronic medical record, using standard templates. Printed educational material from the electronic medical record program is given for both problems, medication handouts are given via electronic medical record files, and prescriptions sent via e-mail to pharmacy with diagnosis codes. Patient is instructed to return in 3 weeks for follow up and to call if problems occur sooner.		Idem	

Step 4 Patient #1—Assessment and Plan: As the visit progresses, the use of Instant Medical History makes a clear difference in the outcome of the patient care. The time saving is obvious because the information is gathered earlier in the encounter. The clinician gets the information earlier so he can begin the treatment plan earlier. In addition, in-office patient education is possible by the nurse on screen and patient education handouts are allowed.

Routine Office Visit

A. *Inexperienced Physician*
B. *Experienced Physician*

Comparison Cost/Time CPT/RVU

Breakdown (Any provider)

Comparison Cost/Time CPT/RVU

Time/Cost/ Reimbursement Analysis
(No computer screening)

A.
Production: CPT Codes for Billing 99203 + 99212 + 99213

Revenue: RVUs 1.4 + 0.72 + 1.0 = 3.12

Medicare Relative Value Unit is $35.88

Reimbursement: 3.12 RVU × $35.88 per RVU = $111.95

Expense: Overhead is 40 percent of revenues × $112 = $44.77

Labor cost for inexperienced physician: $24.00 + $7.20 + $12.00 + $14.40 + $14.40 = $72.00

Nurse cost: $5.00; Receptionist cost: $2.40

Other unnecessary care: $150.00

Total Costs = $266.77

Time: Physician: 20 + 6 + 10 + 12 + 12 = 60 min

Nurse: 15 minutes

B.
Production: CPT Codes for Billing 99204 + 99212 + 99213

Revenue: RVUs 2.59 + .72 + 1.0 = 4.31

Reimbursement: 4.31 RVU × $35.88 per RVU = $154.64

Expense: Overhead: 40 percent of revenues × $154 = $65.85

A.
Costs = $266.77.
Physician time: 1 hour; patient time: 2 hours.
LOSS ($154.83)
Medicare Payment: $111.95.
RVU 3.12

B.
Cost: $160.88.
Physician time: 1 hour 13 minutes; patient time: 2 hours
LOSS ($6.24)
RVU 4.31
Medicare Payment: $154.64

Time/Cost/ Reimbursement Analysis
(With computer)
Any provider

Production: CPT Codes for Billing 99205 + 99212 + 99213

Patient meets criteria for a New Patient Comprehensive Evaluation and Management Code because of the dual diagnoses. Additional CPT codes: 96100 + 90718

Psychological Screening is administered and preventive tetanus immunization is given

Revenue: RVUs 3.22 + 0.72 + 1.0 = 4.94
Medicare Relative Value Unit is $35.88
Reimbursement: 4.94 RVU × $35.88 per RVU = $177.25

Additional revenue $58 + $19

Expense: Overhead is 40 percent of revenues × $177 = $71.88

Labor cost for any physician: $12.00 + $7.20 + $12.00 + $14.40 + $12.00 = $57.6

Nurse cost: $10.00

Receptionist cost: $2.40 Total Costs = $129.48

Time: Physician 10 + 6 + 10 + 12 + 10 = 48 min

Nurse 27 minutes

Profit: Using comparable codes without additional codes, the profit is $47.77. Making use of the valid additional codes for

Costs = $129.48
Physician Time: 48 min
Nurse time: 27 minutes.
Patient time: 1½ hours
Medicare Payment: $177.25.
RVU 4.94

(continued)

Routine Office Visit A. Inexperienced Physician B. Experienced Physician	*Comparison* *Cost/Time* *CPT/RVU*	*Breakdown (Any provider)*	*Comparison* *Cost/Time* *CPT/RVU*
Cost for experienced physician: $20.43 + $7.20 + $12.00 + $14.40 + $33.60 = $87.63		performed procedures increases profit to $125.27	
Nurse cost: $5.00		INSTANT MEDICAL HISTORY TOTAL PROFIT $47.77	
Receptionist cost: $2.40		TOTAL PROFIT	
Time: Physician 17 + 6 + 10 + 12 + 28 = 73 minutes		WITH ADDITIONS $125.27	

Step 5—Better Quality Care, Enhanced Revenue for the organization, and Improved Patient Satisfaction: Finally, patient-interview software allows health care to be better both for the patient and for the provider because (Drucker, 1986):

- The patient is empowered and has more input and control over his or her care.
- The patient receives in-office patient education.
- The patient sees a seamless flow of data between all parties concerned and knows that all of his or her problems were addressed.

It also allows the receptionist to focus on duties of patient reception, patient soothing by phone, and eliminating confrontations with the nursing staff because data has not been put into the computer.

The patient's complaint is appropriately addressed at an early stage of disease. The depression is treated, improving control of the headaches. The patient is given adequate handouts on a complicated medication program and medical problems so that the patient is comfortable with the diagnosis. The treatment plan is clear and set out for the patient, thus avoiding multiple calls back to the physician's office taking telephone time with staff. The patient knows his or her care is better.

The organization benefits because the losses from missed depression that cost the organization money are eliminated. When the diagnosis of depression is missed, complications often develop later and cost more money. The case demonstrates that quality of care is actually cheaper. Because the physician has the information to make the proper diagnosis, not only are fewer unnecessary tests ordered, but the accuracy of the diagnosis is increased. Early diagnosis reduces morbidity. Lower morbidity for the health care system translates to lower costs of providing care. Greater accuracy in diagnosis improves outcomes. Better documentation allows the provider organization to bill properly for work done.

Case Study 2

Translating Surgical Language into Codes
By Dr. James Weintrub and Greg Brownell

Dr. James Weintrub, a plastic surgeon, and Greg Brownell, a software expert, have worked together for more than five years to develop an Internet-based coding system that is more convenient for doctors to use.

In 1998, Dr. James Weintrub, a plastic surgeon, and Greg Brownell, an Internet expert, both residents of Providence, Rhode Island, set sail on an ambitious project: to reduce the complexity of disease and procedure coding to its simple elements so that doctors could code quicker, more easily, and more accurately. It was not to be as simple as they thought. This is their story.

Weintrub and Brownell were not naïve:

- They knew the codes were contained in large paper volumes used by the coding industry, professional coders, health plans, and payers.
- They knew the American Medical Association played a central role in developing and licensing the codes.
- They knew everyone who had tried to unravel the codes found coding logic baffling, Byzantine, and bewildering.
- They knew doctors themselves rarely bothered to try to understand and apply the logic to their daily practices.

In any event, for years, Weintrub and Brownell labored on their Web site, www.dpnx.com to consolidate the contents of the coding books and manuals into one Web site. The goal was to reduce the complex coding system into a Web form so that physicians and their coders could access the precise and appropriate code easily and quickly at one site.

But according to Weintrub, "It was a lot harder than we thought it would be. We wanted to teach coding to doctors—what the logic was, how to code quickly, and how to pick exactly the right code."

Why was that difficult? They ran into a couple of unexpected obstacles.

- One, doctors were not all that interested in the whys, whats, and hows of coding. Sure, they wanted the right code, but they wanted someone else to figure it out; the office or hospital coders, for example.
- Two, surgical jargon, the technical jargon of surgeons, kept getting in their way. Surgeons wanted to use their own language, the patois of the operating room suite, to find the code. They underestimated the importance, the variation and the complexity of language, the multiple variables of any common procedures.

When a surgeon, for example, removes the gallbladder through a laparoscope, he may call the procedure "a laparoscopic cholecystectomy," "a lap chole," or a "gallbladder chole." Consider too an appendectomy. It may be dubbed "an appy," "an incidental appy" secondary to some other procedure, or a "ruptured appy with an abscess or peritonitis," or a "lap appy," if removed through a laparoscope. It gets even more complicated with other procedures with more variables. Surgeons preferred to find the right code by using familiar technical jargon, rather trying to understand the proper terms in coding manuals.

Therefore, Weintrub and Brownell found themselves in the role of translators of surgical jargon. Toward this end, they developed a Web site, appropriately designated as www.dpnx.com. What they do, they say, on their Web site is simple:

- The site is about one thing: CPT codes for surgery.
- Their goal is to help translate operative procedures into CPT codes.
- Their search tools and drilldown technology are lightning fast and easy to use.

For the first time, surgeons can use their everyday language to find the right procedure codes using clinical abbreviations, clinical shorthand, and colloquialisms.

Primary care practitioners, who are now doing more office procedures for the convenience of their patients and for more office income, may find www.surgerycodes.com just as useful as surgeons. Before the Web site, just learning how to find the right code to submit an appropriate claim may have dissuaded primary practitioners from performing office procedures.

Case Study 3

The Story of the National Procedures Institute
By Dr. John L. Pfenninger, President and Director, The National Procedures Institute

Dr. John Pfenninger is a family practitioner who passionately believes his compatriots in their office scan do more procedures and do them well with more conveniences for patients and less cost to the health system.

• •

The story of the National Procedures Institute (NPI) is quite simple. I was born and raised on a farm, so I was used to, and enjoyed, working with my hands. Surgical specialties interested me, but the time needed to finish a residency program and the lifestyle afterwards were not very enticing. Subsequently, I chose family practice, so that I could "do everything like the old country doctors."

Family Practice Residencies Deficient in Teaching Office Surgical Skills

It didn't take long to see that family practice residency programs really were quite deficient in teaching office surgical skills. Initially, physicians that were in private practice as "GPs" became residency directors. They tended to do many more of the surgical procedures. They delivered babies, performed appendectomies, set fractures, and so forth. As time went on, however, experienced faculty became few and far between. Salaried physicians had a tendency to do less and less with their hands. Hospital credentialing processes and liability concerns from insurers further limited interest in procedures.

Learning to Do the Simple Things

Still, there were many of us who wanted to learn how to treat hemorrhoids, inject veins, do vasectomies, put in IUDs, apply casts, do dermatological surgery, perform the procedures needed for emergency and hospital care, and more. However, there was no formalized training available to learn these procedures! Although state and national academies offered a small smattering of selections once or twice a year, there just wasn't enough quality education being offered in the procedural skills area.

Doing Office Procedures Makes Sense

Doing procedures makes so much sense. Many things can be performed in the office as opposed to the hospital. Surgeons are trained to do everything in the operating room but this markedly increases cost. Sebaceous cysts, lipomas, hemorrhoids, and many other conditions can be treated in an office setting. Patients appreciate this, as do the insurers, because costs are kept to a minimum.

Other Advantages

Other advantages of doing procedures include a reduction in the delay of diagnosis. In other words, if a skin lesion looks atypical and the clinician is comfortable doing a skin biopsy, it is biopsied on the spot. The alternative is referring the patient away. This may take 6 to 8 weeks before another evaluation. In the case of melanoma, this puts the patient at increased risk.

Physicians who do procedures have a tendency to know more about the disease process. Describing what a rose smells like or what an orange tastes like is difficult. How does one explain the color red to a blind person? Similarly, it is difficult to explain various disease processes.

However, if the clinician becomes involved with seeing, feeling, and exploring the innuendoes of a disease process, the diagnostic acumen becomes more accurate. Doing procedures can also break up the monotony of the day-to-day practice.

In addition, reimbursements still are greater for surgeries and procedures, versus nonsurgical areas. Numerous studies are available showing that those who perform procedures have a significantly higher net income. For most family physicians, they chose the specialty not to be case managers and paper pushers, but rather, to provide comprehensive care. Doing procedures makes this more likely.

NPI Born in 1989

Thus, in 1989, NPI was born with the purpose of teaching procedural and surgical skills for primary care clinicians. It has grown from teaching two courses the first year to over a hundred in 2006. Over 15,000 clinicians have trained with the National Procedures Institute. After 17 years of teaching procedural skills, NPI remains the leader for educational opportunities in the field of teaching primary care physicians to perform appropriate procedures in their offices.

Along with the text, *Pfenninger and Fowler's Procedures for Primary Care*, NPI seminars have changed the way physicians deliver medical care in the United States. NPI can be accessed at www.npinstitute.com.

Chapter 5

Physician Office Dispensing Stages Comeback

Prelude: Other ways of looking at prescribing in the office—its economic impact on doctors, costs and convenience for patients, and increased patient compliance.

Too often a prescription signals the end to an interview rather than the start of an alliance.

Barry Blackwell, 1973

Something old,
Something new,
Something borrowed,
Something blue,
A silver sixpence in her shoe.

Victorian wedding saying

Physician office dispensing is like the Victorian wedding saying:

- Physician office dispensing is something old. It was common before the modern pharmacy came on the scene.
- It is something new because it has only resurfaced in the last 10 years.
- It is something blue because critics consider it unethical for doctors to profit from prescribing.

- It is something borrowed because its software is borrowed from the computer world.
- It is something that puts money in the doctor's shoe.

New software makes it possible for doctors to internalize prescription writing rather than sending prescriptions to local pharmacies. This creates greater productivity and profitability. Furthermore, doctors can prescribe prepackaged drugs at the point of care, cut costs, and increase convenience for patients. Patients have become more cost and convenience conscious with health savings accounts and high-deductible health plans.

An added benefit is greater patient compliance in taking medications as prescribed. Studies indicate that noncompliance—by not picking up drugs at the pharmacy, not taking drugs as prescribed, stopping the drug on their own—may drop as much as 70 percent (Nystrom, 2006).

Prescribing software also allows doctors to manage their drug inventory, maintain accurate medication records, check for drug interactions and allergies, and, in many instances, more readily route prescriptions directly to pharmacists.

Primary care physicians are in a low-margin business. To increase margins, they are performing more office procedures, upgrading coding, delegating history taking to computers, hiring nurse practitioners and physician assistants, doing more ancillary procedures, and dispensing drugs. Collectively, these activities are often called *point-of-care medicine* and generally require more information-technology applications.

Typically, doctors seeing 20 patients a day write one and a half prescriptions and one and a half refills per patient, or three per patient. This amounts to 60 prescriptions a day. If these doctors average about $6 profit per prescription, that is an extra $360 per day of profit.

For multiphysician practices, a pharmacy technician is usually hired to handle the prescription program, the technician's salary more than offset by the increase in revenue generated. With office dispensing, hard-pressed primary care physicians can respond to downward economic pressures from decreasing reimbursements, mounting overheads, and competition from retail clinics located in pharmacies.

Office dispensing, however, is not for everyone. In 43 of 50 states, a physician's license allows doctor office dispensing, but in 7 states office dispensing is forbidden or limited. The seven states are: Massachusetts, New Jersey, New York, New Hampshire, Texas, Utah, and Montana (Physician Total Care, Inc., 2006).

There may be other reasons not to dispense as well:

- hesitancy to change existing practice patterns
- fear of being labeled as "commercial"
- lack of office space to store drug inventories
- reluctance to buy required inventories
- reservations about upsetting cordial relationships with local pharmacists

Appealing to harassed and hurried consumers—who may not welcome one-stop prescription shopping for lower-priced drugs at the doctor's office—often overrides these concerns.

Office dispensing creates controversy. Nay-sayers argue dispensing for profit is unethical and results in overutilization. Yea-sayers say office dispensing bolsters compliance. An article in the *Archives of Internal Medicine* indicates nearly two thirds of patients who underuse prescription drugs never tell their doctor about the underuse.

When patients leave the office with prescription in hand, compliance soars and software makes refills easy, again increasing compliance. Dispensing champions also say office prescriptions end illegible handwriting errors or confusion over sound-alike drugs, cuts prescription costs by as much as 50 percent, and ends many of the dangers of noncompliance (Nystrom, 2006).

Why Office Dispensing Is Rare

Currently, only about 10 percent of doctors dispense prescriptions in their offices. This low rate may be resistance to change, fear of antagonizing the local pharmacy, or regulations in some states prohibiting office dispensing.

Doctors may not want to keep large inventories on hand. They may simply not have the space to store these inventories. On the other hand, once physicians buy their own inventories, they become acutely aware of drug costs and may cut back on the volume of drugs they dispense. They also please patients who are short on time and money. Consumer-driven-care advocates commonly criticize doctors for not knowing the costs of drugs, tests, or health aids or devices they prescribe. When doctors know the price of drugs they dispense, this objection is overcome.

Among proponents of drug dispensing are members of the Physicians Total Care in Tulsa, Oklahoma, and Allscripts Health Care Solutions in Libertyville, Illinois.

Physicians Total Care, Inc.

Physicians Total Care (PTC) facilitates office dispensing by purchasing prescription medications in bulk and repackaging them into individual prescription sizes for physicians, who then dispense the medications by using the company's software. PTC software provides convenience for patients, lowers prescription costs by as much as 50 percent, processes refills, provides all generic and brand pharmaceuticals, including over-the-counter products, and allows physicians to earn up to $6 per prescription.

Allscripts Health Care Solutions

Allscripts Health Care Solutions is a market leader in electronic health systems. Its system, Touchworks, contains a dispensing module. Its EMR automates most physician activities—prescribing, capturing charges, dictating, ordering lab work and viewing results, providing physician education, and taking clinical notes. The software enables the doctors to produce a complete medical record.

Will Office Dispensing Become Common?

Will the efficiencies, safety, convenience, and potential revenue produced by companies like PTC and Allscripts lure doctors into dispensing? Perhaps. Squeezed by managed care and Medicare, doctors are seeking additional sources of revenue—and they are searching for ways to provide more value for consumers.

What's more, if new software makes it easier to handle inventory, label prescriptions, manage medication, increase compliance and convenience, and cut costs, it may simplify serving assertive baby boomers and other patients who demand more value-added services.

Innovation Talking and Action Points

Office dispensing using prescription-generating software is an example of a technology innovation that potentially benefits both doctor and patient. The old saying "Necessity is the mother of invention" applies here. *Need* is a source of innovation. In the case of primary care physicians, there are these needs:

1. for more revenues to prop up a low-margin business
2. to please the new consumer, who is seeking time-savings conveniences
3. to avoid the hazards of illegible handwritten prescriptions and sound-alike drugs
4. for a way to help patients comply with doctor orders

There is no sure way to ensure compliance, but doctors handing patients the prepackaged drug and instructing them how to take it helps patients comply more readily. Satisfying these needs may seem like rationalization to critics, but as I have said, "One man's innovation is another man's aberration."

Case Study 1

Physicians Total Care Medical Director Tells of Benefits of Office Prescribing

By Dr. Scott Nystrom

What follows is a company profile of Physicians Total Care. The author, Scott Nystrom, MD, FACP, is medical director and a practicing oncologist. Like most oncologists, he is acutely aware of the prescribing and costs of drugs and their impact on practice.

He is certified by the American Board of Internal Medicine and subspecialty boards in oncology and hematology. He has had over 35 years clinical experience in hematology and oncology. He has held academic positions at the University of Southern California, the University of Connecticut Medical Center, Wayne State University, and Tufts School of Medicine and Tufts New England medical center.

He has practiced actively in both academic and private practice settings during his career. He has written numerous articles and has been the recipient of many awards, including being twice named as "best doctor" in hematology and oncology by *Detroit Monthly* magazine.

He currently serves as the medical director for CancerExpertsMD, a Web site providing expert case review in oncology and hematology. In addition, he functions as medical director for Physicians Total Care. Its software enables physicians to dispense at the point of care.

• •

In my capacity as chief financial officer for the Great Lakes Cancer Management Specialists (GLCMS), I realized in mid-2004 that the negative impact of the Medicare Modernization Act (MMA) was going to be significant. Our practice needed a method to prescribe, dispense, and bill for oral medications and injectables at the point of care within the office setting to offset Medicare cuts.

After considerable research, we decided Physicians Total Care (PTC) was the strategic partner we needed. Simply put, PTC repackages and distributes wholesale pharmaceuticals. The company developed a proprietary drug-dispensing software, the PTC9000 Medication Management System (PTC9000). This system enables physicians to inventory and dispense any prescribed medication directly to patients while in the doctor's office (or via mail for refills).

This is accomplished by providing practices with sealed single unit of use medications. This eliminates any need for open bottle pill counts. With the PTC9000, there was no additional liability risk. Prescription error rates were nil. The PTC9000 minimized the need for retail pharmacy. In addition, PTC provided patient medications more accurately and cost effectively. While at GLCMS, it became clear that there was no equivalent software in this market segment. The physicians at GLCMS quickly recognized point-of-care physician dispensing could potentially and permanently alter the current prescription distribution landscape.

Our practice was very similar to any typical practice. Each of us spent one half to one hour per day addressing pharmaceutical issues for payers and pharmacies. For every three doctors, we had one full-time employee addressing these issues. This overhead produced no revenue. Dispensing at the point of care using the PTC9000 converted this dead overhead into a profit center. At the same time, we were providing better health care at a lower cost.

The two major reasons patients never fill their prescriptions are cost and convenience. Surveys have found that over 20 percent of all prescriptions never get filled. Dispensing at the point of care increases the fill rate and enhances compliance.

For each dollar invested in improved compliance, hundreds of dollars of long-term health care costs are avoided. At GLCMS we were able to immediately address reasons for noncompliance. If a patient has trouble with cost, we found it could be remedied by prescribing either generic or therapeutically equivalent.

By so doing, GLCMS physicians lowered the average cost of a prescription by 50 percent. To give some perspective, in 2005, PTC physicians averaged less than $30 per prescription while the national average was over $60 per prescription. In addition, PTC physicians dispense at a 75 percent generic rate while the best managed-payer programs only reach 50 percent generic prescription rates (Nystrom, 2006).

The patient convenience is obvious, but the improved patient care is incalculable. PTC system allowed GLCMS to reduce spiraling medication costs, provide more convenient care, and improve patient compliance and promote healthier outcomes.

Since joining PTC as medical director in 2005, the prospective magnitude of point-of-care dispensing soon became apparent.

An estimated 400,000 community practicing physicians write over $750,000 annually in prescriptions (Nystrom). All are potential PTC customers. PTC estimates that its total market potential is over $200 billion and is currently growing $20 billion per year. PTC's statistics indicate physicians using the PTC9000 manage costs better and the total cost of prescriptions written can be reduced to $375,000 from $750,000 while maintaining equivalent or better medication therapy.

The patient, the physician, and the payer drive demand for the PTC9000. Besides the spiraling costs of medications, even patients with insurance coverage are facing ever higher co-pays. High co-pay provokes greater noncompliance.

Many newer brand-name drugs rapidly exceed the patients' total annual prescription drug allowance. Once this annual prescription benefit payment has been breached the patient becomes 100 percent liable for all subsequent prescription costs. Payers are on a mission to lower pharmaceutical costs. Physicians' income is being squeezed and substantial time is required to deal with pharmacy issues for no revenue.

The PTC9000 supports physicians by increasing revenue without incremental cost to the practice, patient, or payer. In addition, PTC9000 can potentially yield cost savings through more efficient handling of prescription-related tasks. Most patients welcome this service and PTC believes that over time, virtually all physicians will dispense pharmaceuticals directly to their patients.

PTC has averaged 170 percent in revenue growth over the last 3 years; the customer base increased over 400 percent in 2005. Greater growth in terms of numbers is expected in 2006 and beyond.

Physician-income compression has caused the entire physician market to pursue ancillary income sources. Physicians using the PTC9000 can make from $20,000 to $100,000 annually in additional income while delivering better and lower cost health care.

With the advent of retail pharmacy (Walgreen's, Costco, CVS, Wal-Mart, etc.) now offering walk-in physician-based services that compete directly with physician offices, soon all practices will take notice. The PTC system provides a simple response to this competitive threat.

I strongly believe that the old retail pharmacy distribution model is about to undergo a tsunamic transformation. Through capitalistic incentives, the PTC system creates a new pharmacy distribution model. This model reduces cost, improves patient convenience, compliance, and care while providing a competitive response to retail pharmacy's "walk-in–doc-in-a-box" strategy. This industry stands at a pivotal inflection point. A tidal wave of change is about to wash over the medical industry.

Case Study 2

The Role of Electronic Prescribing in Lowering Physician Drug Expenses

By Dr. Craig Marrow and Michael Coleman, MBA

Dr. Craig Marrow and Michael Coleman, MBA, are medical director and chief operating officer, respectively, of the Southwest Medical Associates, a 225-physician group, in Las Vegas, Nevada. Here they describe how electronic prescribing using the Allscripts EHR has lowered prescribing costs, increased safety, and enhanced practice efficiency.

• •

This case study examines a successful electronic prescribing program at Southwest Medical Associates (SMA) of Las Vegas, the largest multispecialty physician group in Nevada with 225 physicians and 650,000 annual outpatient visits. SMA, which is a subsidiary of Nevada's largest managed care organization, publicly traded Sierra Health Services (SHS), hoped electronic prescribing would help its physicians better identify opportunities to prescribe generic drugs as alternatives to more costly brand-name medications. Doing so would help reduce the group's pharmacy benefit costs.

After 3 years of using the TouchWorks Rx+ ePrescribing solution from Allscripts, by December of 2005, SMA's generic fill rate (GFR) had achieved a 4.8 percent lead over a controlled group of physicians in other SHS network groups that do not use electronic prescribing.

Because every one point increase in GFR equals a cost savings to the organization of 1.5 percent, SMA's increased generic utilization saves $4.75 million each year, or 7.2 percent of its 2005 drug spends of $66 million. TouchWorks, which is a full EHR, also greatly streamlines the process of approving prescription refills, in the process creating indirect financial savings to SMA of $208,640 a year through increased nurse productivity.

Taken together, TouchWorks' positive financial impact of $4.96 million annually has netted SMA a reduction in costs of $5.17 per prescription on average. SMA's solution also has increased formulary compliance for the group's physicians and enhanced patient safety. Thanks largely to its electronic prescribing initiative, SMA now has a generic utilization rate of 73.2 percent, one of the highest rates in the country.

Early Steps Toward Electronic Prescribing

SMA began looking for an electronic prescribing application for its more than 200 physicians in 2002. Executives at Sierra hoped electronic prescribing would help reduce pharmacy expenses by speeding the prescription process, increasing generic utilization and formulary compliance, reducing pharmacy callbacks, and streamlining the refill process. At the same time, SMA executives were looking for a new EHR for the practice.

In searching for an electronic prescribing solution, SMA selected Allscripts. The company not only had a long record of success with electronic prescribing, its customers generate almost as many prescriptions as the rest of the industry combined, but its modular, Web-based TouchWorks EHR included a full electronic prescribing module called TouchWorks Rx+ that could be implemented as a stand-alone solution. Allscripts also was closely integrated with IDX Systems Corporation, now part of GE Health Care, the maker of SMA's Groupcast practice management system. The strategic partnership between the two companies delivers clinical and financial applications that are tightly integrated, enabling customers to streamline billing, improve cash flow, provide detailed financial practice analysis, and simplify patient record keeping. SMA implemented the TouchWorks Rx+ ePrescribing module as a stand-alone system beginning in February 2003. In the third quarter of that year, the group began to implement the full TouchWorks EHR, gradually giving its physicians instant access to each patient's medical chart, including their medication history.

The EHR was deployed in every exam room via "thin-client" computers, which are stripped-down machines with little or no application logic that communicate directly with Allscripts' secure, Web-based servers. By putting thin clients in every exam room, SMA ensured that Rx+ and the rest of the EHR would be as ubiquitous as pen and paper.

Physician Incentives Ensure Utilization

SMA launched the new electronic prescribing system with a highly effective financial incentive program to encourage its adoption by physicians. Long before this, SMA already had begun to base physician bonuses on the entire group's performance against Sierra's pharmacy budget. The more those SMA physicians prescribed generic alternatives to brand-name drugs, the larger the group's bonus pool grew.

Individual physicians received a higher or lower percentage of the total pool based on their performance against quality and customer service measures.

With the start of the EHR implementation, SMA modified its bonus policy just enough to make a difference. The change mandated that, as of January 2004, only SMA physicians who were 100 percent TouchWorksRx+ compliant would be eligible to receive bonuses (the change applied only to the 180 SMA physicians who prescribe medications; the other 55 doctors were hospitalists and anesthesiologists, who do not write prescriptions). For such a small change, the policy adjustment had a large and swift impact. Within 1 month, 90 percent of all prescriptions written at SMA were generic prescriptions. By the end of 2 months, every last SMA physician was using Rx+ to prescribe medications electronically. During the same time frame, the practice went from zero prescriptions to its current average level of 80,000 electronic scripts per month, making it one of the highest-volume electronic prescribing groups in the nation.

How It Works: Simple, Straightforward

Prior to implementing Rx+, SMA physicians wrote all of their prescriptions by hand. They also manually completed an office visit checklist to document all medications prescribed for each patient that was filed in the paper chart. Physicians were provided educational materials to encourage them to prescribe generic drugs whenever appropriate, but there was no systematic way to remind them about particular drug choices at the point of care. Today, the process is dramatically different. In a typical encounter, the physician enters the patient's name and a direct prescription.

Reduced Staff Time Spent on Refills

Although electronic prescribing saves physicians time in the exam room, its most significant time savings comes in the form of reduced pharmacy calls and far quicker medication refills. Prior to implementing Rx+, SMA's refill process followed a typical pattern for paper-based practices:

- The patient calls the pharmacy or the physician's office to request a refill.
- The patient and pharmacy information is hand recorded.
- The patient's chart is pulled.

- A nurse or the physician reviews the information.
- The prescription is phoned or faxed in to the pharmacy.
- The patient is phoned and notified when the prescription is complete.

With the new, TouchWorks-enabled renewal process, the staff workload is dramatically reduced:

- The patient calls the pharmacy requesting a refill.
- The pharmacy sends an electronic request to the physician via a nurse.
- The nurse (or physician, in the case of a controlled substance) reviews the request and approves it electronically.
- The approval arrives in the pharmacy's computer system.
- The pharmacy fills the prescription and contacts the patient.

The money-saving numbers for SMA are impressive. Every month, SMA's prescribing physicians receive an average of 9,500 electronic requests for prescription refills. Nurse interviews and time-motion studies reveal that, by handling refill requests electronically rather than over the phone, SMA has reduced its daily total nursing time spent on refill requests for each physician by 93 percent, from 5 minutes per phone call to just 20 seconds per electronic request.

Spread over 1 year, that amounts to 8,867 hours in cumulative nursing time savings, time that can now be spent more productively on revenue-generating patient services. Calculated at an average wage of $23.53 per hour for Las Vegas nurses (Fuch and Sox, 2001), the indirect savings to SMA amounts to $208,640 per year in increased staff productivity. "The time savings from electronic renewal of prescriptions is phenomenal," said Dr. Morrow. "After a quick glance at the medication list to confirm that the requested prescription is accurate and appropriate, the refill request can be immediately granted."

Potential for Medical Errors Reduced

More than one in five Americans reported that they or a family member experienced a medical or prescription drug error in 2001. Of the 16 percent reporting a medication error, over one fifth said the error turned out to be a very serious problem (Institute of Medicine Report, 2006).

Fortunately, electronic prescribing has been proven to help prevent medication errors. Physicians are convinced that the system's clinical decision support and automatic drug utilization review prevents medical errors that would previously have slipped by unnoticed. Michael Coleman, the Southwest Medical Associates' chief operating officer, says there is little doubt that Rx+ has made dramatic improvements in patient safety. "We're certain that we've seen error issues go down but we have not been able to collect good data on that because we have no benchmark measuring what occurred prior to e-prescribing," Coleman says. "The happy and sad faces in TouchWorks give instant feedback to doctors, and there are adverse reaction and allergy warnings built into the system. Those two things alone have made a huge difference in reducing errors."

Conclusion

Spiraling drug costs continue to pose a significant challenge for managed care organizations striving to provide health benefits programs at a price employers and patients can afford. By improving generic utilization rates, managed care organizations and physician groups can hold the line against price hikes and help reduce pharmacy benefit expenses. In this effort, electronic prescribing is their most powerful tool. By using electronic prescribing, Southwest Medical Associates and Sierra Health Services documented savings of $4.75 million per year from higher GFR and another $208,640 in indirect savings from reductions in staff time devoted to prescription refills.

Their experience is further proof that, with the right electronic prescribing application, physicians can both improve the bottom line and enhance patient care. A key lesson for other managed care organizations and physician practices is that a group's total GFR can be significantly improved by tying prescription adherence to financial incentives—even to the point of barring noncompliant clinicians from participation in incentive programs. SMA's program has proven so successful that Sierra Health Services decided to adopt it statewide. In October 2005, the managed care organization along with Allscripts and the Clark County Medical Society announced an initiative to provide TouchWorks Rx+ to all 5,000 of Nevada's practicing physicians.

The program will be the nation's first statewide electronic prescribing network and a new testing ground for the effectiveness of electronic prescribing. Allscripts expects other states will follow Nevada's lead and adopt electronic prescribing to enhance patient safety and reduce health care costs for their citizens.

Chapter 6

Innovative New Practices Are Managing Costs, Time, Convenience, and Disease

Prelude: Doctors are rapidly innovating and adjusting to cost, time, and disease demands by creating new types of practices.

The test of innovation is whether it creates value. Innovation means the creation of new value and new satisfaction for the customer. The test of innovation as well as "quality," isn't "Do we like it?" It is "Do customers like it and will they pay for it?"

Peter F. Drucker, 1985

Searching for a New Relationship: A Patient's Point of View

You have a generous income—but you are weary of:

- impersonal health care
- playing telephone tag with doctors
- not finding a doctor when you need one
- not knowing exactly how healthy you are, because your doctor does not have time to give you practical preventive advice
- not having a doctor who makes house calls

- not being able to call a doctor directly 24/7
- not having time to leisurely discuss your health or your disease with a knowledgeable expert

When it comes to your health, money is no object.

A Precious Few, Less Than 1 Percent, Are Leaving

A few doctors are leaving current practices to set up new types of practice more to their liking. I estimate their numbers are less than 1 percent of all practicing physicians. although I can find no single source to document the actual number. Weary of current practice time restrictions, managed care hassles, too little time for patients, and low pay, doctors are turning to innovative forms of practice, inside and outside their offices. The success of these practices depends on your willingness to pay for them.

In 1996, two internists in Seattle, Garrison Bliss and Mitchell Karton, started a *concierge*, or *retainer practice*, also known as a *boutique practice* (Sharpe, 1998). The two doctors created this new type of practice because they were fed up with hassles, busyness, and low economic and psychic rewards of traditional practice. The idea was straightforward: for a yearly retainer fee (in the $1,000 to $2,000 range), the physician, often an internist or family physician, offered patients:

- Unlimited access to the doctor 24 hours a day, 365 days a year
- Unhampered e-mail and telephone access
- Uninterrupted time with the physician
- Wellness programs
- Routine physical examinations (that many insurers don't cover)
- Navigating patients through the medical maze
- Referral to top specialists

The term *concierge* implies someone who greets you when you enter and lavishes attention upon you. The doctors who chose this type of medicine first called themselves concierge physicians and formed the Society of Concierge Physicians. Partly because of controversies (criticisms that they were practicing "luxury medicine," abandoning former patients, and practicing "elitist" medicine), they changed their organization's name to the Society of Innovative Medical Practice Designs (SIMPD).

SIMPD Mission Statement

The Society for Innovative Medical Practice Design is an organization of health care providers promoting a direct financial relationship with their patients in order to restore the integrity of the patient-physician relationship. Our members are innovators in medical practice design, including concierge, retainer, retail, and cash pay physicians, who, along with other individuals, are committed to patient-focused medical practice and to improving the patient-physician relationship. It is our mission to ensure that physicians and patients retain the right to design and implement practices that enhance the effectiveness, efficiency, service, and value of health care.

Concierge practices have come under heavy criticism. In Senate hearings, Representative Pete Stark (D-California) charged, "Concierge care is like a new country club for the rich. The danger is that if a large number of doctors choose to open up these types of practices, the health care system will become even more inequitable than it is today" (Zugar, 2005).

Dr. Troyen A. Brennan, a physician and lawyer at Brigham and Women's Hospital in Boston, asserted, "No matter how innovative and attractive luxury primary care is to some patients and physicians, it poses questions about equity. We should identify ways in which luxury primary care can be regulated by the medical profession (perhaps by mandatory cross-subsidies and careful monitoring of the prevalence of such care), while also addressing other threats to access" (Brennan, 2002).

He continued, "The questions that luxury primary care poses should remind us that as physicians we have a commitment to the equitable distribution of health care and therefore a duty to address market innovations that could leave some patients without access to care" (Brennan, 2002).

Representative Stark and Dr. Brennan are speaking for the political and academic medical establishments. They are not speaking for private practitioners deeply dissatisfied with current practice conditions—nor are they speaking for patients who are tired of the old practices and who frequent these new practices. Patients who pay retainer fees say they are happy with these practices, and practictioners apparently are too. Their reenrollment rates are over 90 percent (SIMPD).

Boutique or concierge practices with annual retainers represent a tiny share of physician practices. Only 300 physicians, about one of every 2,500 doctors, practice retainer medicine in the United States. They serve about 100,000 Americans, or one of every 3,000 citizens (SIMPD).

Boutique practices are a marginal practice phenomenon. Over 50 percent of these practices are concentrated in affluent metropolitan areas in Arizona, California, Florida, and the state of Washington. Here, according to SIMPD, is the number of retainer, or concierge, practices in 28 states (22 states have no retainer practices). (See Table 6–1.)

Physicians in retainer practices profess to be deeply satisfied, saying they are practicing medicine as it should be practiced. By carrying one third to one half of their previous practice load, doctors devote more time to patients, address their concerns, practice preventive medicine, improve quality of care, and help patients weave through the medical maze.

Table 6–1 *Number of Retainer, Concierge Practices in Individual States*

Alabama, 2	Indiana, 1	New Hampshire, 2	Tennessee, 1
Arizona, 8	Kansas, 1	New York, 2	Texas, 16
California, 23	Massachusetts, 5	Ohio, 4	Utah, 2
Connecticut, 1	Maryland, 2	Oregon, 5	West Virginia, 2
Florida, 17	Michigan, 3	Pennsylvania, 3	Washington, 10
Georgia, 1	Minnesota, 3	Rhode Island, 1	Wisconsin, 1
Illinois, 1	Missouri, 2	South Carolina, 2	Virginia, 1

Source: Society of Innovative Medical Practice Designs (SIMPD).

Getting Out of the Rat Race

Many doctors left their former practices to get out of the rat race. In an average year, their patient load was 2,000. Their typical income per patient per year was about $200 per patient for total revenues of $400,000. In many practices, $400,000 barely met overhead, averaging about 60 percent to 70 percent of revenues. According to MCVIP, a Boca Rotan company that organizes and helps set up concierge practices, these are percentages generally cited by practice management firms.

If, on other hand, they are in a concierge practice with 500 patients, they receive $100,000 in fees plus $1,150 a retainer for each patient. Do the math: $1,150 times 500 is $575,000, and $575,000 plus $100,000 is $675,000, a 69 percent improvement over the previous income of $400,000, for seeing a quarter as many patients and devoting more time and effort to each one.

Physicians are a conservative lot, often shunning controversies and risks surrounding these practices. They do not want to be under the political microscope. It is doubtful that these new practices will ever be a significant force in the marketplace; however, you are likely to receive more attention, a better quality of care, and quicker access to specialists if you should choose to become a member of such a practice.

Other Types of Innovative Practices More Likely to Grow

Other innovative practices—cash practices and retail practices—are more likely to grow than the concierge practices, and doctors will be more likely to encounter them in the industry.

SimpleCare is an organization that was created in Renton, Washington, a suburb of Seattle, about 10 years ago. Its operating concept is simple. Patients pay cash for short ($35), medium ($65), and long ($95) visits.

Cash payments at the point of care eliminate the need for third-party reimbursement. Third-party reimbursement requires hiring a staff to submit claims, paperwork to justify claims, and a system—and sometimes outside agencies—to ensure collections. These functions are the principal reasons most physician overheads exceed 50 percent. The founders of SimpleCare say many of their patients are uninsured or on Medicaid and appreciate the convenience and low-fee structures.

Retail Outlet Clinics

Retail medicine, which is now occupying retail spaces of Wal-Mart, drug stores, and grocery chains, has already experienced explosive growth. These clinics may be suited for young and middle-aged two-income family consumers who suffer from time bankruptcy.

In the course of their busy lives, they may seek to combine shopping with medical care for minor problems such as bronchitis, influenza, sinusitis, and upper respiratory conditions. They may also want to visit these clinics at night or on weekends, when their regular doctor's office is closed. Two leading companies backing these retail clinics are MinuteClinic and Solantic, but many more are on the way. Doctors are also organizing companies to treat patients for injuries and illnesses at work (for example, www.onsitedocs.com and through telephone consultations, www.teladocs.com).

Disease Management Companies

The biggest innovations in caring for chronically ill patients by far are occurring in the disease management field. Practicing physicians do not usually have disease management practices. Instead health plans or other organizations that start disease management companies rely on nurses and may only hire doctors as medical directors.

It is not that the physician's role is unimportant. In *Voices of Health Reform* (Reece, 2005c), Dr. William Gold, chief medical officer and vice president of Blue Cross Blue Shield of Minnesota, and Dr. Victor Villagra, president of Health & Technology Vector, a Farmington, Connecticut, disease management consulting firm, discussed the field of disease management.

Both stressed disease management as a huge innovation; the missing piece of health reform and as a fundamental means of transforming chronic disease care. Think about it. Patients with chronic disease spend 99 percent of their time outside traditional practice settings at work or home.

If one can track, treat, and educate these patients, said to consume 80 percent of all health care costs, then complications, emergency room visits, and hospital admissions can be dramatically decreased when nurses use systematic protocols. Furthermore, if any health plan engages physicians in the process, they can refer these patients to doctors when physician skills are most needed; for instance, when true complications require physician knowledge and intervention.

Disease management companies treat and monitor patients with chronic diseases at home and at work, often by personal visits by nurses or by remote video and audio units run by doctors and nurses in remote locations. Some disease management companies are large (for instance, HealthWays), growing rapidly, and on the stock market. Others are affiliated with health plans or big health care systems.

These companies are filling a huge void in U.S. medicine by treating the chronically ill at home and at work when they are outside the reach of physicians in their offices. These companies are not, at present, physician directed; instead they have been created by health plans and disease-managed entities. These organizations rely on nurses to deliver their services.

Innovation Talking and Action Points

U.S. medicine is offering innovative options outside of the traditional practice of medicine, often outside the reach of the usual third parties—HMOs, PPOs, Blue Cross plans and self-care plans offered by companies. For patients, these new practices may involve paying cash at the point of care, paying a yearly retainer fee, paying for being treated at home or at work, or paying while shopping at grocery stores, discount stores, or pharmacies.

Patients with chronic diseases, some of whom are home bound, can be treated at home, either by nurses or remote monitoring devices, or a combination of human and machine-guided care. The important thing about disease management companies, or health plans that employ these companies, is that disease management can be conducted as large-scale enterprises, requires little capital, and fills a desperate need— reducing costs and improving care for a growing segment of the population.

Disease management, because of its ability to mobilize resources to address chronic disease and Medicaid populations, is more promising in the business sense than innovative new practice models for individual physicians.

Consumer-Driven Health Care Spurs Innovation in Physician Services

By Devon M. Herrick, MBA, PhD

Devon M. Herrick is a senior fellow with the National Center for Policy Analysis. He is 43 years old, holds degrees in accounting, has two MBAs, and earned a doctorate in political economy. He worked with the Baylor Health Care System for 6 years and has been with the National Center for Policy Analysis (NCPA) in Dallas for 10 years. The NCPA employs about 40 people and has many contacts with those in academic settings.

• •

Consumer-driven health care (CDHC) is leading to new models for the delivery of medical services. CDHC plans generally include personal accounts—such as health reimbursement arrangements or health savings accounts—that allow patients to directly control some of their health care dollars. Because they have a financial stake in their own spending, patients have incentives to shop for the best price and to make tradeoffs between convenience and cost.

Insurance recordkeeping and claim filing represent a significant expense for physicians. Physicians can speed up their cash flow and reduce billing costs by attracting patients who pay cash or use the debit cards that some plans provide. Thus a growing number of medical providers are offering innovative services to meet the demand of empowered patients.

These new physician services tend to have two characteristics: (1) they offer patients greater convenience, and (2) they step outside normal reimbursement channels—requiring payment at the time of service, accepting insurance reimbursement from only a handful of large provider networks, or requiring insured customers to file their own claims.

Telephone Consultations

Many medical concerns can be resolved with a phone call. However, few insurers reimburse physicians for telephone consultations or e-mail exchanges. As a result, patients may find access to their physician is limited—especially after hours and on weekends. Entrepreneurial providers, on the other hand, are making it easy for patients who pay cash to reach them by phone.

The doctor behind TelaDoc Medical Service is Virginia physician Alan Dappen, who practices medicine almost entirely by telephone and e-mail contact. He charges for consultations based on the time and treatment needed. He bills for 5-minute increments ranging in price from $15 to $22.50. A simple consultation to request medication refills costs from $10 to $15 for up to five medications.

TelaDoc Medical Service offers medical consultations by telephone, nationwide and around the clock. Each call costs $35, plus a nominal monthly membership fee—far less than a visit to the doctor's office at $80 to $100, the urgent care clinic at $150, or the emergency room at $300-plus. TelaDoc has physicians licensed to practice in each state. The subscription-based service keeps patients' medical histories electronically and a doctor usually returns calls requesting a consultation within 30 to 40 minutes (if it takes more than 3 hours, the consultation is free). TelaDoc is not intended to replace primary care physicians, but to provide another avenue of treatment when a patient's regular physician is not available.

With Doctor on Call, available as a benefit through employer health plans or individually as a stand-alone service, subscribers have immediate telephone access to board-certified physicians. According to Doctor on Call, patients can avoid many ER visits by obtaining information over the phone. For about $10 per month ($5 if offered through an employer health plan), an enrolled family can make an unlimited number of calls. Participating physicians do not diagnose or prescribe medications, but they answer any health questions a patient may have.

Convenient Service: Walk-In Retail Clinics

According to a study in the *American Journal of Managed Care*, nearly half of patients wait more than 30 minutes, on the average, to see a doctor in an office or clinical setting (Meza, 1998). However, a new type of walk-in health clinic is conveniently located inside retail stores—often next to a pharmacy, making additional trips to fill prescriptions unnecessary. Waiting is minimal; patients often receive a beeper that allows them to shop for a few minutes until they are called.

MinuteClinic has pioneered retail-based health care in the United States. These in-store clinics allow patients convenient access to routine medical services such as immunizations and strep tests at low prices. MinuteClinics are staffed by nurse practitioners, who are qualified to provide routine medical services. Most office visits take only 15 minutes, and treatment costs range from $28 to $110—with most services costing $49 to $59.

RediClinic, a venture backed by AOL founder Steve Case, plans to open 500 walk-in clinics by 2009. Offering numerous lab tests for prices nearly 50 percent less than traditional physician offices, RediClinic has forged partnerships with Walgreen's, the nation's largest drugstore chain, and Wal-Mart, the nation's largest retailer. Wal-Mart expects to expand the number of stores with walk-in clinics from 11 to 50 in 2006.

Solantic, a chain of free-standing walk-in clinics based in Florida, is staffed by physicians who can provide more extensive services than clinics staffed by nurse practitioners. Solantic aims to provide convenient health care for a low price, offering services ranging from $65 to $165. Patients can register online and fill out their medical history prior to coming to the clinic.

Convenient Service: Laboratory Tests

A number of laboratory services are now available without a doctor's visit. Patients who want X-rays or lab tests may request them online; a physician reviews the request and orders the tests. Results list actual scores, in addition to low and high ranges that might warrant consultation with a physician.

One firm, HS Labs, www.BloodWorksUSA.com, allows patients to register and pay a fee online, then stop by one of a nationwide network of collection points where a technician draws a blood sample. HS Labs offers a blood workup that examines numerous metrics for about $80 plus a $15 order processing fee. A competitor, Direct Laboratory Services, Inc., www.DirectLabs.com, offers a similar battery of tests for $89. The blood profile provides a biochemical assessment of health based on more than 50 individual tests including blood count, thyroid profile, lipid profile, liver profile, kidney panel, profile of minerals and bone, fluids and electrolytes, and tests on diabetes. The company works with more than 5,000 labs, so the service is available in most of the country. Results are available online within 2 to 3 days, by mail within 5 days, and will be forwarded to the patient's regular physician on request.

Lower Prices: Cash-Friendly Practices

Some physicians are seeking alternatives to the high overhead and low reimbursements associated with third-party payment.

CashDoctor, www.CashDoctor.com, is a loosely structured network for physicians, dentists, chiropractors, pharmacies, laboratories, hospitals, and out-patient facilities across the country that are cash friendly. CashDoctor is not affiliated with any insurance company or provider network. Practice styles and fee schedules are available online.

SimpleCare is another physician association designed for patients who pay cash for incidental medical needs and rely on medical insurance only for major medical claims. SimpleCare requires patients to pay in full at time of service. Because its doctors do not need insurance billing departments, they can offer much lower prices.

Higher Quality: Electronic Medical Records

Another innovative feature of many new health care ventures is the use of electronic medical records (EMR). Storing medical records in an electronic medical record improves care coordination by making it easy to access patient information. It also allows the use of error-reducing software to file prescriptions electronically, replacing physician handwriting, a major source of treatment errors. Only about 15 to 20 percent of physicians' offices use electronic medical records (Cortese, 2006).

Higher Quality: Personalized Care

Some physician practices offer concierge or boutique medicine. These doctors care for a limited number of patients but offer virtually unlimited access to their services. Many traditional practices have 2,500 to 3,500 patients per physician; these doctors have only 300 to 600 patients. Some accept insurance plans, some don't. Participating families often pay an annual fee of $1,500 to $4,000 per patient. In return they can make appointments for same-day, hour-long office visits. Patients are often given their doctor's personal cell phone or pager number for 24-hour-a-day access.

Conclusion

As patients manage more of their own health care dollars, they will begin to seek care that is both convenient and low cost. Empowered consumers will compare medical services and shop for care the same way they shop for other goods and services.

Chapter 7

Stopping the Bleeding in the Clinical Trenches

Prelude: How primary care doctors can stay ahead of the game.

Many primary care doctors are leaving the profession to become sub-specialists or to retire prematurely. Some are sacrificing their standards by speeding up their office visits. Some are selling their clinical independence by joining large companies. All are frustrated.

Joining our cardiology, radiology, pathology, gastroenterology, and OB/GYN colleagues in providing ancillary services is one potential and palatable solution to the problems caused by a system in which primary care physicians earn a fraction of what their specialty colleagues make.

Dr. Rich Kirkpatrick, 2006

Massachusetts is facing a "severe" lack of primary care physicians for the first time, driven in large part by low pay and the Bay State's high cost of living, according to a new study.

The long-term effect could leave patients with longer wait times, fewer choices and tougher challenges picking a physician willing to take on new patients as older doctors retire or leave the field.

"Massachusetts leads the nation in patient-care physicians per 1,000 people, but there are substantial and growing shortages in primary care," said Sager, director of the Health Reform Program at the Boston University

School of Public Health. He said that potential or actual shortages are prevalent in areas including Cape Cod, Western and Central Massachusetts and parts of the Merrimack Valley. Sager blames income for causing the gap.

"Statewide, our data indicates doctors' gross incomes are 70 percent of the national average," he said, and "primary care physicians' incomes are simply too low in light of the skills they have and need and in light of how hard they work."

Mark Hollmer, 2006

Clinical trench income trends revolve around three factors: technology, time, and demographics. Physicians who have the technologies, time to deploy them, and patient base on whom to deploy them do very well.

Consequently, physician incomes are bimodal: high among procedural specialists, low among primary care clinicians. Among general internists, income trends and doctor satisfaction has gotten so bad the College of American Physicians issued this recent statement: "Primary care—the basic medical care that people get when they visit their doctors for routine physicals and minor problems—could fall apart in the United States without immediate reforms" (Fox, 2006).

Practice Conditions on the Ground

To capture trends among various specialty groups, let's begin by comparing conditions.

- Procedural specialists make 2 to 10 times more than primary care clinicians and the gap is widening.
- Primary care doctors are seeing more patients and spending less time with each; seeking to become efficient by installing electronic record systems, performing more in-office procedures—biopsies, stress tests, bone density measurements, and the like.
- Doctors are consolidating into larger practices for economies of scale, better market presence, and negotiating leverage with health plans and hospitals.
- Specialists are refusing emergency room coverage without compensation.
- Women patients are flocking to other women doctors for female issues, threatening to make obsolete those male doctors who evaluate and treat these conditions.
- The world of general surgery is shrinking; fewer gastric surgeries, breast biopsies, and exploratory procedures.
- Doctors are approaching hospitals to become hospitalists (doctors who practice exclusively within the hospital) or other hospital employers to avoid pressures to invest in EHRs, practice protocol-based medicine, and deal with soaring overheads.

- Many doctors are saying, "I'm getting a regular job with regular hours."
- Doctor shortages are becoming acute everywhere.
- The locum physician industry is booming (a locum tenens physician is a physician who substitutes temporarily for another physician).
- Hospitals are employing more procedural specialists as malpractice crises intensify.

Primary care physicians are feeling the pain of low incomes, rising costs, and declining reimbursements from health plans, Medicare, and Medicaid. Thus far,

- hiring nurse practitioners and physician assistants,
- consolidating into larger groups,
- sharpening coding precision,
- suing HMOs for unfair downloading and bundling of fees,
- pleading with Medicare not to lower reimbursements,
- installing electronic medical records,
- becoming subspecialists or hospitalists, and
- beefing up ancillary revenues

has only dulled but not relieved the pain.

The public—and congressional—perception that most physicians make too much money does not help the cause of financially beleaguered primary care physicians who may see installing income-producing ancillary equipment as the only way out of the financial "box."

Beating a Dead Horse

Primary care is not dead but is merely waiting for innovations to rouse it (Reece, 2003a, 2004b, 2006a). Primary care physicians simply have to "dismount" from old business models, open their minds and pocketbooks, and invest in new "ponies" (another type of practice) to carry them to new destinations offering more satisfying and rewarding careers.

One Family Physician Who Is Feeling His Oats

Dr. Randall Oates, a family physician in Springdale, Arkansas, is doing just such entrepreneurial and innovative things. In 1994, he founded and continues to be the chief executive officer (CEO) of a software company called DOCS, Inc. It recently changed its name to Soapware, Inc. Its primary product is SOAPware, a low-cost EHR system. His company has installed more systems in physician practices than any other EHR product in the United States. SOAPware is used in 6,000 clinics in

50 states and 22 foreign countries. Oates is widely respected within the EHR field. He is dedicated to designing health information technologies for small medical practices in family medicine and primary care.

In addition to these activities, he has built "boot camp" facilities in Springdale to train physicians to mount the new horse of EHR systems. Doctor Oates's message to his fellow primary care colleagues is: Stop horsing around and pull yourself up by your own bootstraps.

Speaking of Horses

According to Dakota tribal wisdom, when you are riding a dead horse, the best strategy is to dismount and then mount a new one. However, in health care management, doctors have become obsessed with process-based corrective measures—measures based on changing the process of care. Process improvement jargon becomes the enemy of innovation. In the process of dismounting from a dead horse to remount a new one, process-based obsessions may develop. The following saddle-worn list tells the tale of what can happen to those trying to decide whether to change horses. They cannot decide whether to:

1. Buy a stronger whip.
2. Change riders.
3. Say things like, "This is the way we always have ridden this horse."
4. Appoint a committee to study the horse.
5. Arrange to visit other sites to see how they ride dead horses.
6. Increase standards to ride dead horses.
7. Appoint a tiger team to revive the dead horse (a tiger team is a group of aggressive individuals, or "tigers," who bring about change).
8. Create a training session to increase riding ability.
9. Compare the state of dead horses in today's environment.
10. Change the requirements by declaring, "This horse is not dead."
11. Hire consultants to ride the dead horse.
12. Harness several dead horses together for increased speed.
13. Declare, "No horse is too dead to beat."
14. Provide additional funding to increase the horse's performance.
15. Do a cost analysis to see if consultants can do it cheaper.
16. Purchase a product to make the dead horse grow faster.
17. Declare the horse is "better, faster, and cheaper dead."
18. Form a quality circle to find uses for dead horses.
19. Revisit the performance requirements for horses.
20. Say this horse was procured with cost as an independent variable.
21. Promote the dead horse to a supervisory position.

The New Horse: Innovation

Primary care physicians should worry less about the process of reinventing the old horse and just do it. The "new horse" is simply code language for innovation. Unfortunately, innovations may become lost in obsessions with process management. Becoming too steeped in management processes may cause physicians, already drowning in the new economic environment, to forget their original intention was to drain the swamp.

But how, you may ask, can I remount? Here are seven hints:

1. **Study electronic medical record and automation applications.**

   Certain things are evident about the future and will require awareness and expertise in electronic data exchange.

   First, consumer engagement will alter the financial landscape. Doctors will need to bill and collect electronically. They will have to determine if patients have funds in their health savings accounts, and they will be forced to ask for credit and debit cards up front. ATM-like transactions with automatic withdrawal of funds will become common and necessary for practice efficiency.

   Second, physician revenue will be maximized from automated appropriate coding and from total charge capture at the point of service. Many physicians, particularly surgeons but other doctors as well, perform procedures outside of their offices in hospitals and ambulatory care settings. Computer terminals are not ubiquitous in these settings. Web sites are now available that allow these physicians to access the code and transmit it back to their offices, thus allowing total capture of revenues.

   Third, fees will be set by the market, not by health plans. This will lead to a relentless concentration on practice efficiency, a reliance on the consumer as a source of free data entry and to automated history taking, health record entries, and computerized diagnostic support systems.

   Fourth, remote telemedicine monitoring and interviewing units will be placed in the home and at work locations for evaluation of initial complaints and support of chronic disease patients.

   Finally, virtual electronic visits will become routine for nonemergent problems, scheduling, and prescribing and refills.

2. **Focus on outpatient care delivery.**

   During the last 20 years, a progressive shift to outpatient surgery has occurred. Because consumers are demanding shorter stays, more convenience, and full price disclosure in advance, this decentralization to detached outpatient settings will continue.

   This means hospitals, with the help of physician leaders who must organize and deliver the care, will organize in settings far removed from traditional brick-and-mortar settings. These settings will include convenient multispecialty ambulatory care clinics, ambulatory surgery and cosmetic surgery units, preventive and holistic health centers, mobile health evaluation units, and nonemergent care (immunization and routine physicals) in discount store, drugstore, and supermarket settings.

There is a big future for physicians organizing and leading these new care outlets and for marketing customized and targeted services featuring "focused care" for orthopedic, cancer, and heart problems. These new points of service will demand teamwork with specialized nurses, physician assistants, and cross-trained paraprofessional personnel. Because the patient will be the hub of care, outpatient care delivery will extend to the home and workplace.

3. **Consider procedures, money, and lifestyle.**

Young physicians have been quick to recognize certain specialties combine the best in incomes and lifestyle. These include dermatology (no night calls, laser and cosmetic procedures), radiology (CT scans, EMRs, PET scans, and other noninvasive evaluations), and hospitalists (regular hours, readily available technologies, predictable income). These and other like specialties involve performing procedures. The U.S. culture is willing to pay dearly for procedures.

This desire to pay may not extend to the cognitive specialties. Patients are reluctant to pay for preventive commonsensical advice. They can find this advice on the Internet. Recognition that consumers (and health plans) will pay for procedures has spilled over to primary care, where doctors are beginning to offer laser procedures for varicose veins and other cosmetic blights and are performing minor procedures (skin biopsies, vasectomies, cervical biopsies) to enhance incomes and patient convenience.

Something must be done to make independent primary care specialties more attractive economically. These primary care specialties often earn one half to a tenth of what high-tech specialists make.

4. **Know your strengths and weaknesses.**

Medical education and training does not necessarily produce self-knowledge or business knowledge. Indeed, it is crammed with memorizing facts, competing with fellow students, learning from specialists, and sorting out what specialty niches are appealing.

This education and training produces a narrow-minded view of the world. The medical curriculum is so crowded, it leaves little room for garnering practical business skills or an understanding why accountants, practice managers, lawyers, and other professionals are necessary in the present competitive and litigious environment.

The emerging young doctors tend to be compulsive and academically gifted with just enough knowledge to enter the specialty of their choice. However, they may know little of what they are good at; whether they have interactive, leadership, or negotiating skills; or whether they work well within an organization or are best suited for independent practice.

For these reasons, organizations that guide or advise doctors on alternative careers or mid-career changes within the profession put their doctor clients through psychological testing. For example, the Physician Career Network in Denver, Colorado, uses the Birkman method, a tool for evaluating physicians' usual behaviors, underlying needs, stress behaviors, and best career matches. More often, interpersonal understanding is gained from experience in the demands of practice or in the give-and-take of politics or lack of satisfaction within a medical organization.

5. **Make nurses part of your delivery team.**

   Whether doctors realize it or not, making nurses part of the management and treatment team can make or break a practice. Dr. Marshall O. Zaslove, author of *The Successful Physician: A Productivity Handbook for Practitioners* and a leader of productivity seminars for physicians, says many doctors fail because they simply don't listen to nurses or ask them for help.

   Zaslove says simply stopping and asking nurses, "How can I do this better?" or "What would make this practice more efficient?" may enormously increase productivity. To their credit, health plans were the first to recognize and reward nurses. They did so by elevating them to executive positions, making them central players in quality control programs, and employing squads of them to deliver personal, protocol-directed chronic disease care in home and work situations.

6. **Carefully weigh additional degrees.**

   With an MBA degree, doctors presume they can make more money and have greater impact; however, some are skeptical of the effectiveness and job satisfaction of many MD-MBA graduates. As John Ludden, MD, director of the Tufts MD-MBA program, observed, "Doctors would rather be the hammer than the nail" (Shaywitz and Ausiello, 2002).

   It is true, of course, that health plan managers, hospital executives, and staff of other health care organizations such as pharmaceutical companies assiduously recruit MD-MBAs. It is also true there are growing numbers of hospital CEOs with joint medical-business degrees and physician–business people are the preferred leaders of the nation's leading health care institutions.

   Keep in mind there are ways to obtain business skills other than full-time MBA programs. Many community colleges offer health concentration programs taught by experienced health executives. Business schools may have online programs requiring only part-time or weekend attendance, and the American College of Physician Executives and other groups offer a myriad of educational opportunities.

   Some MD-MBAs are disappointed with the outcome. Some even feel they are unemployable, lack job security, or feel they have lost the trust of fellow physicians who perceive that they have crossed over the managerial divide. Although having a business-centered background is helpful when maintaining a practice, it's important to weigh all sides of the education issue before moving ahead with additional coursework.

7. **Know who speaks for your business interests.**

At the practice level, some doctors say individual clinicians can, or should, be innovative enough to overcome intense competition, rising practice costs, and reduced reimbursements. Dr. Neil Baum shares this viewpoint in *Take Charge of Your Practice Before Someone Else Does It for You* (Baum and Zablocki, 1996), as does Michael Gerber in *The E-Myth Physician: Why Most Practices Don't Work* (2004). I suggest these for further reading

Other doctor speakers maintain individual practice managers, practice management firms, and organizations like the Medical Group Management Association, whose members represent over 240,000 physicians. Still others say individual practice associations ably represent doctors' business interests.

Doctor employers are another candidate. Hospitals, integrated health organizations, academic health centers, and multispecialty clinics employ 40 percent of doctors and take care of physician business concerns (U.S. Department of Labor, Bureau of Labor Statistics, 2006). Nationally, the AMA speaks for doctors, but is subdued on business matters lest it be portrayed as a doctor union.

Finally, there are state and local medical associations. They are closer than the AMA to those in the clinical trenches. In the past 2 years, 19 state medical associations successfully sued national HMOs—Aetna, Cigna, WellPoint, and Humana—and may yet win suits against Pacificare, Health-Net, and United Health care. With $150 million won so far from HMO settlements, this group of state societies, representing 700,000 physicians, has formed two foundations—the Physicians Foundation for Health Systems Excellence and the Physicians Foundation for Health Systems Innovation—and is issuing grants to further physician business efficiencies and clinical effectiveness (Reece, 2005c).

Physicians should turn electronic technologies to their competitive advantage while focusing on the outpatient arena. Be realistic and, if necessary, be tested about personal strengths and weaknesses. Make nurses an integral part of the delivery team, and identify and work with those who can best represent your business interests. (Reece, 2006b)

Innovation Talking and Action Points

This chapter covers the health care innovation landscape, changes in how consumers buy and use health care, new technologies making this buying and use practical, and a series of new business models.

A Practice in Evolution: Staying a Little Ahead of the Game in Internal Medicine

By John H. Cook III, MD, FACP

Dr. Cook, a former naval submarine officer, now in his sixties, brings to the table a wealth of experience, not only from serving as a nuclear submarine officer, but as a physician leader in Leesburg, Virginia. Doctor Cook entered medical school after his U.S. Navy duty. He is an internist, but recently also received his boards in geriatrics. As is evident here, Dr. Cook has a management and leadership frame of mind.

• •

Farming looks mighty easy when your plow is a pencil and you're a thousand miles from the cornfield.

Dwight D. Eisenhower, September 11, 1956

Ike's succinct rejection of a staff report guides my description of our evolution. I started 26 years ago as a solo practitioner. Now we are a seven-provider POD (point of care) office embedded within a larger association of PODs (Principles of Database Systems) operating as an limited liability company under a single tax ID number. The following is our bottom-line evolution over the last 4 years.

Differences Between Doctors and Nurse Practitioners Fading

I'll continue to use the term *provider.* In our practice, the line between a physician and an experienced nurse practitioner has blurred to the point it is difficult to tell where it is.

As we look ahead, we see tasks we have to complete to continue to stay a little ahead of a game. A game where rules and reimbursement change suddenly.

Staying Abreast of Revolutionary Advances in Technology

While we are trying to keep up with rules and regulations, we also have to stay abreast of the continuing revolutionary advances in the technology of diagnosis and treatment.

1. We see the need for a practice-wide EMR as so essential that we are willing to book a $20,000 per provider charge to buy the system and integrate it with our scheduling/billing system.
2. The most pressing need is to figure out how to ethically and effectively care for Medicare and Tri-Care patients as Centers of Medicare and Medicaid changes the rules. Limiting Medicare patients or rejecting them entirely borders on unprofessional behavior.
3. We see the practicality of remaining as a training site for nurse practitioner students from four local programs. Not only does it keep us on our toes clinically, but it gives us access to a set of extraordinarily motivated mid-career woman to work within our larger group.
4. We continue to evaluate ancillary services and integrate them if they meet the basic $3 return for $1 of initial expense criterion. So far, in-house laboratory, echocardiography, and ANSAR (Autonomic Nervous System and Respiration) testing have met this criterion.

5. We need to find a way of recovering the cost of new, noncodable dimensions of primary care service. This includes everything from advocacy to the coordination of care of complex patients. Embedded within this is the continuing need to educate our patients in self-care.
6. We need to continue to push back against the abuses of third-party payers especially in their continued imposition of uncompensated administrative requirements. This is the principal reason for creating and expanding a multi-POD group under a single tax ID number. We've learned the power of just saying "no" to new contracts.
7. We need to enter the pay-for-performance arena with the right weapons. The EMR is essential. Internal protocols incorporating the best practices from evidence-based medicine are essential. Patient feedback is essential.
8. We need to continue to upgrade the productivity of each of the clinical and administrative staff. We are evolving toward intraoffice teams of two providers supported by one administrative staff and one clinical staff. The patients like personal service. They like to talk to "Mary" (an LPN) about clinical questions and "Ruth" about scheduling and referrals. They need to know that "their" provider will call them back in a timely fashion. Key to fulfilling this task is developing an internal and external communication system that integrates voice and text with the EMR.
9. We realize that each provider brings a unique set of skills and needs into the POD. We need to support the provider efficiently. Where applicable, we need to develop new skills.

Basic Principles Governing Our Practice

Here are the basic principles that govern our practice:

- We provide same-day emergent care with an available provider and next-day urgent care with the patient's provider team.
- In scheduling, we load level total clinical intensity over 10 hours daily—this means we try to remain as clinically active as possible for 10 hours. We are currently investigating—after the EMR is in place—extending hours to 12 (7 A.M. to 7 P.M.) Monday through Thursday, 7 A.M. to 5 P.M. on Friday, and 9 A.M. to 3 P.M. on Saturday. Load leveling improves staff efficiency. We anticipate each provider increasing clinical services from 34 hours to 40 hours of office clinical work. Those 40 hours will be embedded in the 64 hours that the office is open weekly. In forward planning, it will allow us to add more providers without expanding space.
- We base provider pay on cash derived from E&M activity and individual minor surgical procedures: "You eat what you treat." We track clinical production using relative value units (RVU) using an updated RBRVS (resource-based relative value scale) handbook. Clinicians should get all their cash from the professional component fraction. The POD gets its cash from the facility component.
- Ancillary service–derived cash goes into the general support fund for the POD. It is analyzed every 6 months to see if the $3 cash for $1 expense rule is still operative.
- POD profit is distributed to providers and staff by a formula that changes as conditions change. It is used as an initiative stimulus.
- We limit maximum hours per week to 65 hours per provider. This includes patient contact hours, hospital and nursing home rounds, self-study, administrative hours, 16-hour credit for weekend duty, and a 4-hour credit per day for telephone duty. Currently, we are able to work half that (34 hours) in direct patient care in the office. We believe we can move that up to 40 or more hours a week with the full implementation of the EMR including its pharmacy and remote access components. We continue to try to evolve nonbillable administrative time into charge-producing activity.

Box 7.1   91

BOX 7.1

65-Hour Rule

By John H. Cook III, MD, FACP

• •

I found the 65-hour rule during my previous career in nuclear submarines. We were in the middle of extensive preparations for a special operation. We were working harder and harder, making mistakes and falling behind. A friend of mine, recovering from a helicopter crash in 'Nam, was working in leadership development while he was in physical therapy. He was in a new area called human engineering. He listened to my sob story, then said, "S___, Jack. Your troops are burnt out." He then shared with me the background and details of the rule.

It represents the maximum time that a person who likes his or her work and is trained effectively can work without burnout. It also requires that each man or woman take 1 day weekly away from the job.

I've made empiric additions to the rule over the last 30 years. I believe that woman with children in the home and men with children in after-hour sports need to cut the hours on the job back to 55 hours per week.

Keeping morale, skill, and compassion up also requires a provider to rest at least five full nights a week.

Even God couldn't work more than 6 days in a row.

Chapter 8

Total Knee Replacement: An Innovator's Dream

Prelude: The body parts replacement movement is a powerful convergence of new technologies and demands by aging baby boomers.

Encouraged by doctors to continue to exercise three to five times a week for their health, a legion of running, swimming and biking boomers are flouting the conventional limits of the middle-aged body's abilities, and filling the nation's operating rooms and orthopedists' offices in the process.

Bill Pennington,
"Baby Boomers Remain Active,
and So Do Their Doctors,"
New York Times, **April 16, 2006**

Entrepreneurs dream of scenarios where forces for innovation converge. In the case of knee replacements, these forces are Americans' penchant for quick technological fixes, shifts in demographics and perceptions, and new industry and market structures.

- **Technological fixes.** In 1988, journalist Lynn Payer, who worked in the United States and Europe, wrote that cultural values shaped a nation's approach to health care. She spoke of obsessions of the Germans with hearts, the French with livers, the English with bowels, and the Americans with machines. Americans, she said, think of their bodies as machines. If the front of the machine sags, uplift it; if the plumbing clogs, bypass it; if a part goes out, replace it.

- **Demographics and perceptions.** Baby boomers are turning 60 at the rate of one every 7 seconds (Pennington, 2006). Cartilages of their aging knees pounded daily by jogging or running are wearing out. No matter, the boomers perceive you can have your knees replaced and stay forever young and still function as weekend warriors.

- **Industry and market structure.** The health care industry is rapidly shifting from inpatient to outpatient care, from hospital surgeries to ambulatory surgical procedures, and from hospital-run facilities to doctor-owned or managed facilities. The American Academy of Orthopedic Surgery is aware of these trends. It has launched a national media campaign to educate and promote joint replacements as elective procedures. These surgeons may now only replace joints, but also act as consultants and developers of joint prostheses.

A joint replacement boom is under way, mostly for knees but also for hips and other joints as well. Doctors are operating on younger and younger patients. Statistics from the American Academy of Orthopedic Surgeons show that 418,000 total and partial knee replacements were performed in 2004, 15 percent of them in baby boomers.

At its 2006 annual meeting, Dr. Steven Kurtz of Exponent, Inc., an engineering and consulting firm in Philadelphia, projected first-time total knee replacements would jump to 3.18 million, a 673 percent increase, by 2030. Kurtz said this demand would almost certainly lead to a nationwide shortage of orthopedic surgeons, with long waiting lines for patients. Kurtz, a professor at Drexel University School of Biomedical Engineering, noted, "There are few procedures that return as much quality of life as a knee replacement" (Mann, 2006).

As with any successful innovative scenario, there is no assurance the pace of knee replacements will be sustained. Medicare, alarmed by costs, is cutting back on fees. On July 17, 2006, Medicare announced it would cut reimbursement for hip and knee replacements by 10 percent, to $14,500, a proposal that was subsequently scaled back on August 3, 2006. Private insurers take the Medicare lead, so private fees will also being reduced (Pear, 2006c).

With a freer market, created by consumers holding health savings accounts in high-deductible plans, competition could be accompanied by a drop in prices. Consumers may demand proof of value. This will require orthopedists to invest heavily in outcome databases to prove the value of their particular brand of knee replacement passes muster. There may also be "disruptive innovations" (Christensen, 2000), such as efficient ways to grow knee cartilages or use of injected hyaluronic acid or materials containing hyaluronic acid made of rooster combs or bacterial cultures to lubricate joints (American Academy of Orthopaedic Surgery, 2006). Margins may shrink as more questions have to be answered. Frequent questions may require a larger staff to answer. As George Halvorson, CEO of Kaiser Permanente, said in an interview, "There's going to have to be definitions. What exactly is a successful knee surgery? Does the patient walk without pain after surgery? Can the patient function better?" (Reece, 2005c).

Still, if you were a medical student and had the requisite skills, should you pick orthopedic surgery as a specialty? Well:

- You do good. What patient isn't grateful to walk again without pain?
- You do well. Orthopedic surgeons are among the highest paid specialists.
- Your medical colleagues admire your work. Internists say knee and hip joint replacement is one of the top 10 medical innovations over the last three decades.
- You have the hospital CEOs' undivided attention. You are likely to be the greatest contributor to the hospital's bottom line.

In other words, you have respect from all quarters—consumers, physicians, and hospitals. At least for the present, you will be riding a sustainable wave of technology that shows no signs of abating.

Innovation Talking and Action Points

What has been described here is an innovation based on new technologies (better knees prostheses, superior glues, better imaging techniques, and improved anesthesia) and new demographics (aging boomers who want to remain young and functional). In *Innovation and Entrepreneurship: Practice and Principles* (1986), Peter F. Drucker explains this principle of innovation: "An innovation, to be effective, has to be simple, and it has to be focused. It should do only one thing, otherwise it confuses. If it isn't simple, it won't work. Everything else runs into trouble, if complicated it cannot be reworked or fixed. All effective innovations are breathtakingly simple."

- What could be simpler than replacing a worn-out knee with a new one?
- What could be simpler than ending pain and restoring a person to full function, especially a person who has vowed never to grow old?
- What could be simpler than focusing on one joint?

Nothing. That's why the orthopedist knows what "knees" to be done (poor pun intended). Knee replacement is part of an industry called *implantable medical devices*. Included in these devices are:

- joint replacements of all kinds
- vascular grafts
- coronary and carotid stents
- cardiac pacemakers
- cardiac stimulators
- neurological stimulators
- dental implants
- breast implants

- eye implants
- cochlear implants
- artificial hearts
- drug pumps
- a variety of muscle, nerve, and neurological simulators

Discussing the entire field of implantable devices is beyond the scope of this book, but the implantable device field is a vast playground for innovators and a minefield of safety hazards, as demonstrated in the recent controversies surrounding failures of certain defibrillators.

The safety hazard problem is likely to generate another trend: the formation of safety panels to collect more data about devices and to devise methods to standardize how to notify doctors and patients about any problems (Meier, 2006). Dr. Steven Barchet, a retired naval officer and obstetrician-gynecologist, says that in this age of consumer-driven care with cost shifts to consumers, patients about to undergo a procedure like a knee replacement ought to ask their doctor two questions:

1. If you were to have this procedure, would you be willing to pay for it using your own money?
2. In the event I have this operation and things don't come out to my liking, would you be willing to give me my money back?

Those questions, says Barchet, put the cost/value equation in perspective. Every innovation spawns other innovations and has its upsides and downsides. With total knee replacement, the upsides are no knee pain and return to function. The downside for some patients is unanticipated postoperative pain, and for an unfortunate few, addiction to painkillers.

An unexpected and little publicized innovation is doctor sensitivity to the systematic measurement and documentation of pain on a 1-to-10 basis. It is recorded as another vital sign in many doctors' offices. Forty million Americans suffer from chronic pain (Steinberg, 2005). Measuring and tracking pain has become important in the new patient-centered environment. Prior to knee surgery, osteoarthritis of the knee may be anything from a 4 to a 9; immediately after knee replacement for 48 to 72 hours it may rise to an 8 or a 10, but over time it may drop to zero (Rineberg).

A New Set of Knees, a Story of Short-Term Pain and Long-Term Gain

By Jane E. Brody

Jane E. Brody received her BS degree in biochemistry from the New York State College of Agriculture and Life Sciences at Cornell University in 1962 and a master's degree in science writing from the University of Wisconsin School of Journalism the following year. After two years as a general assignment reporter for the *Minneapolis Tribune,* in 1965 she joined the *New York Times* as a full-time specialist in medicine and biology. In 1976, she was appointed as the *Times* Personal Health columnist, and her widely read and quoted column continues to appear every Wednesday in the *Times* and in more than 100 other newspapers around the country. In addition, her articles on other aspects of science and medicine appear frequently in the *Times* Science Times on Tuesdays. Here Jane E. Brody, a *New York Times* health columnist, describes her postoperative pain after a bilateral knee replacement.

Total knee replacement is now one of the nation's leading orthopedic operations, and it promises to become even more popular as the population ages (and grows heavier) and the body's most vulnerable joints fail to withstand the punishment of decades of use and abuse.

Debilitating wear-and-tear arthritis is the major reason that knee bones are being replaced by 2-pound pieces of metal in people who wish to remain mobile, pain free, and physically active in their later years.

Dozens of people I know who've endured the surgery say it has changed their lives very much for the better. They can walk again with comfort; even play tennis and ski, after years of sitting on the sidelines.

And so, at age 63, I decided to have both knees replaced. I had been nursing my increasingly arthritic knees and bowed legs for two decades—at first with ice packs and ibuprofen whenever I did strenuous activity, graduating to daily Vioxx and Tylenol with growing limits on what I could do without life-limiting discomfort.

The last straw (after giving up tennis, ice skating, and cross-country skiing) was my inability to hike or even join my friends on our morning fitness walk around the park. Even Vioxx (before it was withdrawn from the market) was not keeping me comfortably on my feet.

I consulted one of the world's leading orthopedic surgeons, a man who had done thousands of knee and hip replacements, including 500 double knees. He was very reassuring.

With the aid of physical therapy, he said, I could expect to be driving again in 4 weeks and well on the way to full recovery in 6. Even the reputedly horrific postoperative pain associated with this surgery, he added, is now fully controlled with morphine through epidural anesthesia supplemented by extra doses that the patients can administer.

A neighbor who had one knee replaced last summer had warned me, "The first 4 weeks are hell," but I discounted her prediction, given that I was in good health, top physical condition and slender going into the surgery.

A preoperative education session at the hospital emphasized the importance of good pain control because without it, patients cannot do the physical therapy essential to a good recovery.

I gave two preoperative blood donations (one for each knee), arranged for inpatient rehabilitation after leaving the hospital and thought I was fully prepared for what lay ahead.

I was not prepared for the swelling. When I arrived at the rehab center on the fourth postoperative day, I weighed in at 120, 15 pounds more than I weighed at surgery.

My legs were filled with fluid, hard as rocks, with no visible bones, veins, or tendons. In 4 days I was down to 103, but my legs continued to swell and stiffen for more than 2 months.

As for pain, the surgeon was right on one count: the morphine was bliss—not a bit of pain the first 2 days after the operation. Then it was withdrawn and replaced by two narcotic oral pain medications, which worked pretty well for about 5 days.

But as the various tissues in my knees began to heal and physical therapy got more demanding, the pain grew worse and worse, until at 3 weeks I found myself moaning, then crying for much of the day despite the narcotics and repeated icing of my swollen knees. Sleep was my only relief, but one can't do that 24/7.

Thinking something must be radically wrong, I returned to the surgeon 26 days after the operation, only to be told my knees looked perfect on X-rays and that my mobility placed me in the top two on the recovery scale: I could walk and go up and down stairs, albeit slowly, and I could fully extend my knees and bend them 90 degrees.

As reassuring as this assessment was, it did nothing to control my pain. So he changed my medication to a potent anti-inflammatory drug and suggested that I gradually cut back on the narcotics. That proved to be something of a pipe dream, at least for the next several weeks—and there was no sleeping without a nightly dose of Ambien.

I learned much later that I could have been prescribed a much higher dose of narcotics with no ill effect and much better pain control. No doctor I reported to, however, including the surgeon, even considered that.

The fact is, this operation, which involved cutting my leg bones to straighten my bowed legs, hurts like hell. To the few patients I spoke with who had relatively little postoperative pain, I say, "Count your blessings."

My biggest complaint was not that I was suffering. (The pain at 5 weeks after the operation had definitely eased on most days, although my right knee hurt much more than the left. So much for driving!) My biggest complaint was that I hadn't been warned. I was presented only with the best-case result, not the worst.

I complained to my internist that in the first 3 postoperative weeks all I had been able to do was read three simple novels. Even knitting and crocheting seemed too much for me, let alone the many projects I'd hoped to tackle during my self-assigned 6-week recovery period.

My doctor explained why: "Intense pain is all-consuming. It takes over your life, and it's impossible to focus on much else." In fact, it changes your personality, and now I understand far better why patients with chronic pain can be so difficult to live with. It's hard to be pleasant when all you want to do is chop off the part of your body that hurts so much.

Continuing physical therapy is critical to a full recovery, but at first I overdid it by going three times a week. I have since cut back to twice a week to give my body more time to recover between sessions. It seems to be helping.

Compounding my physical discomfort was the emotional turmoil caused by insane insurance policies. My plan from the outset was to go from the hospital to an inpatient rehabilitation facility, which my policy covers for patients with double-knee replacements.

The insurer, however, wanted me to leave the hospital on the third day after surgery, when I was still restricted to using a bedpan. My hospital-provided case manager (every hospital must have them these days to negotiate with insurance companies) argued for an extra day, but that was covered only because I experienced severe chest pains (due to indigestion, it turned out) on the fourth day, not because my walking was limited to a few steps.

Then the insurer limited me to 4 days of inpatient rehabilitation, not nearly enough in my view, especially since I was going home to a four-story house. After 6 weeks of post-op, I still could descend stairs by bending only one knee.

But the most irritating insanity was the limit placed on my sleep medication: 14 tablets every 23 days. Was I supposed to sleep only every other night? Who came up with such a formula? Certainly not anyone who has ever had major surgery. Although my husband asked, the pharmacy failed to tell him that I could pay for the drug myself, about $4 a pill, far preferable to lying awake in pain all night.

I'm still waiting for that blissful day when I can walk better than I did before the surgery, get through the day without multiple pain pills and sleep without medication. I'm reasonably sure that day will come in the next few months, but I must admit, I'm fast losing patience.

People ask, "Are you sorry you did two knees at once?" Not at all. In fact, I can't imagine going through this twice, and both knees were in horrible shape and needed to be replaced.

I've met several people in rehab who had one knee done and need to replace the other. But having endured the first replacement, they say they are now very hesitant to do it again.

Part Two

Large-Group Practice Innovation

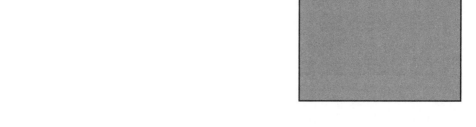

Even small health care institutions are complex, barely manageable places. Large health care institutions may be the most complex organizations in human history.

Peter F. Drucker, 1975

Chapter 9

Kaiser Permanente's Archimedes Model

Prelude: Big health care organizations, such as Kaiser with its $30 billion in revenues, have bigger innovative levers to lift the health care world, such as a comprehensive electronic system connecting all of its physicians.

Give me a lever long enough, and a prop strong enough, I can single-handedly move the world.

> Archimedes, 1267 BC–1212 BC
> From Pappus of Alexandria,
> *Collectio, bk, VIII, prop.10, sec. 11*

The Internet: The Modern Lever

The greatest innovation in the last 30 years is worldwide instant distribution of information. The Internet exemplifies how a small lever can move great weights, like health care. The Internet is a great for leveling, or to use Friedman's term, for "flattening" health care playing fields (Friedman, 2005).

The following is an interview with George Halvorson, chairman and president of Kaiser Permanente.

Reece: An October 2004 *New York Times* article posed this question: Is Kaiser Permanente the model for the U.S. health system? The reporter said the company concentrates on intensive computerization and serves as a model laboratory for addressing how to deal with those 5 percent of chronic diseases causing 70 percent of costs.

I understand you've made significant progress. You have metrics to show you're reducing recurrent heart attacks and heart attack deaths.

Halvorson: Yes, we have. We have dramatically reduced heart attacks and diabetic complications. We're building a database that will be useful at another level—namely, conducting virtual trials.

Let me touch on another point—the Vioxx issue. Were you aware that it was our study that triggered the Vioxx recall?

Reece: No, I was not.

Halvorson: Yes, that was a Kaiser computer follow-up study. That's just the beginning of the type of research you can do when you have a database of 8 million people, and you can track it against age, sex, ethnicity, geography, comorbidity, and you can run all kinds of computer models.

It's almost the equivalent of an 8 million members perpetual clinical trial. The really big clinical trials have thousands of participants, but no more. The ability of what we can do will transform health care.

Reece: Kaiser has something called the Archimedes Project. Isn't that an example of predictive modeling?

Halvorson: Yes, it's fascinating because it computerizes human disease and medical interventions. It allows us to predict consequences of various approaches to care. The program is so good that we have run clinical trials through it. It has predicted outcomes within a couple of percentage points. We can set up to do virtual clinical trials within a relatively short time at a fraction of the expense of real clinical trials.

Reece: You can conduct clinical trials using a computer model?

Halvorson: Exactly. We can take an employer group and identify exactly what kind of care those people are going to need for the next couple of years—and we can predict what differences of care will produce what outcomes. We can also run clinical trials. We have several major drug companies, yet to be announced, who are willing to take test runs through our Archimedes system before putting drugs out into the clinical world.

Reece: Is Dr. David Eddy, that rare combination of an MD with a PhD in mathematics, still the principal investigator and architect behind Archimedes?

Halvorson: Absolutely; he's an amazingly brilliant man.

Enough Talk, Now onto Virtual Reality

The Archimedes model provides a mathematically based lever. It moves and manipulates vast amounts of data, simulating reality. It improves and speeds health care decision making at decision points along the health care spectrum. The model, according to its developers, creates a virtual reality in which virtual people with virtual physiologies who get virtual diseases, go to virtual doctors, get virtual tests and treatments, and have virtual outcomes.

Archimedes, the Kaiser Permanente innovation that now operates as an independent company, has been 10 years in the making. It uses mathematical simulation to create a virtual world. This helps health care organizations make critical administrative decisions. Kaiser has repeatedly tested and validated the model to answer complex real-world decisions.

It's in the Cards

In a disease-modeling test, the Archimedes team conducted a publicly announced, blinded procedure of a major clinical trial. The trial was called the Collaborative Atorvastatin Diabetes Study (CARDS), a trial jointly sponsored by Diabetes UK, the Department of Health of the United Kingdom, and Pfizer. The trial included type 2 diabetics with at least one additional health risk factor for developing heart disease.

On March 26, 2004, Archimedes simulated the CARDS trial using the same data and placed its predictions in four envelopes: one for the principal investigators, one for Pfizer, one for the American Diabetes Association, and one that was kept for the Archimedes team. The outcomes for sudden cardiac death, nonsudden cardiac death, and nonfatal myocardial infarctions including silent MIs were highly accurate. The Archimedes model has also proved accurate in predicting strokes in patients on statin drugs.

Archimedes' great potential exists in the help it provides to organizations targeting and treating chronic diseases. It is common knowledge that these diseases consume 70 percent to 90 percent of health care costs. The model can move simulated people with disease through time, predicting what will happen years ahead.

The model includes everything a physician might do—from checking blood pressures, to weighing effects of laboratory values, to imaging study results, to surgical interventions, to EKG findings. The model has applications for the big chronic diseases: coronary artery disease, heart failure, diabetes, strokes, and asthma.

Innovation Talking and Action Points

Although the company is 60 years old, Kaiser still represents a new business model: an integrated system with a health plan, hospitals, and salaried physicians. It is now busily expanding on that base by focusing on new technologies and improving the health of its 8.3 million members.

The Archimedes model shows how a large organization can innovate. Resources and funding over the long haul make large innovations possible. The Archimedes model could have profound effects, not only in treating patients, but on the clinical trials industry, a big part of the billions of dollars of expenses ($800 million is required to bring a drug to market). Global industry analysts estimate $33 billion was spent in 1997 on research and development (R&D) (Jayashree, 2005).

Archimedes is but one example of the potential artificial intelligence models' impact in revolutionizing support of diagnostic and treatment, in converting invasive procedures into virtual models, and in personalizing drug treatments of cancer and other chronic diseases.

Another company pursuing goals similar to Archimedes is MedAI (Medical Artificial Intelligence) in Orlando, Florida. MedAI has a product, Pinpoint Quality, that is an outcomes measurement application. It enables users to easily identify specific steps to monitor to improve clinical outcomes while reducing health care costs.

Clients can integrate data from clinical and financial legacy systems. This allows companies to undertake quality initiatives. Medical directors, administrative directors, and other members of the organization can create reports of quality indicators. Meeting these indicators can be used to increase payment and practice changes in their organization.

Case Study 1

Kaiser and the Four Pillars of Genuine Innovation
By Dr. Richard L. Reece

Richard L. Reece, MD, is a pathologist, editor, writer, consultant, and author of this book. He resides in Old Saybrook, Connecticut. Part of the contents of this case study are based on an interview with George Halvorson, CEO of Kaiser, which appeared in *Voices of Health Reform* (2005).

According to Peter F. Drucker in *Innovation and Entrepreneurship*, the four pillars of genuine innovation are:

1. doing things differently
2. doing them with efficiency
3. doing them with missionary zeal
4. doing them no matter what the outside world, the traditional establishment, thinks

I became aware of Kaiser's penchant for genuine innovation 25 years ago when I was invited to deliver a speech before Kaiser's medical directors in Laguna Beach. The directors wanted to know the implications of Minnesota's nascent managed care boom. To prepare for that speech, I read Paul de Kruif's little 1943 classic *Kaiser Wakes the Doctor*. De Kruif described how Dr. Sidney Garfield introduced the concept of prepaid medical care for the workers building the Grand Coulee dam.

This led to the official founding of the Kaiser Foundation in 1945. Kaiser now covers 8.3 million members in nine states and the District of Columbia, employs 11,000 doctors and 141,000 other people, and includes the nonprofit Kaiser Foundation Health Plan, the nonprofit Kaiser Foundation Hospitals, and for-profit medical groups.

It was apparent in the beginning that Kaiser innovation was different—so different that organized medicine sought to outlaw prepaid care—the missionary zeal was there from the start. Paul de Kruif declared breathlessly and perhaps a little overzealously, "The Kaiser model proved that good doctors, and especially young doctors, do not insist upon being individual businessmen. They do not mind working on salaries if these are good, and if they have the chance to use the marvelous power of modern medical science—unhampered by the dead hand of no dollars" (DeKruif, 1943).

During my Laguna Beach visit, the late Dr. Jack Gordon, then director of clinical pathology at Kaiser Permanente Medical Center in Los Angeles, made me sharply aware of the efficiencies of Kaiser's approach to care. By centralizing its laboratory operations, including clinical testing, cytology screening, and tissue processing in one location, Kaiser was able to operate with one third the number of pathologists practicing in the outside world. Not only did the Kaiser approach require fewer pathologists, but the pathologists who practiced there were able to see a much greater volume of cases, thereby enhancing their expertise.

In 2005, I had the opportunity to interview George Halvorson, chairman and CEO of Kaiser Permanente, and Dr. Jay Crosson, founder of the Council of Acceptable Physician Practices representing premier multispecialty groups throughout the United States, and chair of the Kaiser Foundation (Reece, 2005c).

Both stressed team-based medicine, setting quality-improvement goals, and investing heavily in information technologies, and basic clinical research. Like the chairman emeritus of Kaiser Permanente, David Lawrence, they believe it takes the resources, teamwork, and commitment of large multispecialty groups "to put it together" (Lawrence, 2002). Kaiser believes the organization, not the individual, is the starting point of excellence; the lever that moves and lifts standards and care delivery.

Dr. Crosson commented, "Our message is that if certain things are put together right—financial incentives, political clarity, spread of information technologies to bind physicians together, standards of best practice, help for physicians to understand governance, and other organization goals—good things will happen." He added, "Physicians in multispecialty practices are the happiest doctors in America because large integrated practices exist only to provide the best care using criteria developed by physicians" (Reece, *Voices of Health Reform*).

Kaiser continues to move forward with its innovative efforts—with Archimedes, its partnerships with the American Diabetes Association and large pharmaceutical firms, its information technology implementations, its team-based efforts to optimize workflow, its group visit concepts, its national learning networks, its population and case management approaches, and its Thrive media campaigns emphasizing that "Kaiser stands for health." By sticking to its principles of genuine innovation, working hard at them, and building on its strengths of size, Kaiser hopes to prove conclusively that one can improve the health of all Americans.

Case Study 2

Improving Health Care Through Artificial Intelligence

By Charles B. Engle, Jr., PhD

Dr. Charles Engle, 56, known as "Chuck," is director of special projects for MedAI, Inc. He received his BS in computer sciences from Bentley College, his MS in computer sciences from Stanford, and his PhD from Polytechnical University in Brooklyn. He served in Vietnam in Military Intelligence for the army and was a pilot. He taught computer sciences at West Point and Carnegie Mellon and has worked at MedAI, Inc., for five years.

• •

Because this chapter focuses on Kaiser's Archimedes project, for balance I have asked another organization, MedAI, Inc., in Orlando, Florida, to share their experience using artificial intelligence techniques for predictive modeling purposes.

In today's world, it is almost axiomatic health care costs are rising. Anything that can be done to contain the costs of health care without impacting the quality of care must be considered. One such innovation is applying predictive modeling to identify patients who have the greatest opportunity for health care costs savings. What is the best way to apply predictive modeling to health care? MedAI has addressed this problem and created and refined an innovative approach to provide accurate predications.

Predictive modeling is the heart of applying artificial intelligence (AI) to health care. Although the government did not publish specific hospitals' prices in its release, assume that in the future your pricing will be public and be prepared to explain it. Know that the uninsured will be looking closely at what you receive, and they will demand the same. As an unintended consequence, insurers may have more power to come to you and renegotiate.

Advantage and Disadvantage of the AI Model

The advantage of a model is the ability to reduce the complexity of a real-world process to a form understandable to humans; the disadvantage is that this necessarily means that some elements of the real-world process are left out or reduced to their most basic form and are thus not truly indicative of their impact on the real-world process as a whole. Choosing how to reduce the real-world process to a model is both a science and an art form in that the modeler strives to retain the essential properties of the process while eliminating the aspects of the process that contribute little to the final outcome. Fortunately, modeling is well established as a discipline and there are techniques and processes available to create models that are useful for the intended purpose; namely, to represent in a simpler form the complexities of a complex real-world process so that it can be analyzed and controlled.

Several Basic Approaches

There are several basic approaches to creating the model to be used for predictive modeling. The spectrum generally runs from rules-based methods on one extreme to pure AI systems on the other extreme. At MedAI, we have perfected a unique approach to predictive modeling. We call it a *blended technology* process. It is this patent-pending blended technology approach that provides MedAI with a significant advantage over other predictive modeling companies using one of the inferior approaches mentioned here.

Which Is the Best Approach for Predictive Modeling and Why?

Rules-based approaches have been around for some time and have proven to be effective within certain limitations. They incorporate a stable methodology that can be supported and communicated to users and they operate with existing IT information infrastructures. However, these models have two serious limitations: They can do no better than the assumptions that went into their design about which factors have predictive value and they do not adapt to changes in the data without expert intervention.

Regression models should also be mentioned here because they are widely used traditionally for predictive modeling and analytics. Regression models are based on statistic techniques that have been around for hundreds of years. For certain categories of problems, when the data is well understood or when it meets certain predefined patterns, the traditional linear regression techniques are easily applied and sufficiently accurate. They do not provide extremely accurate results and they can be applied in limited instances, but when they can be applied and the accuracy is sufficient, they are relatively inexpensive to use. However, they are extremely sensitive to outlier data and missing data, causing undue overemphasis on these items in creating the predictions. Further, regression models are strictly linear and assume as their fundamental basis that the data is uniformly or normally distributed. When this is not true (when the data is not normally distributed or is nonlinear), these methods are once again widely inaccurate.

Pure AI techniques, such as neural nets, are newer and more sophisticated approaches to predictive modeling with greater flexibility and more adaptive capabilities than rules-based approaches. Pure AI approaches avoid the problems just cited because they are nonlinear and have more flexibility.

This allows them to adapt better to data not normally distributed and not linear yielding more accuracy in the predictions. Published research suggests that AI models are roughly twice as effective as rules-based models in "noisy" data. Although they still suffer from the problem of sensitivity to extreme outliers and missing data, their flexibility helps to account for these problems.

The downside in comparison to regression models is this: Pure AI techniques are also more complex and less well understood by the untrained, unsophisticated consumer. Also, it is easy to over-train the model, therefore, limiting its ability to generalize. However, development cost is a one-time cost so complexity can be justified. The consumer can be educated and trained.

Blended technology (as implemented by MedAI) is considered the combination of traditional linear statistical techniques with nonlinear artificial intelligence techniques. By careful analysis of the problem, automated and semiautonomous techniques can be used to blend different analytical approaches to create a predictive model that has considerably more accuracy than either technique alone with safeguards against over-fitting.[1] Also, the

---

[1]In statistics, overfitting is fitting a statistical model that has too many parameters. An absurd and false model may fit perfectly if the model has enough complexity by comparison to the amount of data available. Overfitting can lead to spurious or incorrect associations. Overfitting is generally recognized to be a violation of Occam's razor.

internal dynamics of the process are considerably more transparent, therefore eliminating the "black box" metaphor. This synergy is the essence of MITCH (Mutltiple Intelligent Tasking Heuristics), the predictive engine in use at MedAI.

So Which Approach Is Better Under Which Conditions?

Table 9–1 *Differences Between Various Artificial Intelligence Models*

	Blended Technology (MedAI)	Artificial Intelligence	Regression Models	Rules-Based
Accuracy	Excellent ●	Good ☽	Satisfactory ◗	Fair ☽
Maintenance/ Cost	Excellent ●	Excellent ●	Excellent ●	Poor ▸
Adaptability	Excellent ●	Good ☽	Satisfactory ◗	Poor ▸
Interpretability	Good ☽	Fair ☽	Good ☽	Excellent ●
Scalability	Excellent ●	Fair ☽	Excellent ●	Excellent ●
Speed of Training	Good ☽	Good ☽	Excellent ●	N/A

Source: Abstract of the United States, 2000–2004.

A few reports comparing the predictive accuracy of different vendors and defining an industry standard for predictive accuracy of high-risk prediction models have been published. These include reports by insurers in the United States relating to predictive modeling, which established both actuarial benchmark accuracies and theoretical maximums (or maximum R^2) for such modeling. In addition, earlier publications sponsored by the Society of Actuaries refer to the R^2 accuracy standard as being in the 0.15–0.20 range (Cumming, Cameron, Derrick, Knutson, 2002).

A 2002 study sponsored by the Society of Actuaries compared results across several predictive modeling vendors. All vendors used traditional rules-based modeling. Using a validation set consisting of 61,580 members from the health plan for Sentara Health Care (based in Norfolk, Virginia), R^2 values were calculated and compared. The highest R^2 value among the systems published in this article is 0.15. Using Sentara data, MedAI obtained an R^2 value of 0.31 using AI modeling. This result was further improved to 0.34 by predicting per member per month (PMPM) charges. We were also able to demonstrate another strength of AI: the ability to effectively use and predict outliers in the model. The true R^2 values reflect this ability and place emphasis on the outliers. While many scientists argue this is a weakness of the R^2 statistic, it should be considered a strength of the R^2 statistic in health care, because the high-cost patients are those that require identification and sophisticated care management approaches.[2]

---

[2]This paragraph adapted with permission from *Predictive Modeling in Health Plans* by Randy Axelrod and David Vogel, 2003.

In summary, MedAI has demonstrated significant success in predictive modeling as applied to the health care domain by creating an innovative technique to blend linear and non-linear statistical techniques and AI specialized for identifying and illuminating relationships among data from a patient data set. Using this advanced capability, MedAI has had unparalleled success in forecasting health care outcomes and the need for services.

Chapter 10

The Mayo Clinic Innovates the Mayo Way: Leaving Nothing to Chance

Prelude: Physician consensus: a powerful force for innovation.

Control of medicine will never again belong completely to physicians. If that is true, physician should decide what parts of the system are important, what parts they want to control in the future.

They should look around to determine where doctors have been particularly successful in working out viable relationships with medicine. A good example of successful accommodation, where physicians have remained in charge of what is important to them, is the Mayo Clinic.

Victor Fuchs, 1982

What's Important to Mayo Physicians

Control? Yes. You think that way when you were founded in a cornfield in rural Minnesota in the late 1880s, and when you've succeeded for 100 years by paying attention to detail. Planning? Yes, you plan meticulously when you have over 2,500 specialists working together with 42,000 employees in three locations. With that employment base, you need to plan. Attention to details? You bet. The Mayo Clinic has succeeded on training themselves and their employees to design everything from buildings, to exam rooms, to dress codes, to demeanors to give patients visual and experiential clues to tell the compelling story of the Mayo Clinic (Berry & Bendapudi, 2003).

A good example of the Mayo Clinic's passion for control, planning, dress, design, and visual imagery is their new SPARC (See, Plan, Act, Refine, and Communicate) laboratory. This laboratory has been developed to see how the Mayo can best improve the patient–doctor interaction by studying room architecture, furniture placement, body language, and the behavior of both patients and doctors.

The idea is to observe how patients interact in waiting areas and exam rooms, and how they work with doctors, nurses, and staff to navigate the health care process. The Mayo team wants to create a basic template for facilitating service delivery innovation: a systematic process that includes how to brainstorm new ideas for using the space, rapidly prototype novel service-delivery designs, and use customer observation and direct feedback to refine solutions.

Innovation, Above All Else

Above all else, however, the Mayo Clinic believes in innovation. It's in the Mayo organization's DNA.

- When Dr. W. W. Mayo founded the clinic as an integrated health care group, built upon by his two sons—still known as Dr. Charlie and Dr. Will—it was innovative.
- When the Mayos put multiple specialists in one building, it was innovative.
- When the Mayo brothers hired Dr. Henry Plummer in the early 1900s to design their buildings, surgical and diagnostic instruments, examining room, record system, and pneumatic tube–powered chart-delivery system, it was innovative.
- When the Mayos developed a research division that culminated in two Mayo researchers, Dr. Edward Kendall and Dr. Philip Hench, sharing the 1950 Nobel Prize for their work on adrenal steroids, it was innovative.
- When the clinic founded Medical Innovations, Inc., in 1965, which has designed, patented, and marketed over 1,000 medical devices, it was innovative.
- When the Mayo took its diagnostic reference laboratories national in the 1970s, it was innovative.
- When the Mayo Clinic collaborated with IBM to expand and refine its IT system over the last 20 years, and then worked with IBM, GE, Siemens, and Philips to build and market a better MRI machine in 8 months, rather than the usual 18 to 24 months, it was innovative.
- When the clinic developed its clinic trials service, it was innovative.

Now the clinic has taken their boldest reform innovation to date. On May 21 through 23, 2006, Mayo hosted a national symposium on health reform. Before the symposium, Mayo CEO Dr. Denis Cortese and Mayo administrative director Robert Smoldt staked out the Mayo position on reform in the April issue of the *Mayo Clinic Proceedings*. Cortese and Smoldt said, among other things, that the health system suffered from lack of quality and safety, the uninsured, public unease, rising costs, misaligned payment incentives, and a looming baby boomer retirement (Cortese & Smoldt, 2006).

To fix the problem, Cortes and Smoldt argued, would require national learning organizations, led by physicians with shared visions, professionalism, IT tools, and systems engineering management. Cortes and Smoldt concluded:

> *To achieve this vision of a new health system for America—one that functions as a vibrant, innovative learning organization—we propose a consumer-driven market-based model that delivers universal coverage to all Americans, a model similar to the Federal Employee Health Benefits Plan (FEHP) or the Universal Health Voucher Plan.* (Cortese & Smoldt, 2006)

Federal Government

They then laid out the roles of physician (committing to the shared vision of learning organizations), patients (making intelligent lifestyle choices, getting involved in their own care, accepting more financial responsibility, insuring themselves and their families), private insurers (committing to measuring performance, covering chronic disease, being patient centered, insuring risk), and the federal government (enabling innovation, coordinating and financing care).

At the symposium, the participants, all national leaders, suggested ways to overcome challenges to reform, to generate momentum toward a sustainable system, to take action steps toward more patient-centered care, to create commitment to improve the social climate, and to identify ways to build collaboration and commitment on health care issues. Various panels at the reform forum focused on reducing health costs, universally sharing scientific knowledge, fixing the safety net, relieving pressure on U.S. businesses, paying for quality performance, and creating a chronic care model that works for everyone.

The consensus among the more than 300 national leaders from all health sectors attending the Mayo symposium was this:

- The public expects major health care reform—soon.
- It is morally imperative all Americans have health insurance.
- The United States already spends more than enough on health care.

To meet these expectations and resolve these problems, the participants made these suggestions (in rank order):

1. Build public and business mandate for national change.
2. Effect transparency among systems and physician practices.
3. Define essential health services for all Americans.
4. Provide results-based reimbursement with a patient component to incentivize plans.

5. Encourage formation of integrated systems.

6. Reward consumers for choosing high-quality plans and providers. (Mayo, Clinic National Symposium, 2006)

Innovation Talking and Action Points

The Mayo Clinic is an example of self-contained and disciplined innovation within a closed organization. Those at the clinic believe its model can be extended to the United States as a whole, but Mayo is in no hurry to do so.

Case Study

Just One Innovation After Another

By Dr. Richard L. Reece

Richard L. Reece, MD, practiced pathology in Minneapolis, Minnesota, from 1965 to 1990 and served as editor-in-chief of *Minnesota Medicine* from 1975 to 1990. During his time in Minnesota, he visited the Mayo Clinic often and formally interviewed Eugene Mayberry, MD, who was CEO of Mayo. (See Reece 1988a.)

• •

Innovation is part of the disciplined Mayo style. If I were to characterize the Mayo approach to innovation, I would call it *internal disciplined innovation*. Innovations at the Mayo bubble up from within through an elaborate committee structure used for consensus decision making.

At any given time, about one third of its medical staff is involved in institutional committees and another third in interdepartmental division committees. Its committees turn over every 2 years, and its administrative appointments turn over every 5 to 10 years, so every Mayo physician at some point is involved in the process.

I did not come up with the phrase *internal disciplined innovation* for Mayo decision making lightly, without testing it out on others. I once suggested to the CEO of a competing Jacksonville hospital that the Mayo's success could be attributed in large measure to its tightly vertically integrated structure. "Yes," the CEO said, "but it is monastic integration." By that he meant that the clinic makes little attempts to horizontally integrate into the surrounding community. It tends to be guarded in talking about its methods at national conferences or sharing its methods to the outside world.

The Mayo has mastered disciplined integration. As a fee-for-service institution in a managed care world and with its three missions of teaching, research, and service, it feels it has to be disciplined.

Here are the results of previous interviews with two former Mayo Clinic CEOs: Eugene Mayberry and Robert Waller.

Dr. Eugene Mayberry

This information is based on an interview that took place in 1987 (Reece, 1988b):

In the mid to late eighties, the Mayo Clinic was busy establishing its new sites in Jacksonville, Florida, and Scottsdale, Arizona. These innovative moves occurred because the Mayo's patient base in the upper Midwest was threatened by the managed care explosion in the Twin Cities, the traditional source of nearly half its patients. Minneapolis–St. Paul HMOs were keeping their members in network and the Mayo was not part of that network.

Prospective payment methods and HMOs did not favor the Mayo, a fee-for-service institution. Mayo had its own fee schedule, which did not jibe with HMO fee schedules. Mayo did receive payment on the basis of capitation, a fixed monthly payment per member per month, and therefore was excluded from HMOs with capitated plans. So it sought to grow in the Sun Belt, with its more favorable fee-for-service environment.

The Mayo also was diversifying nationally through its laboratory network, the *Mayo Clinic Health Letter,* Mayo Medical Ventures and other joint ventures, and money-making ventures to support its programs for education and research.

The Mayo prides itself on its efficiencies: its identical examining rooms, its instant communications systems linking its three sites, its records systems, and its emphasis on outpatient surgery, its intimate referral system, and its low hospitalization rates.

The Mayo considers itself very much a fee-for-service business. It is not enthusiastic about accepting nonpaying or low-paying patients. This is hard to do, as Mayo learned several years ago when it elected to stop seeing Medicare patients in Jacksonville. Most of these patients simply stopped coming to the Mayo. The Mayo has been criticized for this attention to the dollar, but says it has bottom lines to meet to support its research, teaching, and innovation programs.

Dr. Robert Waller

This interview was with Robert R. Waller in 1998, then the chief executive at the Mayo. He was, at the time, infuriated with Medicare's declining reimbursements, its fraud investigations, and its 45,000 pages of paperwork. He had this to say:

> Our basic operating strategies are twofold. One is to do our best to remain committed to the principle that the clinical practice of medicine must sustain itself fiscally. With the constant pressure on reimbursement, we must work very hard to keep this commitment. The dollars that used to flow from the practice of medicine to fund education and research no longer do so at the levels they did in the past.
>
> Therefore, we must find other ways to fund them because we believe such programs are essential if we are to improve continuously. To sustain those programs, we compete vigorously for extramural grants and contracts, and we are expanding our fundraising efforts. Mayo Medical Ventures, an entity within Mayo that provides health information for the public, among other activities, generates revenue to help fund research, education, and clinical innovation.
>
> We have an office that focuses on forging strategic alliances with industry. Mayo Medical Laboratories generates revenue for our academic missions by providing reference laboratory services to worldwide markets.
>
> So, our first operating strategy is to try to make the practice sustain itself financially as best we can in a world of declining reimbursement. And then we must find alternative sources of revenue to fund the programs in research and education without which we would not be what we want to be.

> Our second operating strategy is to support the "mixed model" of medical practice. By that I mean we care for fee-for-service patients, patients who have no sources of income, patients from international locations, and the ones who come to us through our own health plans. We also have a direct contract without an insurance intermediary. In addition, we accept patients sent to us from several hundred managed care plans throughout the country. Caring for patients through whatever mechanisms they may choose to come to any Mayo practice is what we mean by the mixed model of practice. (Reece, 1998)

Note the emphasis on Mayo's fee-for-service model and the need to innovate to produce nontraditional sources of revenue to make up for declining reimbursements. Mayo has never believed in capitation models or in HMO-directed managed care, and obviously feels it should be trusted to do the right things for the right reasons without intermediaries dictating what it should do.

Mayo sees itself as a model for efficient care and for innovative leadership in a changing world. A study by researchers at the Dartmouth Medical School's Center for Evaluative Clinical Sciences noted that the Mayo used fewer than nine physicians per 1,000 patients on average to treat patients during the last 6 months of life; in contrast, New York University Medical Center used 28.3 physicians per 1,000 patients (Goodman, Stukel, Chang, & Wennberg, 2006).

To maintain its reputation for efficiency, the Mayo is not only taking a leadership position on health reform but is revising its medical school curriculum to produce future physician leaders. Instead of starting medical students with a week of orientation, the Mayo medical school now has an introductory course for new students consisting of a 3-week session on leadership.

Mayo medical school leaders know young doctors can no longer expect to go into solo or small practices; instead, they will practice as members of interdisciplinary teams. They will have to learn to work within systems that demand real-time current information; safe, effective care backed by evidence; malpractice-avoidance strategies; finding help for patients without insurance; and working with corporate executives to help make clinical decisions. Reaching those goals will take forward-thinking and high-order innovation.

Part Three

Hospital– Physician Joint Venture Innovations

The health care community is entering a new era of partnering as physicians and hospitals continue to search for the right balance in ownership or participation in health care facilities, service lines, and ancillary revenue income streams. The scene has changed dramatically, however, from the surge of mergers and acquisitions in the last decade. Not only have market conditions changed, but new models have emerged in physician hospital transactions and ventures.

Healthcare Financial Management Association, 2005

Chapter 11

From Hospital to Physician: Integrated Facilities

Prelude: Two big questions for hospitals and doctors are: Integration or disintegration? Unified vision or separate divisions? One answer: Join together as equity partners in a large ambulatory care center, a 50,000- to 250,000-square-foot facility, known as a "Big Box."

While ambulatory services typically compose the minority share of the revenues of the larger hospital and health systems, their revenue and growth potential are explosive by comparison to inpatient services.

For certain physician specialties, ambulatory services are their future, plain and simple; for a number of clinical specialties, ambulatory services are the lion's share of their business (e.g., gastroenterology, orthopedics, radiology, ophthalmology, ENT, and others).

These are the obvious. The not-so-obvious is the growing ambulatory service potential for clinical specialties that have historically been inpatient focused, such as cardiology, oncology, and certain sub-specialty surgical services.

Daniel K. Zismer, 2003

The "Big Box" Approach to Specialty Care

A Big Box ambulatory center, which at this stage is a concept rather than a reality, is a 50,000- to 250,000-square-foot outpatient clinical-service site aggregating, consolidating, coordinating, and showcasing specialty-based, diagnostic, interventional, consultative, and rehabilitative outpatient services. A Big Box is strategically and financially focused, achieving its goals through delivering superior clinical outcomes wrapped in an exceptional patient experience.

Big Box centers may be physician owned, health system owned, or structured as a health system and physician partnership (more on the partnership designs and potential later in this section). A well-run Big Box is a high-revenue-per-square-foot strategy, producing return on capital rates at the high end.

Although there may be multiple partners in the Box, the design and management of the clinical service array are seamless to the customer. The strategy is branded and aggressively promoted as a "destination strategy" for superior, high-value specialty care.

What's a destination strategy? An ambulatory health service destination strategy succeeds when target markets (patients) identify as much with the location as their physician (e.g., "I'm going to Great Falls Clinic Specialty Center for my cancer care—my doctor works there").

To the patient/customer, the Big Box is a seamless system of specialty-services delivery; it is not simply a "box" of independent physicians sharing space under one roof. Patients move efficiently from initial consultation to diagnostic imaging to outpatient, invasive therapeutic procedures and surgeries, and to rehabilitation services and follow-up care as necessary, all without accessing a traditional hospital environment.

A Remarkable Series of Newsletters

From 2002 to 2004, Daniel K. Zismer and associates at Dorsey Health Strategies in Minneapolis, Minnesota, published a series of remarkable articles in the *Discovery Dorsey Health Strategies Newsletters*. These newsletter articles called for new thinking by hospital boards and CEOs in not-for-profit hospitals on relationships with specialists.

Zismer said specialists contributing the most to hospital bottom lines were being driven by downward economic pressures—so much so that physicians were disengaging and cutting the umbilical cord linking them to "mother" hospitals. Like Humpty Dumpty, if these specialists fell off the wall, it might be impossible to put the hospital–doctor complex back together again.

Zismer claimed markets had shifted from centralized hospitals to specialist-managed facilities: "Just as not-for-profit community hospital boards stop reeling from slings and arrows of managed care, break-neck consolidation, primary care acquisitions and physician practice management companies debacles of the 1990s, along comes risks of losing loyalties of key physician specialties who fuel more profitable lines of business for most community hospitals," Zismer said (Zismer, 2003b).

When he and his associates wrote the newsletters, he was in Minneapolis, working for Dorsey Health Strategies. In 2005, he moved to Duluth, where he works with Essentia, a consolidated hospital organization preaching and practicing hospital–physician integration.

Ironically, Minnesota is an odd place to be warning about looming hospital–physician disintegration. It is unlikely the Minnesota hospital–physician industrial complex will ever fall completely apart. Based on 25 years in practice in Minnesota, I know the state has an enlightened and constructive approach toward hospital–physician collaboration. Minnesota is a collaborative, consensus-oriented place. As an example, health plans, physician groups, and hospitals joined together in 1993 to form the Institute of Clinical Systems Improvement (ICSI). ICSI facilitates collaboration on health care quality improvement. Today ICSI has 56 group members and is funded by all six Minnesota health plans. The combined medical groups and hospital systems represent more than 7,600 physicians, average 136 physicians in each group, and cover more than two thirds of Minnesota's citizens.

Coalescence Around Common Goals

Of the Minnesota health care establishment's penchant for coalescence around common goals, Dr. William Gold, chief medical officer and vice president of Blue Cross Blue Shield of Minnesota, says:

> *We're problem solvers. We talk to each other. There's a level of trust and openness and a tremendous number of really good thinkers and committed people. We're able to do things other states or other regions think about but very few can pull off.* (Reece, 2005c)

Perhaps the most passionate advocate of Minnesota and its gift for collaboration and constructive corporate teamwork is William Ouchi, professor in the graduate school of management at the University of California in Los Angeles and an international consultant to several *Fortune* 500 companies.

In pointing out the cooperative nature of Minnesota society, Ouchi says of Minneapolis, the hub of the Minnesota business community,

> *It is not a monolith or a centrally directed hierarchy, nor is it a completely atomized amalgam of disconnected actors. It is a city with strong tradition of populism, the home of many socialist movements. It is not a place of do-gooders or altruists but of realistic, self-interested individuals within an institutional network that constrains each person slightly, so that no one can achieve his or her goals by interfering with others. There is, rather, a stable pattern of repeated exchanges over many years that make social choice and collective action possible.* (Ouchi, 1984)

Even in the face of the clannishness of Minnesota's medical establishment or perhaps "corporative-ness," hospital–specialist relationships are strained, even disintegrating.

Specialists' unrest stems from economic pressures and low personal productivity in community hospital settings. Surgeons grow restless and unhappy when they have to wait when an operating room is being "turned around" to accommodate a different type of specialty procedure—neither are they pleased when they learn facilities fees exceed surgical fees.

The Rise of Out-of-Hospital Ambulatory Surgical Centers

This strain between hospitals and specialists is occurring elsewhere in the United States. Over the last 25 years, nearly 4,300 ambulatory surgery centers have sprung up. About 90 percent of these are physician owned, with the other 10 percent being owned by hospitals or corporations, such as HCA. Physicians also own about 100 doctor-owned specialty hospitals (Federated Ambulatory Surgery Association, 2006). Specialists are bailing out of hospitals to found, manage, and own their own facilities.

As one former hospital administrator wryly observed to me, "Old hospital administrators never die, they just lose their facilities" (Coombes, David, Personal Communication, 2006). Dr. Chris Smith, president of the Georgia Association of General Surgeons, asserts there are good reasons for doctors owning their own ambulatory facilities: Ambulatory surgery centers charge 40 percent or less of what hospitals charge with better convenience to patients and to surgeons, and they operate more efficiently" (Reece, 2006a).

Piggybacking Around Specialty Hospital Moratorium

In December 2003, President Bush, pressured by the American Hospital Association and other hospital lobbying groups, imposed an 18-month moratorium on new specialty hospitals. This moratorium and certificate-of-need laws in many states have effectively blocked new specialty hospital construction. However, in 2006, the moratorium ended. Given the entrepreneurial instincts of specialists and the desires of hospitals to be affiliated with specialist-driven centers of excellence, it is only a matter of time before ways around the moratorium will begin to surface.

In Nashville, a group of entrepreneurial neurosurgeons struck a deal "piggybacking" an 18-bed specialty hospital, featuring six operating rooms doing 250 procedures a month, upon St. Thomas Hospital's 683-bed hospital. Molly Guterriez of the American Surgical Hospital Association, the specialty hospital trade group, said of the deal, it was the "correct model" for creative physician ownership through cooperation with a local hospital, of a specialty hospital (Pack, 2006c). It was also a creative example of physician–hospital joint innovation.

To say hospital CEOs and their boards resist joint ventures with doctors understates the case. Hospital executives and their boards reluctantly share revenues and responsibilities with physician upstarts.

Why share revenues when you have always been king of the financial hill? The answer is: Times, they are a'changing—and changing fast. It will no longer be possible for hospitals to control and own most facilities and collect the bulk reimbursement, such as facility fees. These fees usually exceed the surgeons' fees for the procedure itself.

Bundled bills are the combining of hospital and physician charges with hospital components averaging more than 80 percent of the bundled bill (Coombs). The 80/20 hospital/physician fee ratio may not be acceptable for specialists and their business advisors in the new competitive environment. Specialist owners will continue to seek more of the action.

As technology renders complex procedures simpler and as care moves to the outpatient arena, hospitals will have to be open to partnering with physicians or risk facing open adversarial competition from orthopedic, cardiac, and neurosurgical groups. CEOs will have to initiate confidential strategic discussions with specialty leaders and board members to pull off mutually profitable ventures or risk losing lucrative specialty business.

Innovation Talking and Action Points

This chapter features three fundamental innovations taking place between hospitals and physicians:

1. Partnership to adjust to how consumers are buying and using health care
2. New technologies facilitating shifting to an outpatient environment
3. New business models

These innovations are discussed in the case study that follows this chapter.

Hospital CEOs and their boards need to recognize the competitive environment is shifting fast toward specialty-based outpatient practices. The CEO must move quickly to cultivate those specialists who contribute most to the hospital's bottom line and engage them in discussions about win-win partnerships.

An example of where win-win hospital relationships might lead is the "smart hospital," a concept now being developed and implemented by Health Care Management Directions (HCMD) in Nashville, Tennessee. HCMD dedicates itself to developing and managing technologically advanced acute-care hospitals, which it calls "smart hospitals," in the 40- to 60-bed range, using advanced information technologies and designed for greater efficiency, increased patient safety, and superior customer service.

These hospitals function best as facilities affiliated with and as extensions of an existing health care system. Philosophically, Health Care Management Directions believes physicians need to be an integral component of the smart hospital through management participation and facility ownership, or as joint venture partnerships with hospitals and physicians. Health Care Management Directions envisions itself as a minority or majority owner, depending on the wishes of equity partners, or as a consultant, for third-party owners, providing management expertise.

Dr. Kenneth Kizer, a former Navy diver, emergency room physician, and California health official, became the Veteran Administration's undersecretary of health in 1994. Dr. Kizer's *Vision for Change: A Plan to Restructure the Veteran's Health Administration* (1995) is a blueprint for the transition from hospital- to community-based systems. His vision includes, among other things:

- For the hospital to remain an important, less central, part of a larger, more coordinated community network of care
- For the hospital to be restructured around substantive clinical functions and product lines, rather than around specialties
- For the hospital buildings themselves to no longer be the central point of patient services
- For patient care decision making to be carried out as close to the patient as possible
- For the operating framework to be an aggregate of agreements and protocols and the information systems that monitor patient flow

Case Study

Big Box Ambulatory Health Centers Strategies
By Dr. Daniel Zismer

Daniel K. Zismer, PhD, is executive vice president of Essentia Health and CEO of the SMDC Health System. Essentia Health is a multistate health system focused on integrated health care, rural regional health care, and long-term care in eight states. SMDC integrates 390 physicians with four hospitals serving the northeastern regions of Minnesota and northwestern Wisconsin.

What's in the Box?

Clinical services aggregated in the Big Box tend toward diagnostic, invasive, surgical, and rehabilitative specialties, including imaging services, ambulatory surgery, endoscopy, and other therapeutics requiring more complex and invasive diagnostics and related ancillary support services (e.g., laboratory, professional support, restorative therapies, and specialty-focused physician consultative support).

Primary care is included, but the primary care specialties available typically have high referral potential to other services in the Box (e.g., internal medicine, OB/GYN, specialized pediatrics, and urgent care). Retail products and services may be available as well; pharmacy, optical, and cosmetic adjuncts if such services as plastic and cosmetic surgery and therapeutic oncology are available in the Box.

Expansive thinking could lead owners to such services as sports medicine and sports urgent care, specialized athletic training, fitness facilities, and health education. Builders of these centers have included community gathering spaces to encourage nonmedical use; in other words, a community destination gatherer. If more complex surgical services are offered, 23-hour beds may be included depending upon state-regulated licensing requirements.

Looking Beyond the Obvious in Business Strategy of the Big Box

When floor planning the Big Box, there are the obvious and the not-so-obvious opportunities for strategic aggregation. The obvious are services that, on the surface, have overt clinical affinities, one for the other, such as orthopedic surgery and imaging services. There are the not-so-obvious opportunities as well; those that apparently have little clinical affinities such as orthopedics and cardiology. Put both in a Big Box ambulatory center and the business affinities emerge; in the case of orthopedics and cardiology, the business affinities are imaging diagnostics (cardiology is quickly becoming an imaging-based specialty), invasive procedures, rehabilitative services, and physical training, conditioning, and laboratory diagnostics.

Physicians will sometimes see the Big Box business affinities potential before health system executives. This leads to a divergence of interests; for example, a group of specialists goes off on their own to do a Big Box center.

What Is the Financial Productivity Potential of the Big Box?

The financial productivity potential of the Big Box ambulatory center varies according to the collection of services inside the Box. Financial return goals vary as well according to the interests of those who own and occupy the Box. Capitalization costs also vary as a function of the contents of the Big Box and overall design, fit, and finishes. If asked to "ballpark" the net revenue potential, per square foot, the potential can range from $300 to $700, per "usable" square foot. Costs related to capital (facilities, all technologies, furniture, fixtures, and equipment) will generally come in at $275 to $350 per square foot (land costs not included). In other words, a Big Box would cost $265 to $350 per square foot to build but would have potential revenues of up to $700 per square foot. As a general rule of thumb, capital costs of the assets in the Box typically approximate 25 percent of the cost of the Big Box itself, assuming reasonable scale.

Contribution margins can approach 30 percent to 36 percent on specific specialty services in the Big Box, and in the aggregate. Financial returns are modulated by the strategy and service mix and management effectiveness inside the Big Box.

Who Should Own the Facility?

Here, *facility* is defined as the physical structure—the building and the land. A number of larger, well-capitalized health systems have concluded that application of balance sheet capacity to the ownership of land and facilities is not a prudent choice. Moreover, if a hospital (or health system) anticipates partnerships with physicians, the risks associated with being both a partner and landlord can be high. Consequently, specialized real estate developers are frequently brought to the table. Why?

- To provide well-managed, experienced turnkey development
- To assume all or a portion of the financed risk associated with the project
- To involve physicians in ownership (either with or without the hospital as a partner)
- To manage the physician mix in the facility (often too politically "charged" for the hospital to manage)

Ownership of a facility may be syndicated to tenant physicians and referring physicians. Models exist where primary care physicians, who refer to tenant specialists, may own portions of the building, housing the referral specialists. Primary care patients who refer patients may have partial ownership. Lease rates are variable, but must stand fair market tests. Certain ownership models allow physicians to earn equity over time based upon the length of their lease commitment.

What About Primary Care Physicians?

Although the principal focus of this section is the Big Box ambulatory center as a vehicle for specialty physicians, primary care physicians need not be left out. As earlier noted, primary care physicians located in the Box were positioned as important value drivers. They may participate variously in the value they create. Experience would include primary care physicians with the Big Box strategy in one of several integrative models:

- Health systems would be interested in placing their salaried primary care physicians in Big Boxes to attract patients who might then be referred to the hospital.
- As investors in the real estate: Primary care physicians in independent practice may be attracted as passive investors in the facility even if their practice is not housed in the facility.
- "In-office exception" opportunities: Physicians and hospital–physician partnerships that share the same street address and, otherwise, comply with the in-office exceptions and related rules may pursue joint ownership of colocated licensed providers (e.g., an ambulatory surgery center) and/or services provider companies (e.g., imaging or diagnostic services companies) that serve the occupants of the Big Box. The range of partnership options, in this region, is impressive. Specific legal and regulatory requirements apply.

On Campus or Off Campus?

Here the term *campus* refers to a Big Box located on hospital grounds or placed elsewhere. Either can work; it depends upon the goals. On-campus Big Box–centered strategies apply when specialists want the advantages of the strategic and financial returns of the Big Box while maintaining close proximity to a high-tech hospital.

Off-campus Big Box–centered strategies apply when partners agree that other geographies hold greater promise. Some health systems develop both. If a Big Box is placed on campus and is attached to the hospital or otherwise shares the same street address, the opportunities for hospital–physician joint ventures are further enhanced (e.g., application of "underarrangements" relationships).

Making the Big Box Work: Engineering Success in Advance

Big Box ambulatory centers work as high-revenue/high-margin-per-square-foot enterprises if the vision is engineered in advance to meet financial goals.

- Superior patient experience
- Superior provider experience
- Superior revenue production on the fixed asset base
- Superior operating cost efficiencies
- Attractive overall return on capital and the potential of the provider/owners

Effective engineering of the building design cannot be done after the ribbon cutting. By then the potential of the facility is literally set in stone. The potential for optimal design is lost forever. Application of appropriate lean-design methods and models should be "baked" into the design. If the prospective owners think like Toyota, the company that created the concept of the "lean" corporation, a corporation designed for maximum efficiency through work flow design, five goals would apply:

1. Optimize patient flow and diagnostic and procedural throughput.
2. Optimize capital-intensive physical space (e.g., high-cost "production lines").
3. Minimize customer "pain points" (e.g., delays, unnecessary wait points, unavailable information, etc.).
4. Eliminate waste and rework.
5. Optimize the productivity of all staff (e.g., especially high-skill/high-cost staff).

Effective application of lean manufacturing methods and up-front models produce, among other useful tools, a value-stream map. A value-stream map is created from a collaboration of experts in lean manufacturing techniques working collaboratively with users and designers of the facility.

What Is the Psychology at Play?

Jaded health system executives who observe physician specialists pursuing Big Box strategies independently snap to judgment: "It's all about the money—it's greed."

Physicians who have pursued Big Box strategies independently often tell a different story: "Sure financial returns matter, but it is also important to claim some measure of control over our futures: the care we provide and the clinical and patient experience we deliver daily. The hospital folks often forget we accepted substantial financial risk to strike out on such a path. It's not all about the money." Once the risk is taken, physicians will work tirelessly to make the strategy work. There is no shortage of outside talent, experience, and sources of capital ready to help.

To accept the big picture, all parties participating in the Big Box would have to understand its value as a destination for consumers who want to see specialists.

1. More, not less, clinical service will move to the outpatient setting.
2. Patients prefer the convenience, accessibility, and amenities of well-done Big Box centers. Why? Principally because they're not hospitals.
3. Physicians who are owners care more—about performance, the experience, operations, operating costs, and initial and future capital investments.
4. Pressures on capital investment return rates demand scale, economies, and synergies; the future doesn't favor multiple, small, specialty centers operating inefficiently; more "Big Box" centers are likely.
5. It's relatively easy to successfully create and promote a Big Box brand in target markets.
6. Infrastructure costs are scaleable (e.g., common electronic health record, other information technologies, concierge service, common space, etc.).
7. Capital risk is shared, including with third-party facility and technology providers.
8. They can be located strategically, even in competitors' backyards.
9. If the ownership structure is well designed, partners can come and go efficiently.
10. If a hospital is a partner, the spin-off business potential is pursued at a profit; in other words, the Box makes money and profitable patients are referred.

Engaging the Specialists as a "Smart" Health System Strategy

This case study argues for hospitals and hospital-based health systems to aggressively engage select medical specialties as integrated health system partners. *Integrated* is defined here as levels of partnership that bind one party to the other over the longer term by methods that align: roles/responsibilities, accountabilities, and incentives toward the highest levels of "system" performance—clinical quality, patient experience, and market, financial, and economic performance.

The Rationale for the Engagement of the Specialties Now

In the early to mid-1990s, hospital-centric health system strategy was all about the ownership of primary care physicians by hospitals. The strategic theory was based upon predictions of future capitated health care delivery markets that failed to materialize:

- All systems would be paid by way of global capitation contracts; primary care physicians would control the downstream flow of dollars to the specialists.
- Primary care physicians will be the control point for health services consumption rates and use patterns.
- Unnecessary variation in clinical practice patterns and, thereby, costs will be moderated and managed at the specialty levels by primary care physician interventions and oversight.

Consequently, health system strategists believed that to control primary care was of principal importance; the specialists could remain in "free orbit" around the larger "planetary bodies" composed of hospitals and employed primary care physicians.

The specialists would be dependent upon the "downstream" referral of covered lives controlled by these partially integrated systems of health care delivery. Full integration was not necessary. Employment of primary care physicians was sufficient.

It didn't work. Why not? Two reasons:

- *Reason 1*: The theorists wrongly assumed that because patients have primary care physicians, primary care physicians largely control the supply-and-demand curves associated with downstream specialty-services consumption rates.
- *Reason 2*: The specialists are dependent upon these half-integrated systems of care; that is to say they (the specialists) are bereft of strategic and business model reconfiguration potential on their own, rather they will take what hospitals and integrated primary care physicians give them.

The lesson learned (by most) was that absent strategies to engage the specialists as long-term participants in organized, integrated clinical care delivery models, hospitals risk the loss of business through reorganized, specialty-focused business strategies.

Examples in this regard abound: cardiologists, cardiovascular surgeons, vascular surgeons, interventional radiologists, and intensivists join to form a free-standing heart hospital; 40+ gastroenterologists merge and establish free-standing GI labs and imaging centers; specialty-focused, multispecialty "Big Box" ambulatory centers form including outpatient surgery, imaging, and rehabilitation services.

The picture is clear. While primary care physicians serve panels of patients, specialists greatly influence the directional flow of more marginable medical services and, to a greater extent, control the direct-cost structure of the hospital-based care delivery manufacturing processes and ambulatory service processes. As hospitalists and intensivists take control of the U.S. hospitals' inpatient environments, the direct influence of primary care on medical services cost structures lessens further.

This lessening of the influence of primary care physicians over the economics of care should not be confused with being of less importance to patients and patient care, however. Primary care physicians in integrated health systems will continue to play an important role in the overall management of disease as well as patients' access and movement through the continuum of care. Primary care physicians remain important but, perhaps, for reasons other than were envisioned during the early hospital and primary care physician consolidation phases in the market.

What Are the Smart Specialty-Focused Business Models?

Before pursuing presentation of a specialty-focused partnership case study, it's useful to re-visit "the why"; the why is:

- A handful of specialties control (at least influence) a significant portion of health system (and hospital) revenues.
- The practice patterns of specialty physicians strongly influence financial margins and return on capital performance.
- Larger organized groups of specialty physicians can, with relative ease, export profitable revenues from hospitals to facilities and business entities they own.

The U.S. health care provider system, especially the not-for-profit sector, will see more, not less, consolidation and integration of hospitals and physicians, especially the integration of specialties for all the reasons cited previously.

The End Game

The end game is fully integrated health care with the phrase *fully integrated* defined as all providers (hospital and physicians) working for and within a unified business model. Until the end game is achieved, we'll see hospitals and health systems become portfolios of deals—aggregations of a number of partnership models. The information that follows represents the opportunity for several under one roof.

An Urban Health System Strategy

A large, multisite, urban health system establishes a two-pronged strategy: secure new specialty-services markets in a lucrative, growing segment of a competitor's backyard and secure the longer-term loyalties of high-profile and high-quality physician specialists.

The health system is already well on its way with the employment of primary care physicians located at multiple strategically placed sites. Hospital-based specialty "marquis" programs were prominent as well: heart and vascular, bone and joint, neurological and neurovascular, cancer care, and women's services. Specialists associated with these centers of excellence are largely independent and vulnerable to become competitors of the health system or employees of competing health systems.

The next strategy on the way to a more fully integrated health system is a Big Box ambulatory center; a 150,000-square-foot outpatient specialty center branded with the health system's name and reputation; a visible, high-profile, outpatient strategy—a highly visible market attractor. The strategy is as follows:

(a) Pursue competitive strategies on their own or in partnership with other specialists, or

(b) Align with a competing health system; vulnerable relationships as just cited.

In as much as the independent specialists had no interest in employment (at least not initially), the preferred strategy became the Big Box outpatient or ambulatory center. The clinical care and market goals are:

- A highly visible, integrated center attracting patients to a comprehensive set of specialty-focused diagnostic and therapeutic services delivered from an integrated, "seamless" ambulatory delivery platform
- A simple, but effective method to lawfully integrate operating economics and capital risk while aligning incentives toward market and financial goals
- An integrated clinical care platform operating on a single, unified electronic health record and related support systems to provide a superior ambulatory patient experience
- Targeting specific specialty services markets for movement from the competition's geographic marketplace to the partnership (ambulatory center) with efficiency

Chapter 12

Making Rooms for Boomers

Prelude: Rumors that making rooms for baby boomers will dictate how hospitals are built may be true.

Convenience of care and perceived amenities make up an important dimension of care, and measures of these items can reflect individual patients' preferences in technology, people, facilities, and coordination behaviors.

Regina Herzlinger (Professor of Business Adminstration at Harvard Business School) has stated that there are two market segments of new consumers: Those who want convenience and those who demand more information. Today's hard-working patients lead busy lives. They demand and deserve convenient and comfortable access to medical services. One could argue that technological advances in minimally invasive surgery were spurred by these demands.

Jon A. Cilingerian, 2004

Hospital Building Boom

The greatest hospital building boom in 50 years is under way in the United States. The boom anticipates growing baby boomer hospitalizations.

- The building boom has generated $100 billion since 2000. It may surge another $100 billion by 2009. (Cannon & Appleby, 2006)
- The building boom is replacing old facilities and constructing new hospitals in suburbs. (Cannon & Appleby, 2006)
- The building boom concentrates on medical technologies for boomers. (Cannon & Appleby, 2006)

- The building boom supplants wards with private beds. (Cannon & Appleby, 2006)
- The building boom is rapidly expanding in major metropolitan markets. (Galewitz, 2005)

Everything from outdated facilities to an aging population fuels new hospital building construction. "We're in the middle of the most significant period of hospital reconstruction and expansion in the past 50 years," says Rick Wade, senior vice president of the American Hospital Association. Earl Swensson, ESA, a Nashville, Tennessee, architectural firm, designed a record number of hospitals in 2005. The associates in the Swensson firm expect business will soon spike 10 percent to 15 percent.

Detached Facilities

New facilities are often detached facilities removed from main hospital campuses. These detached facilities contain operating suites, imaging centers, laboratories, pharmacies, physical therapy units, and diagnostic centers. Many of these facilities are going up in suburbs, where paying consumers live and play. The new facilities offer ample parking lots with free parking, spacious reception areas, one-stop medical shopping, and easy access by Internet, telephone, and walk-in traffic.

Making room for baby boomers is mainly about two things: (1) hospitals planning and (2) hospitals building to attract a huge new generation of aging patients and implanting new technologies into new facilities to keep pace in the medical arms race. Hospitals and specialists are planning how to accommodate the rising gorge of aging baby boomers and their children. Members of these generations will want convenience, access, amenities, proof of value in terms of cost and quality, and a "healing environment." Hospitals and specialists alike will have to develop databases and Web sites to demonstrate to information-hungry consumers they are qualified to play the quality game.

Hospital CEOs and their boards should recognize specialists are ready and prepared to go it alone. Hospitals should do whatever is necessary to placate these specialists. Although these specialists may be "lone rangers," they can move with incredible speed when motivated or threatened.

New, innovative hospital design and hospital cultures will appeal to future health care consumers, be they baby boomers, echo boomers, or those of generation X. Innovative hospital designs fall into these design paradigms that overlap in many instances.

- **Hospitals designed for safety.** The 1999 Institute of Medicine report *To Err Is Human* reported 44,000 to 98,000 patients died needlessly in hospitals. Since then, the hospital industry has been focusing on designing safer hospitals. New designs include one-bed hospital rooms, better lighting, rounding sharp corners off all objects in hospital rooms, installing no-slip floors, making all walls sound proof, and placing handwashing basins in every room (Naik, 2006). The Center for Health Design, an advocacy group, says its main purpose is to provide "researched and documented examples of health care facilities whose design has made a difference in the quality of care." The group has identified at least 35 health organizations building such new facilities.

- **Hospitals designed for rapid information transfer.** Lack of speed of information transfer leads to many hospital errors. Closing the time gap between the writing of an order and the carrying out of that order, the transfer of medical records from a doctor's office to the hospital administrator's office, and even the transmission of data from the operating room to the recovery room, can improve care substantially.

  In future hospital design, expect to see information kiosks in every hospital room for both patient and hospital staff use. Hospitals are already vying for the honors of being one of the country's "most wired hospitals," for being innovators in digital imaging and information management, and for setting up community-wide information systems linking hospitals and doctors' offices.

- **Hospitals designed to create a culture of caring and healing.** This is rapidly becoming a big deal among hospitals that want to be viewed as patient-centered, patient-caring institutions, filled with the touches of home that foster healing. New designs will include spacious receptive atriums, colorful decorating schemes, pastoral paintings on walls, entertainment and information centers, roof-top gardens, plants in the room, gourmet menus, and beds for relatives—even quarters for favorite pets.

  Dr. Leland Kaiser, a professor of business at the University of Colorado in Denver, often addresses hospital and physician audiences as the "architects of the future" and says the 21st century will be looked back upon as the "century of design" in shaping a new environment for patients.

  One of the leaders in this approach of designing hospitals to create a holistic patient environment is the Planetree hospital system. This system originated in San Francisco in 1978 and now has 20 affiliated hospitals. Planetree is a nonprofit holistic system "dedicated to personalizing and demystifying the hospital experience and creating patient-centered care in healing environments." The Planetree model empowers patients and families through information and education and encourages healing partnerships with caregivers. Planetree's holistic approach encompasses healing in all dimensions to satisfy and pamper high-end patients. Other hospitals are becoming known as "luxury hospitals" (Japenga, 2000), because they offer patients luxury accommodations similar to those found in five-star hotels (Pallanto, 2006).

- **Hospitals designed for convenience.** Designs for these hospitals will include such cherished consumer conveniences as ample free parking; electronic check-in sites; Web sites featuring medical staff backgrounds, nurse/patient ratios, and outcomes for major procedures; detached centers of excellence; and one-stop shopping for doctors, lab tests, X-rays, imaging studies, and retail sites for 24/7 care manned by hospital-employed nurse practitioners.

Another development is the emergence of patient-focused hospitals. In these hospitals, everything is designed from the patient's point of view. However, this development is nothing new. From its inception, the Mayo Clinic has designed its buildings, its examining rooms, its reception areas, and its physician–patient encounters with the patient's view in mind.

Case Study

Right Rooms for Boomers for Right Reasons
By Dick Miller, FAIA, President of Earl Swensson Associates, Inc., Nashville, Tennessee

Dick Miller is a veteran architect, author, and president of Earl Swensson Associates, a premier architectural firm in Nashville. Besides hospitals, his firm designs commercial buildings and such structures as the Opryland Hotel in Nashville, which is known for its lush, beautiful, and expansive indoor gardens.

• •

Many major innovations fulfill a demographic need. Here Dick Miller describes how the country's architects are doing this by designing new hospitals to replace old facilities, to build new ones to accommodate aging baby boomers, and to meet the new demands imposed by rapidly changing technologies.

Boomers Can't Be Separated from the Boom

A number of factors continue to drive the hospital building boom. Some of these include the need to:

- replace or renovate 30- to 50-year-old hospitals that were constructed under the Hill-Burton program
- accommodate technological advances
- create improved operational efficiencies
- accommodate a focus on outpatient procedures
- create more healing, hospitable environments that lead to patient satisfaction

Boomers: More Discerning and Demanding

A significant force behind the current building boom is baby boomers who are more discerning and demanding than previous generations. Key trends stemming from a need to satisfy this group of health care consumers, speed positive outcomes and healing times, and also create staffing efficiencies in view of the nursing shortage are:

- Increased patient privacy

- Attention to logistics of illness
- Attention to patient safety
- More accommodation of family members
- Improved way finding
- More attention to patient-friendly interior design
- Efficient layouts that minimize staffing requirements

Toward More Hospitable Hospitals

For more than a decade, as patients become more attuned to exerting their preferences in consumer selection of health care facilities for their needs, design of these facilities has reflected a swing toward an obvious hospitality influence to capture market shares.

Functionalities more associated with the hotel industry are now finding a natural translation into the medical setting—much of it being made possible through available technology. In an almost chicken-or-the-egg scenario, it becomes difficult to define whether technology is allowing the efficiencies of the hospitality industry to adapt to medical settings or if the need for increased patient satisfaction and comfort is driving the development of associated technology.

Future Directions

- *Emergency Department Bedside Registrations.* There is a growing commitment to bedside registration in emergency departments (ED). Two such examples of projects designed by our firm are the ED renovations and expansions at Riverside Regional Medical Center, completed in 2004 in Newport News, Virginia, and Broward General Medical Center, which opened in December 2005 in Ft. Lauderdale, Florida. While both hospitals have small registration desks for backup, they are now able to process more patients in a timely manner by quickly registering them at bedside, thus utilizing all of the ED staff more efficiently and avoiding the creation of bottlenecks common to ED lobbies.

   The old model typically holds registration staff captive to perhaps four registration rooms while patient rooms sit empty and the waiting room is clogged. Bedside registration allows staff to flex up and down, with some cross training, without being captive to the floor plan.

- *Room Service.* A hospitality makeover of the traditional hospital cafeteria provides patients options of being served different times during the day when they are hungry and from a menu allowing for their diet limitations. Their companions also have the option to order meals. Methods of placing meal orders include touching a television screen or using a spoken menu. The idea is to improve the hospital food experience for patients.

- *Decentralizing Imaging to Points of Care.* There is a move to decentralize a concentration of imaging services, such as CT scans and MRIs, to points of care for invasive-oriented departments within hospitals. St. Anthony Hospital in Denver is one of those leading the charge into decentralization through including CT scanners adjacent to trauma and operating rooms.

   Viewed as a lifesaving decision leading to better patient outcomes with less risk, many hospital owners are committing expensive equipment resources to points of service, which eliminates both loss of time (when having to transport a patient to another floor) and added trauma with moving a patient. To offset a loss of utilization, many of these imaging rooms are being made accessible to their contiguous corridors as well as to the treatment room they serve. The CT scanner can also be utilized on other patients without interrupting an operating room or trauma case. This is one of the more patient-centric care philosophies—bringing care to the patient.

■ *Less Need for Sightlines from ICU/CCU Nursing Centers Allows Flexing of Rooms.* The traditional intensive care (ICU) or critical care unit (CCU) layout in which all patient-bed placements are configured so that they can be visualized from the nurses' station is now giving way to acuity management via audiovisual equipment with a monitor for every bed. Utilization of electronic visualization allows more creative configurations of bed units that are acuity adaptable and more efficiently controls large geometrics that accompany rectangles or long oversized nurse stations. (Advancements in telemetry monitoring also allow monitoring of patients outside the ICU setting.)

Direct nursing contacts with patients are being ensured with alcove work spaces adjacent to patient rooms. When ICU/CCU patients are ready to transition and step down to medical beds, pressure is taken off immediate visualization from a central station so that the beds can flex to the patients' needs.

■ *Flexing of Beds.* Additionally related to efficiency of operations, bed towers are being designed for flexing of beds. For example, a 12-bed unit could flex up to 16 beds when needed during peak census without being constricted by a plan layout. A way to achieve this is by designing more angled corners rather than hard geometries, allowing some ebbing and flowing between wings and eliminating hard corners.

■ *Continuing Quest for Sustainability.* As expected, there appears to be a growing increased desire for hospital owners to incorporate sustainability into their facilities. This move toward "green" buildings will continue to grow more and more in the future as owners begin to realize that the short-term, upfront costs of becoming more environmentally friendly will be offset by long-terms gains.

Through research conducted by the Center for Health Design with its Planetree hospital system, hospital owners are learning of the advantages these particular models have over the traditionally designed hospitals regarding patient outcomes, patient and family satisfaction, staff satisfaction, and, importantly, the bottom line.

A Common Denominator

A common denominator in the design of any medical facility, no matter where it is located, is deinstitutionalizing the health care experience for consumers to create a patient-friendly and family-friendly environment. With the introduction of natural light, natural materials, texture, calming sounds, and live plants, apprehension can be alleviated and healing can begin the moment a patient enters a facility. Through the incorporation of this principle and adhering to needs of quality, flexibility, and cost effectiveness, hospitals can be designed for longevity well into this 21st century.

Chapter 13

New Partners for Building and Financing Big MACCs

Prelude: In North Carolina, a doctor and a real estate firm have teamed to build multi-specialty care centers near retirement communities across the state. This might be called "Innovation in the Old Confederacy."

Being "Fustest with the Mostest" was how a Confederate Calvary General in America's Civil War explained why he consistently won his battles. In this strategy, the entrepreneur aims at leadership.

Two completely different entrepreneurial strategies were summed up by another battle-winning general in America's Civil War, who said: "Hit Them Where They Ain't.

Peter F. Drucker, 1985

Health facilities development will accelerate. The next wave will likely be larger and more clinically and programmatically sophisticated. The economic potential will be significant. Innovative facilities design will allow for target clinical service, and geographic strategies will facilitate business partnership between parties who may not have considered partnership in the past.

Physicians, particularly the specialists, hold the potential for innovative and creative partnerships and have potential as partners, providing they don't cling too fast to the paradigm of hospitals and physician collaborators. The given here is the proliferating of new health care facilities over the next several years. The dollar potential is clearly in the tens of billions.

Daniel K. Zismer and Mark Hamel, 2003

What It Takes to Build New Facilities

- In real estate, "It's location, location, location!"
- In hospitals, "It's capital, capital, capital!"
- In construction, "It's health care, health care, health care!"
- In real estate, the suburbs are where it's at.
- In hospitals, it's facilities to attract patients, physicians, and capital.

National construction firms like Turner Construction and HBE, and regional firms, like DeWitt Corporation in Raleigh, North Carolina, are providing capital to hospitals and to doctors to free up money for other uses. New capital can make or break new projects. Hospitals now use their campuses to maximize returns, leverage existing real estate, create cash, and free up capital to maintain hospital–physician relationships. Competition, Medicare reimbursements, and profitability requirements are causing hospital CEOs to reevaluate real estate portfolios. Hospitals are spinning off neglected buildings to create needed capital. Two types of facilities have existed in health care: hospitals and physician clinics.

Tax-exempt debt, government support, and philanthropy have traditionally financed hospitals. Physician owners, sometimes with hospitals as passive investors, have financed clinics. Explosive growth and profitability of ambulatory services compared to inpatient services are changing capital equations. This is especially true for multispecialty ambulatory care centers.

Partnerships and Big MACCs

Several years ago, Robert J. Zasa, partner and cofounder of Woodrum Ambulatory Systems Development, coined the term "Big MACC" as a phrase for multispecialty ambulatory care centers. Besides bricks and mortar, Zasa says partnerships between hospitals, specialists, realtors, and construction firms, propelled by consumer demands and expectations, make Big MACCs a powerful trend. Big MACCs take $325 per square foot to build but generate revenues of $545 per square foot (Zismer and Hamel, 2003). These handsome returns attract construction firms, hospitals, and physicians.

Being "fustest with the mostest" and "hitting them where they ain't" are entrepreneurial strategies dating back to the Civil War. Wal-Mart perfected and practiced these same strategies beginning in the 1960s. Wal-Mart placed its initial stores in rural areas and remote suburbs untouched by Sears, Montgomery Ward, and other retailers. That approach, with its low-price strategy and its disciplined computer-based system for low-priced bidding by its supply-chain contributors, proved to be unbeatable and has assured it of a leadership position among the world's retailers.

Basically, two innovations are in place: (1) moving facilities to where consumers work, play, and live, and (2) finding new partners to help finance the move.

The health system is at a point reminiscent of the department store industry in the 1950s and 1960s. Were department stores going to stay downtown or relocate to suburban shopping malls? In the 1960s, 1970s, and 1980s, Wal-Mart moved its low-cost stores where others feared to tread. Peter F. Drucker calls this innovation strategy "entrepreneurial judo" (Drucker, 1985). In health care, one cannot win by competing with the leaders, large academic centers, big hospitals, or integrated systems—but rather can succeed by becoming a market leader in areas where these big systems do not exist, before health care leaders are even aware of the competitive change (Drucker, 1985).

One example of this "Hit them where they ain't" strategy has been pioneered by Dr. Lucien Wilkins, managing medical director of the DeWitt Health Care Division, a construction and real estate development firm located in Raleigh, North Carolina. In his former career as a gastroenterologist practicing in Wilmington, North Carolina, Dr. Wilkins observed many patients from remote rural areas of North Carolina arrived in his office with late-stage cancers. Wilkins surmised this late-diagnosis issue stemmed from rural patients having no access to doctors or medical centers.

Wilkins persuaded the DeWitt Corporation to hire him as their medical director. He and the company, he argued, could build convenient care centers for the medically underserved in high-growth areas of North Carolina. These areas were rapidly becoming magnets for retirees seeking low-cost retirement communities near golfing, fishing, and mountain retreats. Says Wilkins, "The reason I chose to work with the company was to move my ideas faster. The DeWitt Corporation has a construction company, a development arm, a real estate arm dealing with land acquisition, leasing, and sales. They also have an air conditioner company, an electric company, and other resources including property management. The company offered me all of the capabilities of the company to help accomplish my dream, my mission" (Reece, 2005c).

Over the last 5 years, DeWitt has planned and is building six ambulatory care centers and is in the process of preparing to build three more. These centers feature access to major highways, nearby retail outlets, and specialty care with associated laboratory, X-ray, imaging, physical therapy, and pharmaceutical services. These Big MACCs are built where people work, live, and play, with an unusual, creative partnership with a real estate development company possessing capital and other wherewithal. In his new position as medical director of DeWitt Healthcare, Dr. Wilkins is creating and executing major health care innovation.

The main force hindering the development of new health care facilities—principally new hospitals, but also ambulatory surgery centers and imaging centers—are certificate of need (CON) laws. These laws vary from state to state and are largely created by state hospital associations who fear new facilities will siphon off business from existing facilities. CON laws may become a point of political controversy between hospitals and physicians, with hospitals favoring retention of CON and doctors pushing for reform.

Case Study

Building Them Where They Ain't—DeWitt Health Care Multispecialty Ambulatory Care Centers (MACCs) Models

By Dr. Lucien Wilkins

Lucien Wilkins is a retired gastroenterologist who is pursuing a career as managing director of DeWitt Health Care in Raleigh, North Carolina. His mission and that of DeWitt Health Care is to bring quality health care to medically underserved neighborhoods where those neighborhoods are, even if they are in remote rural areas.

Dr. Wilkins is partly driven by his experiences as a gastroenterologist when he often saw patients in the late stages of their disease because patients from rural North Carolina delayed visiting doctors until it was too late.

Mission

"The mission of DeWitt Health Care is to bring MACCs to medically underserved neighborhoods, suburbs, and rural areas. Our facilities are of quality construction; are easily accessible in highly visible, convenient locations with abundant parking; and feature covered entryways and diagnostic and treatment services in the same medical office building as the physician office suites."

Design of Facilities

Our facilities are designed to be patient centered and physician friendly. We bring together medical services and care providers under one roof so each can benefit from the other yet remain autonomous. Whether diagnostic and treatment services are provided by private enterprise or public hospitals, we promote excellence, timeliness, and value for the patients.

DeWitt Health Care provides need-determination services, acquires the real estate, finances the project, develops, constructs, and manages the facility as well as assembling diagnostic services, physicians, and other providers for the outpatient medical facility.

Conveniences for Doctors and Patients

By providing the diagnostic services adjacent to the medical office suites, physicians and other providers in urban or rural locations can practice in the way they were trained and are accustomed, and the patients can enjoy the convenience of one-stop medical care.

Six Freestanding Models

As of June 2006, DeWitt Health Care has developed six MACC models that are now open or under construction. All are freestanding full-service outpatient medical centers located in North Carolina. They are similar in format. Diagnostic services, mobile imaging pad, urgent care, specialty center, and medical/dental office suites are part of each model. There are three more centers in the works for 2007.

These centers differ in a number of ways. Some have public hospital–provided services, while others have privately provided diagnostic services. Some facilities are owned by physicians, some are owned by DeWitt Health Care; some offices are for lease, and others are office condominiums for sale. Medical campus facilities have offices for lease and land or offices for sale. We offer a variety of lease and sale options to suit the needs for physicians, dentists, and medical service and other providers.

Strategic Locations

All facilities are purpose-designed outpatient facilities with quality construction at strategic locations with emphasis on location, accessibility, and convenience for the patient. All have the diagnostic and treatment services located near the office suites for patient and physician convenience. DeWitt Health Care understands and addresses the practice, business, and real estate needs of the physician, and the safety, comfort, and convenience of the patients.

Details of Models

The DeWitt Health Care MACC models are:

- The Rocky Point Medical Pavilion is a 22,500-square-foot, one-story medical office building, located in rural but rapidly growing Pender County. Located in one facility will be an imaging, mobile imaging, laboratory, urgent care, physical therapy/cardiac rehab, and conference center. The central facility will be provided by Pender Memorial Hospital/New Hanover Health Care Network. The specialty center, fitness center, and medical office suites are occupied by private providers. Outparcels are available for a pharmacy and medical-compatible retail and other medical-related users.
- The Pavilion at Carolina Beach is a 22,500-square-foot one-story medical office building with imaging provided by a private user and lab services provided by a private user. In this office building will be services for urgent care, internal medicine, bariatrics, orthopedics, specializations, physical therapy, a coffee shop, and durable medical equipment provided by private users. The location is highly visible and easily accessible with abundant parking at a lighted intersection. There is a pharmacy and physician and dental offices across the street. Over 15,000 residents and over a million visitors yearly have access to this facility.
- The Waterford Medical Center is a 33,000-square-foot, three-story medical office building located in rural but rapidly growing Leland in Brunswick County with 25,000 residents who previously had virtually no health care, no diagnostic services, and left the county for health care. The outpatient medical center provides imaging including a mobile MRI, lab, urgent care, orthopedics, durable medical equipment, physical therapy, internal medicine, pediatrics, specializations, dentistry, and other private services for the community. A national pharmacy and medical-compatible retail/food service are adjacent to the medical center.
- The Brunswick Medical Campus is a 22-acre medical campus located at Supply in Brunswick County with a 38,000-square-foot medical office building with private users providing imaging, laboratory, urgent care, a specialty suite, durable medical equipment, orthopedics, vein center, allergy, nephrology, pediatrics, cardiology, dentistry,

physical therapy, psychiatry, and OB/GYN services. A second 15,000-square-foot, one-story medical office building on campus has a local pharmacy and medical/dental office suites. A medical transportation company is located on campus. A planned endoscopy center, vascular center, oncology center, bank, food service businesses, and medical office buildings will round out the campus.

- The Health Express, a 26,000-square-foot outpatient medical center with an additional 12,000 square feet of medical-related retail space, is now located on a shopping center property. It will be a full-service medical-destination facility located conveniently adjacent to retail, food service, and commercial services. The health care services are geared to provide the best services and care in an environment sensitive to the time and distance restraints on health care. The center includes a full-service diagnostic center including imaging and two mobile imaging pads, urgent care, fitness, physical therapy, cardiac rehabilitation, family medicine, pediatrics, vision, and dentistry services. Wrapped around the center are retail shops and food service. Excellent visibility, access, and parking will make seeking and receiving care easy and convenient.

- The Falls Ridge Medical Center is a 15,000-square-foot MOB located next to existing medical offices, a pharmacy, and retail center in a rapidly growing urban location adjacent to an interstate beltway for convenience and access. Falls Ridge Medical will have imaging and mobile imaging provided by a regional hospital seeking to provide community outreach and urgent care, physical therapy, and medical and dental care provided by private physicians and dentists.

Chapter 14

From Independent Specialty Practice to Hospital Employment

Prelude: Medical and hospital practice isn't what it used to be. Physicians are now leaving private practice to become salaried hospital employees.

What is the tipping point? It's the thought that ideas and behavior and products behave just like the outbreaks of disease. They become social epidemics. Things happen all at once, and little changes make a huge difference.

The phrase "tipping point" comes from the world of epidemiology. It's the name given to that moment when the virus reaches a critical mass. People who understand the tipping point have a way of decoding the world around us.

Malcolm Gladwell, 2002

An old saying goes, "One cannot run a hospital with doctors, and one cannot run one without them." Similarly every university administrator has said, if only to himself, "One cannot run a university with the faculty but one cannot, alas, run one without it either."

This applies to all modern organizations, including the business enterprise. All enterprises are becoming "double-headed monsters," which depend for their performance on professionals who are dedicated to their discipline, rather than to the institution, who are the more productive the more dedicated they are, and who, at the same time, have worked toward the accomplishment of the goals of the whole.

The emergence of the "double-headed monster" is also the result of population dynamics. It is yet another example of turbulent times that managers have to learn to manage.

Peter F. Drucker, 1960

Are Hospitals at the Tipping Point with Specialists?

Historically, hospital organizations and specialty practices have run on separate tracks. Hospital leaders run the facility, provide the beds, and provide the staff, and specialists use the facility as their workshop to perform procedures, do diagnostic workups, conduct treatment, and place ill patients. Hospitals and doctors traditionally charge separately. With doctors as employees, the billing function may be consolidated.

- Have relationships between specialists and hospitals reached the "tipping point"?
- Will hospitals, rather than specialists, float the health care boat?
- Is there an epidemic of specialists rushing to be employed by hospitals to escape managed care hassles, malpractice expenses, and mounting pressures to computerize every aspect of their practices?
- Are more specialists seeking to become employed by hospitals rather than going through the tedious legal and regulatory process required for ownership or strategic partnerships?

Could be. As will be shown here, physician employment is proliferating out there, and it may be approaching critical mass: the tipping point.

Evidence of the Physician Employment "Virus"

A virus is a contagious agent and may be applied to sociological phenomena as well as disease. The hiring of formerly independent specialists is a distinct change in direction in American medical culture.

- The *Puget Sound Business Journal* (Neurath, 2005) carried an article that opened, "Tacoma orthopedic surgeon Dr. Nick Rajacich is one of an increasing number of doctors who, faced with intolerable financial pressures, has given up independent practice and gone to work for a hospital." Rajacich said five Tacoma orthopedic surgeons, a third of Tacoma's orthopedic workforce, had become hospital employees.
- Stefani Daniels, RN, MSNA, CMAC, founder and managing partner of Phoenix Medical Management, has observed an "epidemic" of specialist hiring by hospitals. She sees an explosion of hospitals' employment of general internists. She says, "Doctors are fed up with malpractice and regulatory pressures."
- Louis Joseph, HCA, vice president of Physician Services for Central Group Operations in Nashville, commented, "I've never seen anything like it. Suddenly, specialists from all over our system, from Florida to Alaska, are approaching us about going to work for us."

- Phillip Miller, director of communications at Merritt Hawkins & Associates, notes, "Hospitals are hiring more specialists to lock them in. Hospitals are using employment to retain specialists as competition heats up. What's different now is that doctors are driving hospital employment."

In 1968, in *The Age of Discontinuity*, Peter F. Drucker defined *discontinuity* as a sudden shift changing the "structure and meaning of economy, polity, and society." The United States may be at the point where the discontinuity virus is spreading, infecting, and transforming hospital–physician relationships. External forces on the hospital side (medical arms races, critical need for specialists to provide high-tech services, demand for multi-million-dollar technologies) and on the specialist side (downward economic pressures, expenses of running practices, worries over costs of malpractice, and electronic information systems investments) are changing the structure and meaning of hospital–physician relationships.

This doesn't mean, however, that hospital CEOs are kings or queens of the hill and specialists are sycophants; rather, it means new relationships, new understandings, and new responsibilities.

According to the Merritt Hawkins & Associates' *2005 Review of Physician Recruiting Incentives*, the demands for and average pay of specialists have reached an all-time high: cardiologists ($320,000), radiologists ($355,000), orthopedists ($361,000), and internists ($161,000)—yet these specialists are seeking hospital employment, frequently at lower pay levels than in independent practice. Phillip Miller, communications director and a vice president at Merritt Hawkins, says three reasons may drive this paradox:

1. Medicare reimbursement cuts for procedures and for fees in freestanding ambulatory and imaging centers
2. Emotional burnout from overwork, long hours, malpractice fears, and mounting premiums
3. A new generation of doctors, often married to other doctors, who seek a balanced lifestyle and more family time

Innovative Opportunities for Hospitals and Specialists

For hospitals and physicians alike, these trends may open innovative opportunities. The hospitals can now engage specialists as employees in creating hospital-owned outpatient-focused centers of excellence, and doctors can gain managerial experience and exert clinical control while being subsidized by the hospital.

True innovations can be "win-win" opportunities, but it will take time, successes, and setbacks for hospital executives and specialists to get used to their new roles as business partners with new accountabilities and responsibilities.

Case Study

Emergency Rooms, Hospitals, and Innovation
By Stefani Daniels

Stefani Daniels is the managing partner of Phoenix Medical Management, a national consulting firm exclusively devoted to hospital-based case management programs since 1994. She has held faculty appointments in Columbia University, the University of Pennsylvania, and Nova Southeastern University's School of Business and Entrepreneurship in Ft. Lauderdale, Florida.

She serves on the editorial board of Lippincott's *Case Management Journal* and the Credentialing Advisory Board for the Center for Case Management.

Daniels is a graduate of Stockton State College in New Jersey and Villanova University in Pennsylvania and spent the majority of her career in the executive suite of hospitals in New York, Pennsylvania, and Florida. She is a frequent guest speaker at regional and national health care meetings and is the coauthor of the textbook *The Leader's Guide to Hospital Case Management.*

• •

In 2003 when the Centers for Medicare and Medicaid Services (CMS) issued a revision to administrative rules governing the Emergency Medical Treatment and Active Labor Act (EMTALA), emergency department medical directors with whom I worked predicted a shortfall of on-call medical specialists. Thomas Scully, CMS administrator at the time of the rule revision, anticipated that the new language would give greater flexibility to the hospitals to provide for specialty availability. "It is consistent with the recommendations of the Secretary's Advisory Committee on Regulatory Reform to help hospitals focus less on unnecessary requirements and more on providing quality care to their patients," he said.

As the managing partner of a hospital case-management consulting firm (Phoenix Medical Management, Inc.), I often work with emergency department medical directors to establish case management programs to help physicians channel patients to the most appropriate level of care. In that role, I hear their laments about emergency department (ED) overcrowding, lack of critical care beds, the growing numbers of uninsured visitors, and the difficulties in accessing medical specialists especially neurosurgeons, orthopedic surgeons, and obstetricians.

EMTALA requires every emergency department to provide a medical screening exam to any person who comes to the hospital emergency room and requests treatment. If the exam reveals an emergency medical condition, the emergency department must stabilize and administer transfer to another facility. In the past, stringent EMTALA requirements gave emergency departments considerable power over a specialist's time, diminishing the specialist's incentive to be on call. However, under the revised rules, physicians are permitted to be on-call simultaneously at more than one hospital and have the discretion to schedule elective procedures during on-call times.

In essence, the new rule gave them permission to limit the amounts of call time they are willing to take. Dr. George Molzen, president of the American College of Emergency Physicians (ACEP), said that the rule could potentially allow specialists to opt out of being on call to the ED.

To assess the effect of the new rules and the current practice climate, the Robert Wood Johnson Foundation underwrote a grant to the American College of Emergency Physicians to survey emergency medical directors. The study findings, coupled with the growing demands for ED services, confirm further strain on an already frayed system. Two thirds of the respondents reported inadequate on-call specialist coverage in all U.S. geographic regions (Gore, 2004). Seventeen percent noted that some specialists had already negotiated with their hospital for fewer on-call coverage hours. Based on several subsequent confirming studies, it appears that Dr. Molzen was correct.

Historically, ED on-call coverage was an opportunity to grow a practice for a new physician. Patients they treated in the emergency room were often then referred to their specialty service. In addition, "taking call" was seen as part of a physician's obligation in return for hospital privileges.

With the growth of freestanding outpatient facilities and specialty care centers, however, they became less dependent on having privileges at general hospitals. At client hospitals, emergency medical directors speak of several major environmental forces that are creating the scarcity of specialty physicians. Among them are:

- a limited number of specialty training spots
- the costs of medical malpractice liability insurance
- uncompensated services or minimal reimbursement
- lifestyle balance

An emergency medical director at an Ohio hospital told me that 5 years ago he had over 20 specialists whom he could count on to respond within 30 minutes to a call for emergency service. Now he has just five. Located outside a major metropolitan area, in a predominantly rural agricultural area, the hospital especially depended upon their specialists for hand surgery and plastic surgery emergencies. As a result, the number of transfers from the hospital has grown to over 25 percent.

A few years ago, another client hospital had to downgrade their trauma center from level 1 to level 2 due to inadequate specialty services. The ED medical director reported that both the cardiologist and vascular surgeon members of the trauma team joined with other cardiac and pulmonary specialists and opened a specialty hospital before the moratorium was issued.

We have seen trauma centers close in many cities including Los Angeles, California, and Sherman, Texas. In a report issued by the Washington State Hospital Association, 30 trauma centers closed between 2000 and 2004 as hospitals faced volume increase, higher costs, liability concerns, and low or no payment for trauma services.

The growing reluctance by specialist physicians to provide emergency or trauma team on-call coverage has prompted a number of hospitals to resort to an incentive system to encourage specialist participation. Some report that they pay stipends for emergency or trauma on-call services or they guarantee certain levels of reimbursement. One chief financial officer even reported that he offers some measure of medical liability relief in exchange for on-call commitment.

However, when the annual costs of incentives escalate, hospital executives seek a more practical alternative by hiring full-time specialists. A CEO at a New York hospital explained that employing full-time specialists not only gives them ED coverage, but also supplements hospitalist services. "It's a win-win situation for the hospital and the physician," he said, and has had the additional serendipitous outcome of significantly reducing the waiting time for consultants' response. In turn, this has reduced the hospital's average length of stay by nearly 1 day.

The steady growth in ED visits, the increase in uninsured patients, the unfunded mandates of EMTALA, the dramatically rising liability insurance premiums for all physicians—but especially so for orthopedic surgeons and neurosurgeons, and the erosion of physician participation in emergency service provision have all contributed to the growing trend in specialist-physician employment.

What began as a minor blip on the radar screen in about 2003 has escalated into a growing trend. This trend is attracting young physicians who are eager to avoid the pressures of private practice in exchange for a healthy balance of life and work schedules and a reliable and rewarding paycheck.

P.S.

Anytime two or more hospital execs get together, talk will eventually turn to the "tremendous" or "dramatic" change the industry has undergone in recent years. However, the speed of change is relative. Yes, recent years have brought considerable change—increased competition, advances in technology, reimbursement reductions, safety and quality requirements, and regulatory oversight, to name a few—but change in organizational culture and operations moves at glacial speed compared to most other industries.

In some companies, innovation and change are ingrained into their culture and huge resources are devoted to new ideas. World-class innovators such as 3M, Sony, and HP do not need any prodding to innovate. However, many hospitals have historically preferred the relative comfort of the status quo, which reflects a monumental investment of financial and emotional resources. One often hears the plaintive plea: "Don't change just for the sake of change." It's a logical statement but also a potentially fatal one if it is allowed to lull a hospital into a false sense of security.

Innovation in case management is reflected in the degree to which the organization has anticipated changes in the environment and adapted their programs in accordance with those changes. If the hospital effectively employs innovation, then the legacy case management models dependent upon chart review and Deceased Client Profile and Utilization Review activities would be a thing of the past.

As the need for innovation and transformation grows, execs and program leaders are challenged in ways to which they are not accustomed. The skills and traits of rapid change leadership are quite different from the skills of those who lead continuous process-improvement initiatives. Moreover, the change agent will undoubtedly encounter tremendous resistance from within as people cling to the familiar past and struggle to think outside the contextual boundaries within which they have operated for years. However, here are a few ideas that you may find helpful to get started:

1. **Change what you measure.** Nothing communicates priorities more than the metrics used by the case management program, how they are shared, and the degree of outcome ownership. While many case management metrics measure the degree to which quality is absent such as complication rates or infection rates, to spawn innovation in case management, use metrics that measure how the stakeholders have benefited over time from case management interventions.
2. **Unleash your inner entrepreneur.** Innovation means behaving in an unorthodox manner. Yes, we know that many hospitals tend to be complex, bureaucratic organizations in which orthodoxy is rewarded and entrepreneurial actions are discouraged. One way to shake things up within case management is to think of the program as a semi-

autonomous business. What fresh ideas will be generated if team members started to think of case management as their own business?

3. **Revamp reward systems.** Case management programs typically reward compliance with standards and compliance. However, to create a vibrant, agile program that takes advantage of opportunities that arise over time, a reward system must demonstrate that innovation is not only acceptable but strongly encouraged through both economic and noneconomic recognition.

4. **Get closer to your customers.** Every case-management program should have a detailed understanding of the people most impacted by any potential change. Key stakeholders for case management include patients, physicians, insurers, and colleagues. Determine what they want, need, are willing to do to get what they want/need, and think of your program's value proposition. It will take time to truly connect with key stakeholders, but anything less will produce nothing but window dressing and will fail to deliver the critical insights needed for successful case management transformation.

5. **Boldly go.** Case managers must first understand, then clearly and persistently communicate, the three critical elements of change: a burning platform, a compelling vision for the future, and a way to bridge the two. Communicating these messages becomes an everyday task of the leader and every case-management team member.

Part Four

Employer and Health Plan Innovations

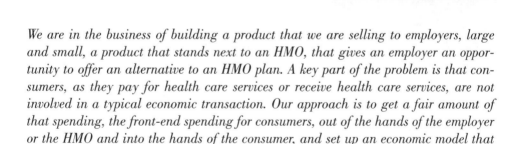

We are in the business of building a product that we are selling to employers, large and small, a product that stands next to an HMO, that gives an employer an opportunity to offer an alternative to an HMO plan. A key part of the problem is that consumers, as they pay for health care services or receive health care services, are not involved in a typical economic transaction. Our approach is to get a fair amount of that spending, the front-end spending for consumers, out of the hands of the employer or the HMO and into the hands of the consumer, and set up an economic model that makes sense.

Chip Tooke, president of Lumenos, 2006

Chapter 15

From High Tech to High Tech/ High Touch

Prelude: High-tech/high-touch care maximizes care potential by educating patients about disease and alerting them to complications by recording their health measurements and by putting them in immediate contact with doctors and nurses.

High tech/high touch is a formula I use to describe the way we have responded to technology. What happens is that whenever new technology is introduced into society, there must be a counterbalancing human response—that is, high touch—or the technology is rejected. The higher tech, the more high touch.

John Naisbitt, 1982

Facing growing cases of chronic illnesses amid continuing nursing shortages, the health-care industry is increasingly turning to home-based medical devices to keep tabs on patients.

A growing array of "telemonitoring" gadgets and video equipment is allowing patient to transmit weight, blood sugar, oxygen levels and other health data electronically to hospitals and nurses who may be far away.

The system scan is costly, but the aim is to lower long-term costs by heading off serious medial problems that crop up between doctor's office visits.

Device makers say the systems allow health-care providers to care for larger numbers of patients with conditions such as diabetes, asthma, and congestive heart failure, who must stick with specific regimens, and be monitored closely.

Elena Cherney, 2006

Forced High Tech/High Touch

In *Megatrends*, John Naisbitt (1982) predicted that the theory of forced high tech to high tech/high touch would come into its own. In recent years, high-tech/high-touch solutions, through use of remote monitoring devices, direct measurement of vital signs, and audiovisual contact with patients, have inspired disease-management companies that train nurses to monitor patients at home and at work.

Managed care plans rapidly gravitated to disease management to cut costs for those 20 percent chronic disease patients who account for 80 percent of costs. In the world of economics, as well as health care, this is known as Pareto's Law, which states that 20 percent of events cause 80 percent of results. Whatever the exact number, care of just a few chronic diseases—heart disease, hypertension, diabetes, asthma, cancer, and depression and other mood disorders—comprises more than half of all health care spending (*National Committee for Quality Assurance*, 2004).

However, these patients, when carefully educated and monitored outside the usual health care settings, can be taught to avoid common complications of their diseases and can be headed off emergency rooms and hospitals encounters. In many cases, companies are developing bedside audiovisual devices for home-bound patients in a successful effort to cut costs by improving care, reducing complications, and decreasing hospital readmissions.

In *Voices of Health Reform* (Reece, 2005c), I interviewed four physician leaders who tied together high technology with high touch and better outcomes: William Gold, chief medical officer of Blue Cross Blue Shield of Minnesota; Victor Villagra, a Connecticut-based disease management consultant; Randall Moore, CEO of American Telecare in Eden Prairie, Minnesota; and Lucien Wilkins, managing director of DeWitt Health Care in Wilmington, North Carolina.

These innovative doctors have implemented technologies and concepts reaching and improving care of consumers where they live, work, and play. Specialists are not only building facilities in previously remote locations, but are deploying telemedicine to evaluate patients no matter where they are. While remote care is now possible technologically, payment for these services is sometimes complicated by state and national regulations and turf battles between providers (Reece, 2004a).

In his book, *The World Is Flat: A Brief History of the Twenty First-Century*, Thomas Friedman (2005) demystifies electronic transmission of texts and image around the world. The chief impact of Internet-based medicine will be decentralized care: from hospitals to outpatient facilities, from doctor's offices to patients at home and at work, and from the United States to countries such as India.

Innovation Talking and Action Points

Telemedicine enthusiasts, particularly entrepreneurs, have anticipated a gold rush toward remote care, virtual office visits, home care, and transmission of financial, claims, diagnostic, and clinical data. Unfortunately, for many of these things, there has been no gold (Reece, 2004a). That may be about to change, as costs rise, staff shortages grow, the chronic disease population explodes, and hospitals and doctors look for more efficiency and revenues.

So, hospital chief information officers, physician leaders, and practice managers, be prepared. Lay the groundwork for remote care, experiment with virtual office visits, transmit images, create personal health records, resolve those turf payment issues, take down those regulations impeding remote specialist care, and flatten health costs. In other words, prepare your organization for a future already here. Telehealth-enabled, consumer-empowered, provider-powered disease and care management has arrived.

Case Study 1

High-Tech/High-Touch Results
By Randall Moore, MD, CEO of American Telecare, and
Erin Denholm, MSN, CEO of Centura Health

Randall S. Moore, MD, MBA, is the president, CEO, and chairman of American Telecare, Inc. (ATI). His experience includes more than 20 years working as both a physician and an executive in the medical industry, with a focus on system-level change, integrating advanced business and clinical models.

Moore graduated from the Johns Hopkins School of Medicine, before completing his training in internal medicine at the University of Minnesota where he served on the faculty for 9 years. His education also includes study at the University of London and earning his MBA from the Kellogg Graduate School of Management at Northwestern University.

As president and CEO of Centura Health, Erin M. Denholm, MSN, is responsible for home-based service lines including home care, hospice, home infusion, and oxygen and home medical equipment. Denholm has been in home care most of her professional career. She has channeled that passion into a 20-year career in home care.

In 2003, Denholm was one of 20 nurses in the country selected for a 3-year fellowship with the Robert Wood Johnson Foundation, the nation's largest philanthropic organization devoted exclusively to health care. During her fellowship, Denholm collaborated with a team of coaches and instructors from within the health care industry to bring about change in the areas of access, disparity, and prevention.

In 2004, she launched an extremely successful 6-month pilot study using telehealth to manage congestive heart failure patients. As a result of this groundbreaking study, a bill was signed in June 2006 that earmarked $150,000 in funding for a statewide pilot study to determine if the telehealth program would garner similar results among the chronically ill Medicaid population.

• •

Ms. D was 81 years old, emerging from her 13th hospitalization in less than a year for exacerbation of her heart failure. Lengthy intensive care readmissions with ventilator support were

interspersed with periods at home, requiring daily nursing visits, wheelchair assistance, and oxygen treatments. Her local internist had the support of a consulting cardiology group within the broader health care system, as well as case management. Nonetheless, Ms. D continued to deteriorate, as is commonplace with advanced heart failure and the care processes of the acute care disease system.

Discharged on January 2, Ms. D reluctantly agreed to utilize an audiovideo-enabled telehealth solution. This supported not only teleconferencing across normal telephone lines, but also integrated a high-quality stethoscope, blood pressure meter, pulse oximetry, and a medical-grade weight scale. Ms. D was one of the early participants in a telehealth pilot for this leading broad health system.

Designed to catalyze a disruptive solution integration into the care of the highest complexity/ need/cost people with chronic disease, the telehealth-enabled solution promised to be effective, efficient, and patient centered, bringing 24/7 real-time care and support to the patient. In the following 3+ years, Ms. D required only one hospitalization, related to dehydration secondary to a case of the flu. Early, real-time interventions by her care team led to simpler interventions to reverse acute exacerbations of her heart failure. Added patient education through the telehealth system significantly enhanced Ms. D's education and subsequent control of her disease. She was able to replace her frequent hospitalizations and wheelchair with a lifestyle that included normal activities, including going out with "the girls" and volunteering 5 days a week at the local community center.

The Allina health system in Minnesota experienced similar results as telehealth virtual care was applied to other patients, filling a key gap as patients with high needs and costs could have care delivered prospectively, on a real-time basis. Similar results were seen in a more systematic manner through the Centura Health at Home program. Centura Health at Home launched a program focused on Pacificare Secure Horizon patients with heart failure. Secure Horizons is a Medicare risk-managed care product managed by Pacificare.

The goals of the program included lowering rehospitalization and ED visits/costs by 60 percent, as well as improving patient satisfaction and knowledge of their disease and self-management. In the 6-month pilot, Centura hospitalization costs dropped 95 percent and ED costs 100 percent, leading to a net health care cost reduction of 73 percent after paying the costs of the added telehealth program. Patient and physician satisfaction were high. The number of home care nursing visits dropped from 11 per episode without telehealth to 3.5 live visits with 9.5 telehealth visits per patient per month.

Adding the efficiency of telehealth reduced home nursing expenses by about 50 percent. Clinical personnel experienced increased satisfaction in knowing more timely and effective care was delivered.

The Difference: Reengineering the Patient–Provider Relationship

Ms. D and the Centura experience are among a growing cluster of dramatically improved clinical outcomes in which telehealth solutions play a key role, but only insofar as enabling reinvention of clinical care to fit the needs of the highest need/complexity/cost patients.

In *Crossing the Quality Chasm: A New Health System in the 21st Century* (2001), the Institute of Medicine stated the need for care to be safe, effective, patient-centered, timely, efficient, and equitable. They also presented 10 rules for care system reinvention, translated into patient terms in the following exhibit.

Telehealth-enabled care empowers skilled clinicians and patients to transform their entire experience, creating a continuous healing relationship, customized around patient needs and preferences, incorporating evidence and supercharging CQI, proactive care, and prevention replacing reactive interventions.

Telehealth solutions can bring the expertise of interdisciplinary teams together and eliminate waste as the needs of the patient with complex disease are met earlier. With much simpler interventions, delivered 24/7, medical expertise comes to the patient, instead of the patient needing to find delayed medical care.

Current disease-management programs and strategies attempt to fill gaps in the care and education of people with chronic disease, separate from what the provider team might do. The highest need (top 5 percent of the population who consume over 50 percent of all health care resources) benefit from telehealth-enabled disease management supporting a new level of care and relationship between clinical team members and the patients they serve.

Clinical processes must be reengineered to optimize the application of health care resources to maximize the health of a population. When data continues to show that the top 1 percent of the population consumes approximately 25 percent of all health care resources and the top 5 percent uses over 50 percent, the high burden of chronic illness within the top 5 percent suggests we need radical reinvention of our care processes.

Building more hospital beds, at costs exceeding $1 million per bed, is not the answer (Moore, 2006). Throwing technology at people is not the answer. Our system's historical approach of assuming there was not much that could be done to change the course of our highest need/cost members is also not the answer.

Medical leadership understands our acute illness systems do not meet the needs of the small portion of the population who consumes so many resources. Reinventing care processes that enable a 24/7/365 continuous healing relationship between a care team and highest-need patients can and will radically change the course of many people just like Ms. D or the patients served by the Centura team.

Technology solutions must support teams and their programs as they bring patient-centered care to the patient—as they empower patients to take control of their disease. Delivering dramatically improved outcomes while lowering costs may demonstrate a model for health care purchasers to fund alternative care models that support passionate innovation to meet the needs of patients we serve.

WHAT PATIENTS SHOULD EXPECT FROM THEIR HEALTH CARE

1. **Beyond patient visits:** You will have the care you need when you need it— *whenever* you need it. You will find help in many forms, not just in face-to-face visits. You will find help on the Internet, on the telephone, from many sources, and by many routes in the form you want it.

2. **Individualization:** You will be known and respected as an individual. Your choices and preferences will be sought and honored. The usual system of care will meet most of your needs. When your needs are special, the care will adapt to meet you on your own terms.

3. **Control:** The care system will take control only if and when you freely give permission.

4. **Information:** You can know what you wish to know, when you wish to know it. Your medical record is yours to keep, to read, and to understand. The rule is: "Nothing about you without you."

5. **Science:** You will have care based on the best available scientific knowledge. The system promises you excellence as its standard. Your care will not vary illogically from doctor to doctor or from place to place. The system will promise you all the care that can help you and will help you avoid care that cannot help you.

6. **Safety:** Errors in care will not harm you. You will be safe in the care system.

7. **Transparency:** Your care will be confidential, but the care system will not keep secrets from you. You can know whatever you wish to know about the care that affects you and your loved ones.

8. **Anticipation:** Your care will anticipate your needs and will help you find the help you need. You will experience proactive help, not just reactions, to help you restore and maintain your health.

9. **Value:** Your care will not waste your time or money. You will benefit from constant innovations, which will increase the value of care to you.

10. **Cooperation:** Those who provide care will cooperate and coordinate their work fully with each other and with you. The walls between professions and institutions will crumble, so that your experiences will become seamless. You will never feel lost.

Source: Adapted from Institute of Medicine Report, *Crossing the Quality Chasm.* National Academies Press, Washington, D.C.

Case Study 2

The Disease-Management Market
By Brooks O'Neil, Senior Analyst Avondale Partners

Brooks O'Neil has been in the investment business for nearly 20 years. Much of that time was spent at Piper Jaffray, a growth company investment bank based in Minneapolis, Minnesota. At Piper Jaffray, O'Neil was an institutional salesperson covering the Boston market, an all-star research analyst, and the leader of the health services investment banking effort. O'Neil has also enjoyed success as a research analyst and investment banker at ThinkEquity Partners, TripleTree, and Dougherty & Company.

O'Neil joined Avondale Partners as a senior research analyst in January 2006.

He follows disease management and other rapidly growing sectors of the health care services market for the firm. He graduated from the University of Connecticut with a bachelor's in English and has an MBA from the Amos Tuck School of Dartmouth College.

Healthways is the nation's largest pure-play provider of comprehensive disease-management and care-enhancement services. As a disease management analyst, I follow Healthways' activities closely. The company's programs are sold through health plans in all 50 states, the District of Columbia, Puerto Rico, and Guam. Healthways was founded in 1981 and went public during 1991. The programs are based on up-to-date, evidence-based clinical guidelines. As of February 2006, Healthways had over 2.0 million lives under management nationwide. This is a tiny fraction of the addressable market.

Healthway's integrated product line currently includes programs for people with diabetes, coronary artery disease (CAD), heart failure (HF), asthma, chronic obstructive pulmonary disease (COPD), end-stage renal disease (ESRD), cancer, obesity, acid-related stomach disorders, atrial fibrillation, decubitus ulcers, fibromyalgia, hepatitis C, inflammatory bowel disease, irritable bowel syndrome, low-back pain, osteoarthritis, osteoporosis, and urinary incontinence. In addition, Healthways offers programs that identify and provide care to individuals at high risk for incurring substantial health care costs in the next 12 months. The company offers high-intensity services for more than 160 disease conditions for the 1 percent or less of the population facing the imminent risk of hospitalization or another high-cost health episode.

Chronic care management is an approach that offers much promise in addressing the cost and quality of health care for critical segments of the population. In a paper published in *Health Affairs* during 2001, Marc Berk and Alan Monheit showed that 10 percent of the U.S. population accounts for almost 70 percent of health expenditures annually. According to the Centers for Medicare and Medicaid Services, total spending for personal health care in the United States was $1.936 trillion for 2005. This suggests that health expenditures for the 10 percent of the population that constitutes the heaviest utilizers were greater than $1.3 trillion.

Berk and Monheit concluded,

> Although we have seen enormous efforts over the past decade to control rising health care costs, relatively little effort has been targeted toward those who account for the majority of service use.

Disease-management programs such as Healthways offers are designed to identify high-risk patients as early as possible and coordinate and integrate a patient's care to achieve a more successful health outcome. Typically using sophisticated technology and a team of highly skilled, caring health care professionals, disease-management companies work closely with patients, physicians, hospitals, and health plans to encourage adherence to evidence-based standards of care that generate significant improvements in health and significantly reduced costs of care.

Table 15–1 *Distribution of Health Expenditures for the U.S. Population. Selected Years 1928–1996*

Percentage of U.S. Population Ranked by Expenditures	1928	1963	1970	1977	1980	1987 Payments	1996 Payments
Top 1%	—	17%	26%	27%	29%	28%	27%
Top 2%	—	—	35	38	39	39	38
Top 5%	52%	43	50	55	55	56	55
Top 10%	—	59	66	70	70	70	69
Top 30%	93	—	88	90	90	90	90
Top 50%	—	95	96	97	96	97	97

Source: Health Affairs, 20(2).

Industry sources estimate disease management will become a $20 billion market in the United States, up from less than $1 billion during 2005 (O'Neil, 2006). Today, Healthways and Matria Health Care, Inc., are the major established, freestanding, publicly traded players in this space, although there are a handful of private players. Many of these are growing rapidly, and one (Health Dialog) generates revenues over $100 million (Lawlor, 2006).

Disease-management initiatives in Medicare and Medicaid are coming. CMS, which administers both Medicare and the federal portion of Medicaid, recently has made a significant commitment to disease management.

Combined, in 2005, government programs, state and federal, accounted for 46 percent of annual health care expenditures in this country, or $891.5 billion (ASPE, 2005). Statistics indicate both Medicare and Medicaid serve populations that are particularly susceptible to chronic illness. To date neither program has done much to incorporate efforts to improve care or manage cost for those receiving therapy for chronic illness.

The benchmark for successful chronic care management programs is return on investment (ROI). In recent years, there has been considerable debate about the ROI potential of many chronic care management programs. However, there is a growing body of credible, documented evidence that indicates immediate, substantial ROI and patients who are receiving better care because of such programs. The ROI is achieved by reducing unnecessary visits to the doctor or hospital and minimizing costly complications.

Importantly, the science of chronic care management as practiced by Healthways and others is in its infancy. For the first time, health care professionals are developing a documented and analyzable record of care for a broad base of geographically diverse, chronically ill individuals over time. The data collected will allow Healthways and others to rapidly advance the science of chronic care management and improve our approach to treating a wide variety of expensive, debilitating diseases.

Interestingly, in the opinion of this author, today employers want:

- a suite of services that can be delivered on an a la carte basis or as a more comprehensive health enhancement offering
- a total population management solution delivered in a cost-effective manner
- sophisticated, flexible, and scalable information systems

As a veteran health analyst, I will tell you the data suggest that for about 50 percent of the population, annual spending for health care is next to nothing. (See Figure 15–1.) Typically, the needs of these people can be addressed very effectively through broad-based demand management products that include patient education, 24/7 nurse triage, health system navigation, pricing information, and decision support. This is essentially the first line of contact for individuals seeking to access the health system. Over time, we expect these offerings to become increasingly robust as information on specific providers will become much more valuable going forward.

For 40 percent or so of the population, health care spending can be more significant (several hundred to several thousand per year) and appears worth managing immediately. More importantly, the spending pattern for these individuals suggests they may be at-risk for expensive health issues in the future. Getting these people involved in a health enhancement program(s) now will generate a positive outcome for the individual and for whomever is at-risk for the cost of care.

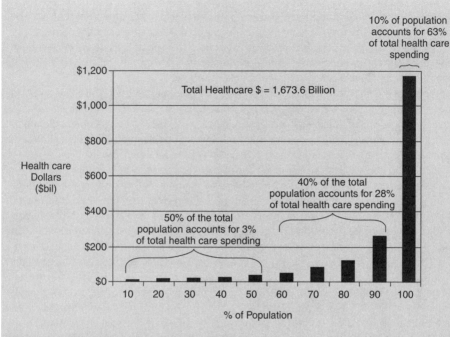

Figure 15–1 *Distribution of Health Care Spending*

Source: Avondale Partners, LLC

Programs for these individuals generally fall into the wellness/prevention categories. The individual may be overweight and could benefit from support to help develop a more sensible diet, a fitness program, or from programs designed to address stress. Others may smoke or have other unhealthy behaviors.

Although there is still considerable debate about the importance of these risk factors and what to do about them, employers are increasingly willing to at least test programs that may be proven effective in controlling the rapid growth in health care spending. In addition, there is growing awareness that the cost of absenteeism can often be several times the direct medical spending for these individuals.

The data clearly suggests 10 percent of the population will be among the highest utilizers each year. Many of these will be chronically ill. Most of these could benefit from participating in a chronic care management program focused on their condition. Others may experience some type of acute health episode such as a premature birth, a heart attack, or a serious accident. These individuals and/or their caregivers can benefit from the case-management programs Healthways offers related to intensive care, trauma, disabilities, and complex or rare disorders.

Healthways has developed a set of proprietary capabilities that are strategically important and in short supply. These capabilities will be difficult and time consuming to replicate. Health care data can be used proactively to identify and manage the health of most individuals today. Healthways receives such information from a wide variety of sources including health care claims (medical, lab, pharmacy), patient self-reported information or from a health risk assessment tool, or information from care providers such as doctors and other sources. All of this information is brought together and stored in easily accessible (and analyzable) formats.

However, winners in this business will need more than data. They need state-of-the-art care management protocols and clinical professionals with the ability and willingness to meet the needs of increasingly mobile patients over time.

Some of the effort can be managed remotely via the mail, telephone, and Internet using nurses, pharmacists, and other care providers in coordination with an individual's physician(s). Other elements must be delivered locally, including directly in a patient's home. Ultimately, it will be the combination of information and tools to help people improve their health (and a company's to improve their benefit structures) that will create the best outcomes.

Thus, the company now has a knowledge-based business that is readily scalable and that can become significantly more profitable as it matures. The business is also portable, making expansion into new geography relatively manageable. Although many of the types of players identified as having a strategic interest in the space have some of the capabilities needed to be successful, few have them all and almost none have been in the business long enough to develop a track record of performance.

The market to serve these individuals is evolving. Clearly, doctors and hospitals will play a central role. However, both the physician and hospital markets remain highly fragmented. In both cases, reimbursement for services is largely oriented around payments to treat illness rather than prevent them. Most participants in each market remain undercapitalized and have been extremely slow to integrate information technology in care management.

Winners in this business will need sophisticated information technology (IT) systems and access to information; state-of-the-art care management protocols; the ability to purchase, distribute, pay for, and manage drug therapy for an increasingly mobile population; and clinical professionals with the ability and willingness to deliver care to these patients over time.

We are not suggesting care by doctors is not necessary. Rather, once a diagnosis is made, care management can often be delivered more effectively and efficiently by care support professionals over the telephone or via the Internet. When direct care support is necessary, it is often most effectively delivered in the patient's home. Thus, unless physicians change both their approach to care and what they charge for it, they will not be central to this component of care management.

Healthways typically sells its programs through health plans. Matria has built its model by selling both through health plans and direct to self-insured employers. There are pluses and minuses to each model. Bottom line is at this point in the evolution of disease-management services both work well in most cases. By selling through health plans, Healthways avoids any competition with an insurer and assures itself of unfettered access to much of the claims data necessary to conduct its business. In addition, most health plans contract with multiple employers. By selling one new plan client, Healthways can potentially add a large number of new employer relationships at one time.

On the other hand, there are few truly national health plans. Any employer that operates in multiple locations (particularly across state lines) may need to deal with two or more different health insurers.

The odds that each contract with Healthways today are low. By contracting directly with a disease-management vendor, an employer can arrange for services from one vendor wherever that employer has operations. In this situation, it may be more difficult for the disease-management vendor to access key information from multiple insurance companies and third-party disease-management administrators.

Chapter 16

Pfizer Innovates

Prelude: A major pharmaceutical company explores the outside world.

A current buzzword, "unsiloing," mangles the word silo to make an important but simple point: Managers must cooperate across departments and functions, share revenues, and cross-sell products to boost the bottom line.

Carol Hymowitz, 2006

In 1995, Pfizer, now the world's largest pharmaceutical corporation, made an innovative decision. It created Pfizer Health Solutions, a wholly owned subsidiary, to promote health, prevent disease, manage it, and coordinate it. Pfizer also sought to increase access to care for patients suffering from chronic disease while reducing overall health costs.

Pfizer recognized a world existed beyond selling pills; medications are just part of the process of preventing and treating disease. Once patients have been prescribed medications, they pass through a health care gauntlet traversing pharmacies, health plans, Medicare, Medicaid, hospitals, rehabilitation units, outpatient surgeries, and chronic disease care at home and at work. The true costs of care lie beyond prescriptions. The pharmaceutical industry has traditionally functioned by creating "silos." These silos launch specific product lines, market them, manage them, and concentrate on them.

This silo mentality is logical. It focuses the attention of executives, managers, and sales representatives on what needs to be done; selling the product. Unfortunately, it creates a myopic vision of a complex world. Specialists live within their own world, and cross-specialty care may not be coordinated. That is why critics say health care in "fragmented." Overspecialization may distort health care's true business: to heal patients, before and after, they develop the disease.

"Siloship," to coin a phrase, misses another point: Health care may be overly specialized and fragmented. It suffers from individual and collective tunnel vision. Tunnel vision, that is, overspecialization without regard to the total picture of patient care, may be a degenerative disease of the U.S. health system. Pfizer set out, in its own way, to heal that disease and to restore the system to health by collaborating, integrating other silos, and creating and using proprietary clinical software programs.

The Pfizer Health Solutions View

Competitors may see the world differently, but what follows is perhaps an overly idealistic view of how Pfizer Health Solutions (PHS) sees the world. PHS is dedicated to improving health and health care delivery through innovative personalized, coordinated, and accessible health care services. Pfizer seeks to create positive examples of constructive health system changes that lead to structural changes in health care around the world—and, of course, along the way to better health, Pfizer would like to sell more drugs to those who need them.

PHS plans to achieve these results by developing and implementing community-based health-improvement projects. These will focus on helping individuals and populations living with or who are at risk for developing chronic diseases such as obstructive lung disorders, cardiovascular ailments, and diabetes. Working in partnership with government, health plans, physician organizations, and advocacy groups, PHS hopes to create customized care management and health-improvement programs for the commercially insured, Medicaid or Medicare beneficiaries, and the medically underserved. These programs now operate throughout the United States as well as internationally.

Fruits of Collaboration

Through these collaborations, PHS hopes to:

- Give people the tools and guidance they need to better manage their health and navigate the health care system.
- Improve communication and coordination between patients and health care providers.
- Create replicable examples of positive change including improvements in health and, as a result, reductions in health care costs.
- Break out of the "siloship" mentality.

The Seven "Cs"

PHS goes about its new business outside its former silo in these ways:

1. **Collaboration** with the multiple players and health care stakeholders delivering care: Medicare, Medicaid, health plans, hospitals, physicians, community health centers, and chronic-disease-management firms.

2. **Collection and analyzing** data across the health care spectrum in partnerships with sophisticated data mining firms like Geriatric Health System, Inc., whose predicted insurance expenditure survey (PIE) allows PHS to identify high-risk individuals and to predict future health expenses, and IX Match, Inc., which provides a knowledge management tool for gathering and tracking business development trends.

3. **Creating and testing** innovative care delivery models that will assist in fundamentally changing fragmented U.S. health care delivery.

4. **Concentrating** on and promoting health and wellness education to help prevent the pain, suffering, and cost of debilitating medical conditions.

5. **Coordinating** care for patients with medical conditions among all stakeholders who will assist in promoting care-management initiatives while improving outcomes.

6. **Committing** resources to information technologies to implement evidence-based guidelines, improve process efficiencies, and reduce costs.

7. **Cooperating** with community and political leaders to launch health initiatives for improved health in high schools, health clinics, hospitals, and neighborhood pharmacies.

One cannot implement these seven Cs without help, so PHS seeks innovative business partners who wish to increase health levels of communities, employees, or even the citizenry of their states or nations.

PHS looks to collaborate with other organizations and entities that share its goals of promoting progressive models of health care delivery and improving total patient health.

This vision, by definition, means their partners are also operating outside of the silo model and are interested in creating a cross-functional health care world. Additionally, PHS seeks partners who strive to help control total health care costs, deliver a positive ROI for their client partners, and publicize a population management and/or health care improvement story. In this manner, PHS strives to create a multiple winning experience for all participating parties as well as patient participants.

Innovation Talking and Action Points

What has just been described is hard to do. Competitors say beneath these noble goals hides a hard-edge strategy to gain an edge for selling its drugs, but one salient feature is obvious. The opportunity for health system improvement lies outside the silo. By venturing outside its silo, PHS is testing the waters of the health system at large, not just mining and minding its pharmaceutical component.

Pfizer Health Solutions seeks to reduce health costs of the chronically ill in its Medicaid program in the state of Florida's Medicaid program and in other similar programs. One may talk of community-wide prevention and health promotion, but the greatest proof lies in improving health and outcomes of the chronically ill, particularly those in the Medicaid population, which covers 53 million Americans (Rowland, 2005).

Through an unrestricted educational grant from PHS, the Faqua School of Business at Duke University issued a March 2005 report on the results of PHS's Florida: A Healthy State program, a program that started in June of 2001.

Here in brief is a summary of the Faqua evaluation.

> *The program exceeded its target number of beneficiaries by three-fold, enrolling over 150,000 Florida Medicaid enrollees. Care managers conducted intensive case management with 19,000 high-risk beneficiaries. Medical Scientists, Inc., an independent third-party organization, calculated that the program saved the state $41.9 million in medical cost savings during the first 27 months of operating, according to methodology calculations agreed upon by the AHCA (Agency Health Care Administration) and PHS. AHCA accepted these savings calculations, but the Office of Program Analysis and Governmental Accountability (OOPAGA), an oversight agency that reports to the Florida legislature, criticized the methods used to calculate the savings and argued that ACHA had not sufficiently assessed whether the program had improved health outcomes.*

AHCA and PHS responded to the OOPAGA report by saying that tracking Medicaid outcomes had inherent limitations. Still, AHCA said the program had reduced inpatient days by 12.6 percent and emergency room visits by 1 percent ("Florida," 2004).

More recently, PHS reported that inpatient days and emergency room visits were reduced (respectively) by:

- 7 percent and 18 percent for congestive heart failure patients
- 17 percent and 4.6 percent for patients with diabetes
- 4 percent and 8 percent for diabetics
- 4 percent and 1 percent for asthmatics

In 2004, the Florida legislature discontinued the PHS program, which continues to be operative for contracting reasons. Both AHCA and PHS representatives have expressed interest in continuing the programs (Florida, Pfizer urging state, 2004).

Although the PHS program has been temporarily discontinued, CMS leaders, state budget and Medicaid directors, and competing disease-management companies are intensively watching, gauging, and judging PHS's beyond-the-drug silo Medicaid performance in Florida for these reasons.

The national stakes for effective disease management are enormous. Forty years ago, Congress created Medicaid to pay for 4 million low-income people's medical needs. Today, Medicaid covers 53 million people and costs $338 billion a year in federal and state funds. The federal and the state governments share Medicaid expenses, with the states paying 40 percent of the load. Medicaid expenses are quickly outrunning the ability of states to pay for them. Medicaid now outspends Medicare, a wholly unexpected development. Medicaid accounts for one third of some states' budgets and will escalate to one half if present trends continue. Medicaid pays for 60 percent of nursing home bills. It covers 8 million disabled people and 25 million children. Medicaid costs can make up 40 percent to 50 percent of some hospitals' budgets (Lueck, 2005).

Chronic disease management is key to saving Medicaid costs. In the study by Duke University's school of business it was noted that 61 percent of national Medicaid enrollees had a chronic disease or disability. That is where the money goes, and that is where the money will be saved. Less than 20 percent of costs go to drugs (White, Fisher, Mendelson, & Schulman, 2006), a significant but not overarching or overwhelming cost element. When PHS initiated its Florida disease-management program in 2001, the deal was that PHS would provide disease management in return for a preferred discounted status for its drugs.

Medicaid care has special problems. States must cover many types of care, such as pregnancy care for low-income women. One cannot cut off beneficiary numbers, as one could do in the private sector, because patients have nowhere else to turn. Furthermore, Medicaid is a fee-for-service program. It pays doctors and hospitals every time for every encounter, making it difficult to encourage efficiency. Finally, because Medicaid enrollees pay little or nothing to see a doctor, they have no incentive to ration care—and doctors, because Medicaid fees are low or because they may not want their other patients exposed to waiting rooms full of poor Medicaid recipients, may choose not to see Medicaid patients.

Medicaid cost reductions, whether for drugs or outcomes, are difficult to measure. Outcome metrics, in short, are hard to document. The Duke University study gave these reasons for these adverse metrics:

1. *Medicaid patients are mobile and unlikely to have home phones, making accurate contact information often impossible.*
2. *Medicaid enrollees distrust unsolicited calls; they fear bill collectors and care managers who want to know about their health status.*
3. *Lower health literacy and language barriers make communication more difficult and interfere with telephonic coaching and educating through written materials.*
4. *Inflexible work schedules minimize ability to address personal issues during business hours.*
5. *Medicare enrollees are more likely to seek treatment in the ED, making follow-up tracking harder to conduct.*
6. *The Medicaid population has higher rates of mental illness and more social/ psychological issues and may be unable to understand health issues or have more poignant life crises to address.*
7. *Medicaid patients distrust doctors and hospitals because of past experiences.*
8. *Medicaid is an entitlement program so the state cannot refuse to pay for covered services.*
9. *Medicaid programs are unable to use financial incentives to alter utilization behavior.*
10. *Medicaid recipients often live in areas were environmental factors outside of their control exacerbate their health condition.* (White, Fisher, Mendelson, & Schulman, 2006)

Florida is rapidly becoming a laboratory to test effectiveness of Medicaid consumer-driven care. Governor Jeb Bush continues to restructure Florida's Medicaid program. During the year 2006, it was serving 2.2 million low-income people at an expected cost of $14.7 billion (Review and Outlook, 2005). Bush's plans are to provide incentives for better service by giving consumers more choice and by reining in spending. These moves could make Florida a model for other states and, if successful, could lead to widespread Medicaid reform.

Over the past 6 years, Florida's spending on Medicaid has grown by 13 percent a year. One quarter of the state budget already goes to Medicaid, a figure projected to hit 59 percent in 10 years. Bush's proposal would transform the system into one based on consumer choice, starting with letting participants decide how to spend the money allocated on their behalf. Each participant would be assigned a premium with which to purchase coverage for basic and catastrophic care.

Another feature of the Florida plan would allow those who follow the medical plan laid out for them by their doctors—take their medication, have their children vaccinated, stop smoking—to earn extra money to deposit for them in flexible-spending accounts.

National competition for Medicaid contracts in other states is under way. Controlling Medicaid costs is a huge potential market. This potential was highlighted in May 2006 when Healthways, Inc., a disease-management firm in Nashville, spent $307.5 billion to acquire LifeMasters, a smaller disease-management firm. LifeMasters' business included an ongoing demonstration project for 30,000 dual-eligible Medicare-Medicaid beneficiaries in Florida and contracts for services to portions of the Medicaid populations in Florida, Georgia, and Texas (Pack, 2006a).

The push of major health plans into the consumer-driven Medicaid market will likely follow. More than 3 million Americans now own Health Savings Accounts and six million are in high-deductible plans. United Health, Aetna, and Humana, among other plans, have reported significant cost reductions among consumer-incented members (Newton, 2006).

Furthermore, in the *Wall Street Journal,* Regina Herzlinger of the Harvard Business School and her coauthor Tom Nurney have been writing about how consumer-driven care is being extended and tested in states other than Florida, states such as Arkansas, Oklahoma, and South Carolina (Herzlinger & Nurney, 2005; Herzlinger, 2006a).

Case Study

Florida: A Healthy State
By Jennifer Hillyer, Vice President, Public Relations, Pfizer Health Solutions

Florida: A Healthy State (FHS) was launched in 2001 as a partnership between the state of Florida and Pfizer, Inc. It was a model health care program whose goal was to reduce rapidly growing health care costs by improving the health of chronically ill Medicaid beneficiaries.

Design of Program

The FHS program was designed to reach its goals by teaching people to proactively manage their chronic disease, increase their healthy behaviors, to drive overall health improvement, and reduce risk factors before they become complications. Through the provisions of education, personal counseling, and health-monitoring devices and tools, beneficiaries have been better able to change their behavior.

This initiative has touched over 183,000 Medicaid beneficiaries in the primary care case-management program (called MediPass) who have asthma, diabetes, hypertension, and/or heart failure among their conditions. The program links 10 of the state's critical safety-net community hospitals together, employing 60 specially trained care managers who provide education, support, and establish an ongoing relationship with high-risk, chronically ill beneficiaries.

Community Organizations and Advocacy Groups

Additionally, more than 350 community organizations and advocacy groups have been involved. Over 600,000 culturally relevant and literacy-appropriate education materials have been distributed to the targeted populations. Over 35,000 home health tools such as blood pressure cuffs, peak flow meters, and scales, have been distributed to participants, enabling them to self-monitor their conditions. Over 24,000 participants with the highest disease risk and burden of illness have been paired with specially hired and trained nurse care managers. All participants have been actively using 24-hour access to triage nurses and health advice.

New Insights

New partnering approaches yield important insights. Of the many lessons learned, the following four guiding principles have given the program greater value and supported its success:

1. *People need tools and education to become proactive in their care.* People often lack the knowledge necessary to manage their disease; they may not even know they are sick. They must understand their condition, the impact of their behavior, and have access to the tools they need to effectively manage their conditions.

2. *Real change requires a local support network.* A committed network of care managers and local organizations that help people in their own languages and communities is essential to success.

3. *Health care delivery is only one part of the health equation.* The path to better health and higher quality of life is driven strongly by social, cultural, family, and financial issues and access to care. Understanding and overcoming these barriers are vital to avoiding and improving medical conditions. Medicaid beneficiaries may, for example, need help with transportation, nutrition, and other social services. FHS care managers help people better connect with the health care system and address problematic barriers in other aspects of their lives, so that their health can become a more important part of their daily routine.

4. *Motivated people can directly impact the cost of their health care.* Educated and engaged people can be healthier and delay the onset of complex chronic conditions. Although they may interact with health care professionals more frequently, their need for acute and costly services such as emergency services and hospital care can be significantly reduced.

Results

Through the help of the FHS care network, participants have changed their behaviors and improved their health, which has led to improved clinical measures such as lower blood sugar in diabetics, lower blood pressure in hypertensive patients, and improved heart function for those with heart failure.

From these clinical improvements people are using emergency rooms and hospitals less and going to routine doctor visits more. The program continues to help people change the way they use and interact with the health care system as they become healthier and consistently seek care in the physicians' offices, rather than costly visits to the ED or hospital.

FHS has exceeded expectations in medical cost reductions to the state of Florida—and while the immediate savings of the program are significant, the program's influence on people and communities will continue to make a profound impact into the future as people manage their health properly.

Lessons Learned

FHS had to take a fundamentally different approach to enrollment, education, and health maintenance when addressing the Medicaid population. The key lesson is that any disease-management program must consider how lower health literacy, limited mobility, language and cultural barriers, and distrust of the existing system all play a large part in dictating how a person responds to help. With the extensive limitations put on Medicaid-affiliated disease-management programs, a complete solution such as FHS can effectively manage the complex needs of a large and difficult Medicaid population.

	7/01– 6/02	7/02– 9/03	10/03– 9/04	*Total*
Medical cost savings*	$12.0**	$27.3	$30.7	$70.0
Program operating expenses and direct investment in Florida health care services	5.6	11.2	8.2	25.0
Health Literacy Study and product donations*	.9	1.5	—	2.4
Total Financial Guarantee	**$15.0**	**$22.5**	**$19.2**	**$56.7**
Total Savings	**$18.5**	**$40.0**	**$38.9**	**$97.4**

Note: Data for year 4 will be released when available.

*Medical cost savings were validated by a third-party organization, Medical Scientists Inc. Actual expenses were compared to expected expenses for the four disease categories and two population groups—TANF (Temporary Assistance for Needy Families) and SSI (Supplemental Security Income) recipients—computed using a combination of the state's budget, actuarial estimates based on historic trends, and epidemiologic models predicting health service utilization and disease progression.

**All numbers are in millions.

Implications

The implications of this groundbreaking program are far-reaching and may provide guidance to policy makers and legislators for the future. This model can be applied to other states (with aspects of it also being applicable to Medicare, commercial, and employee populations) looking to not only find a strong fiscal solution to stretched Medicaid budgets, but also make a tangible and lasting positive effect on the health of the population. Chronic disease is on the rise worldwide, and as the U.S. population ages, it will become a more acute problem. A proactive solution that seeks to understand the individual both physically and emotionally is the only way to change behaviors and put people on the path to better health.

Chapter 17

Restless and Rebellious Employers

Prelude: Not only the natives are restless. America's private employers, who pay for more than half of the nation's health benefits, are increasingly restless about shouldering the burden of rising health care premiums.

The innovations that employer-sponsored insurance has sparked, however, have not proven to be sufficient to ameliorate our nation's fundamental problems of cost, quality, and access to services.

. . . employers may pay the piper but they have been unable to call a consistent tune, for many reasons.

First, with rare exceptions individual employers lack sufficient number of employees in any one market to impress providers with the need to follow their leadership in changing how health care is organized and provided.

Innovative employers tend to be large, and large firms tend to be national. Second, local business coalitions, which may have sufficient market power, have proven difficult to form and sustain for reasons that speak to underlying weaknesses of employer-sponsored insurance in promoting health care reform. Employer-sponsored insurance has proven unable to contain the ferocious forces driving cost increases in the United States and seems to be ill-constructed to do so in the future.

David Blumenthal, 2006

Two trends emerge.

First, American employers are no longer going to play the role of passive consumer. Whether through participation in Leapfrog or other cooperative efforts to drive quality, employers are willing to dirty their hands in the push to improve the health care system.

Second, if the system does not improve and costs continue to rise, employers may no longer share the ride and will start to look for ways to legally and strategically bail out. This is a not a bluff that payers and providers dare to call.

Philip Betheze, 2005

U.S. employers are lowering costs by shifting risks and costs to employees. These shifts take many forms:

- from rewards for exercise
- to stopping smoking
- to losing weight
- to transitioning from HMOs and PPOs to high-deductible plans
- to paying more to hospitals and physicians who adopt quality incentives
- to disease management at home and at work

The Employers' Last Stand

In the December 2005 cover story of *HealthLeaders* magazine, Philip Betbeze describes employers' attitudes as their "last stand." Perhaps he's right. The percentage of employees covered by insurance dropped from 69 percent to 60 percent since 2000. To become globally competitive, GM and Ford cut 60,000 workers (Dingel says Bush ignores, 2006). Employer-based insurance may be in jeopardy because employers feel they can no longer afford to pay for rising health costs of employees.

Stuart Altman, professor of national health policy at Brandeis University, questions "whether it (the health system) can survive the next 10 to 20 years, without something being done to moderate premium increases" (Betbeze, 2005). Brian Klepper, president of the Center for Practical Health Reform, adds, "It's clear employers are reducing health care coverage. They're offering fewer and slimmer benefits. Non-health care CEOs are apoplectic about possible deterioration of their workers' health and declining productivity" (Klepper, 2006). Klepper also maintains that only U.S. businesses have the motivation and clout to pressure Congress to reform health care in a rational fashion (by restructuring the system and putting into place management and control systems needed). Klepper explained his comments in a newspaper article that he authored:

Last September the CEOs of several Fortune firms—Costco, Verizon, Honeywell, Starbucks, Drugstore.com—met in Washington to register alarm over unrelenting health-care cost growth.

The meeting sent two important messages.

First, if not restrained, health-care costs will trump every firm's profitability and competitiveness. No commitment to generous benefits can withstand them. Over the last five years health-care premiums—where all health-care costs converge—have risen 5.5 times as fast as general inflation, four times as fast as workers' earnings and 2.3 times as fast as business income growth.

Second, rather than sending subordinates, the CEOs went to Washington themselves. This conveyed the crisis now warrants the focus of our most influential business leaders and immediate attention on the national policy agenda.

The considerable human implications aside, the economics of health care's cost explosion are profound. Skyrocketing premiums are pricing individuals, corporations, and governments out of coverage. U.S. Bureau of Labor Statistics data show fewer than 45 percent of private sector jobs now offer health benefits, and that number is dropping every year.

Erosion in government-funded coverage is next. As health care takes bigger bites of local, state and national budgets, we can expect reduced allocations for Medicare, Medicaid, public employee and retiree health benefits and public health programs.

Fewer people with insurance will mean fewer financial inputs to the health-care system, a gathering storm for an industry accustomed to always getting more. For example, America's safety net hospitals now operate at paper-thin margins.

Cut back on safety-net reimbursements and increase their load of uninsured and underinsured patients, and many will collapse. Even worse, because health-care is the nation's largest business sector—one-seventh of the economy and one-eleventh of the nation's jobs—its increasing instability could threaten the national economic security.

So far, we've had little real leadership on this crisis. Aware that change will compromise profitability, the health-care industry continues to resist collaborating on meaningful reforms.

The Bush administration's recent proposals—high deductible plans and more individual responsibility—are ideological, not structural solutions.

They will do little if anything to get costs under control.

Meanwhile, Congress is beholden to health care's many powerful special interests and is seemingly paralyzed by the problem's complexity.

Only the larger business community is strong enough to initiate the course correction. By mobilizing, America's non-health-care business interests could pressure Congress and the health-care industry to rapidly implement the standards, transparency, performance incentives and other disciplines required to re-stabilize health-care and that other progressive industries already take for granted. (Klepper, 2006)

As Brian Klepper noted, "Business leaders are, whether they choose to think of themselves as such, in reality, 'health care business practitioners.' For every day of their lives, these leaders and their surrogates insure, broker, purchase, finance, supply, deliver, and support health care" (Klepper, 2006). By this definition, U.S. businesspersons, their purchasing agents, and their health care surrogates are very much health care practitioners.

RHIOs

However, as much as business leaders seek to control and rationalize health care and its costs, their task as health care business practitioners is not easy. Getting a handle on controlling costs can be a snake pit of competing interests. Take the case of regional health information organizations (RHIOs). Supposedly these proposed information entities will form the heart of community data sharing.

What Is a RHIO?

According to W. Holt Anderson, executive director of the North Carolina Health Care Information and Communication Alliance, a RHIO exists when you see an organization consisting of multiple competing enterprises. These enterprises collaborate, build connections, move information among themselves to serve patients, and share agreements and policies allowing patients to get information at the point of care.

RHIO progress, however, remains elusive and slow. Why? What are the problems that slow their establishment?

- Money is a problem. How much will they cost? Who will pay? Will they save money or cost money? Who will they benefit—health plans, employers, hospitals, doctors, or patients?

- "Friendliness-of-use" for doctors using electronic health records (EHRs) is a problem. Will doctors accept them, use them, resist them? Will they regard EHRs as just another bureaucratic boondoggle? As a threat to their clinical sovereignty? As an unneeded, unwanted expense?

- Replication and public domain exposure are problems. Can RHIOs be replicated in different settings? Is the information generated available for public consumption and for use and abuse by government and private entities?

- Patient issues are a problem. Does the data invade their privacy; do you need their consent? Do patients understand RHIOs are necessary for efficiency, safety, and cost effectiveness? Will they become involved and insist on data transfer? (Blair, 2006)

Hospital and physician payment is another problem.

- Will hospitals and doctors be given financial incentives to install EHRs?
- Will the government and private insurers demand EHRs be installed for the purpose of generating compliance with quality indicators, or else providers will not be paid?

On August 6, 2006, the Bush administration took a step in this direction when Secretary Mike Leavitt announced that the U.S. Department of Health and Human Services will launch an ambitious effort to ensure quality. It will require all providers of federally funded health care to adopt quality-measurement tools and uniform information technology standards.

Bush then signed an executive order setting the new requirements. Leavitt said by year's end, the 100 largest private employers will sign similar contracts with the hospitals and doctors they use to care for their workers.

The Evolution of RHIOs

Depending on how you define RHIOs, there may be as many as 300 RHIOs already in existence. Business models are founded on centralized repositories of patient information and decentralized databases owned by RHIO-member organizations. RHIOs may evolve out of single organizations, multiple membership health care organizations (HCOs), community origins, individual practice associations (IPAs), state-level mandates, and multistate collaboratives. Whatever the genesis of these organizations, the entities that make them up compete with each other. Let us be clear: Data sharing among hospitals, clinics, and physician practices entails "competing" organizations. These organizations will require formal and legal partnership agreements.

When speaking about RHIOs, transparency, and data sharing, keep these points in mind:

- Those who say they want to share data compete with one another.
- They may therefore be slow to come to the table.
- They are reluctant to share and show data revealing their strengths and weaknesses, strategic advantages and disadvantages, and profits and losses—anything that can be used against one another.

However, as costs soar and as payers develop more sophisticated aggregating software, aggregated costs around disease episodes involving hospitals, outpatient facilities, ambulatory surgical centers, and physicians' offices will be what counts; not what an individual entity charges. As consumers demand bundled costs for each care episode, business leaders will demand data sharing, aggregation, and upfront cost transparency.

At the point at which aggregated data becomes the focal point of negotiation with payers, data showing improved health and better outcomes may overwhelm mutual distrust among competing parties. To overcome this distrust, neutral third parties are stepping into the void by forming data depositories stripped of name recognition or by creating data collection techniques that do not require expensive electronic health records or hospital–physician systems that communicate with each other.

The role of those trying to put together corporate payers, insurers, hospitals, and patients is a difficult one. In the end, the cooperation of patients is essential. It is them who will:

- benefit most from data sharing
- demand hospitals and doctors share data
- pay more of the costs in a consumer-driven environment

Putting together RHIOs takes the skills of a contortionist. RHIO leaders must keep their finger in the wind, their nose in the air, their eye on the horizon, and their ear to the ground. In other words, leaders must use all of their senses to achieve consensus while meeting with competing parties.

Angst, Anger, and Anguish

Business leaders have a hard time expressing their distrust over the intractabilities, irrationalities, and irresponsibilities of the health system. For one, they may cite the cases of GM and Ford, American auto companies that are now reaching junk bond status because of $1,500 per vehicle health costs (Johnson, 2006). In addition, they may quote Howard Schultz, the chairman of Starbucks, who says the cost of his employees' health coverage exceeds the costs of coffee (CNNMoney.com, 2006). In the end, however, they are not yet capable of pinning physicians and hospitals to the money mat.

How bad are the business problems of paying for health care when it comes to competing internationally? It can best be explained by using the "tale of the tape" technique. This is a time-honored approach used by sports writers for comparing the physical measurements of competing fighters. Here is the tale of the tape for American health care.

The tape, namely the measurement of money U.S. businesses pay for health care, demonstrates, beyond reasonable doubt, that U.S. businesses that pay for 54 percent of total health care costs face a tough fight against foreign competitors, where the government picks up more of the costs of health care (Freudenheim, 2006c). In the United States, health costs are still rising twice as fast as inflation. The following measurements capture the monumental and so far losing struggle of U.S. business-people to reduce health costs.

- According to an April 2006 Commonwealth Fund survey, the United States spends $5,635 per capita for health costs, versus $3,003 for Canada, $2,996 for Germany, $2,903 for Australia, and $2,231 for the United Kingdom.
- In 2005, employer health premiums went up 9.2 percent, again more than three times general inflation, with an average premium of $4,000 for an individual and $11,000 for a family of four.
- In 2004, total spending was $1.9 trillion, $6,280 per person; total spending is expected to rise to $2.9 billion by 2009, and $4.0 trillion by 2015, 20 percent of the GNP compared to the present 16 percent.
- Health insurance expenses are the fastest-growing costs of business, up 143 percent since 2000, and are projected to exceed profits by 2008.

Unsustainable health costs will not be sustained unless the United States chooses to be in a losing global fight. Moderating costs may be beyond the reach of business and may require, as Emanuel and Fuchs speculated, that it would take a depression, natural disaster, or an international war to achieve universal coverage, which might shift health costs from business to government.

Managing, Monitoring, Modeling, and Living Another Day

Restructuring U.S. health care; using management platforms, computer monitoring, and mathematical models for rationalized costs; and ensuring quality as used by other industry sectors may be a partial answer, but it will do little to quench the desire of humans everywhere to live another day in the best possible health.

Dr. John Najarian, a University of Minnesota transplant surgeon, once said to me, "I have never met a patient who didn't want to live another day." That is why patients seek heart transplants and timely access to the other wonders of medical technology. Wanting to live another day is a universal desire and a difficult emotion to contain no matter what the cost.

Case Study

RHIOs as Instruments of Market-Based Reform

By Brian Klepper, PhD

Brian Klepper is the president of the Jacksonville, Florida–based Center for Practical Health Reform, a non–partisan national effort to reestablish stability and sustainability in U.S. health care. Klepper is an acknowledged expert on the subject of national health reform—but he is also a realist. He believes reform will require management tools deployed by U.S. corporations to rein in costs, improve care, and select and reward hospitals and physicians who deliver that care.

Can regional health information organizations actually bring off the kinds of reforms we need? I think so. They'll be good at doing a couple things very well.

First, they'll provide more complete information that will allow everyone touching health care to make better decisions.

Second, they'll create pricing and performance transparency—and that will set the stage for more robust changes, as purchasers demand performance-based reimbursement. But imagine how these structures can work at the outset.

You've just changed health plans and your child's pediatrician isn't in the network. So in the throes of an asthmatic episode, you take him to a new doctor's office. In the exam room, a nurse asks you to list his medications. Flustered, you recite the ones you remember. Then, she enters his name into the computer.

Up comes a list of his drugs—there's one you missed—as well as all health information about him that's available in the computers of the region's doctors' offices, hospitals, labs, and diagnostic centers. With knowledge of the extra drug, the doctor takes a different course of action than she otherwise would have.

You didn't have to (yet again) fill out your son's personal information and history, because it is already in the system. The doctor can check notes made by other physicians and immediately see previous test results and images. She needs to do some tests, but she does not need to redo others. Another doctor ordered those recently on him. This new physician can use that information.

The doctor writes her notes in your son's chart and, when they're completed, his test results are entered as well. This information is now also available to any clinician in the region who sees him.

This was better quality, safer care. It was cheaper, faster, and more convenient. The doctor had complete information, so she could make the best decisions possible. The patient and the insurance company did not have to pay to get information that was already available. State-of-the-science privacy and security protections were in place, so your son's information was available only to other clinicians, and only if you've given written permission.

In this new world, everyone on the network—physicians, nurses, hospitals, long-term care facilities, pharmacists, diagnostic centers and social workers—has access to at least a basic electronic medical record and can get the patient's most recent and important information before making a care decision.

What's more, changes made to the patient's electronic medical chart (the one used by the clinicians) can automatically update your son's personal health record (a "lite" version for patient's use) as well.

You, your doctors, and possibly a family representative are the only ones with permission to see that one. You can enter information into your personal health record, so that you can track your health over time, and so the medical professionals will see it. As we continue to move toward consumer-directed health plans with high deductibles, these new tools can help every patient monitor and manage both the care and costs of his or her own health.

Most health care professionals now take it for granted that linking health care organizations and professionals through the Web would create tremendous quality, safety, and cost improvements. New tools can make sense of the Babel of different computer systems and formats. Implementing them will require the collaboration of health care's different players.

However, there is every reason to believe that, once available, they'll enhance the overall experience for everyone involved, making access to the delivery of quality care less stressful, less complicated, and less expensive.

In government jargon, the organizations that facilitate the exchange of local health information are called RHIOs and they're popping up all over the country. The most practical RHIOs are designed to be "community healthcare utilities." These are not-for-profit organizations supported by the larger community (and potentially hosted by a neutral party, like a local university). A RHIO creates value by linking health care professionals and organizations, and by delivering information that supports better health care decision making by all health care constituencies within the community. The RHIO must demonstrate to its participants that it is a worthwhile investment; only then can it achieve financial stability, independent of external funding from government or philanthropies.

RHIOs are a profoundly new and important development. By facilitating information exchange across professional and institutional boundaries, they should streamline out-of-control health care costs—but equally importantly, the health care crisis is rooted in an inability to see and act on problems and opportunities that exist in the health care marketplace.

Employers are the key to realizing the RHIO's enormous potential, which includes substantial cost savings and quality improvements. Employers pay about half the bills in health care and so have every reason to become actively engaged in a health care information network. Only if they do can they enforce the disciplines of transparency and accountability and bring about performance-based reimbursement to make health care stable and sustainable again.

Chapter 18

Understanding Complexity, Consulting, and Clinical Boundaries

Prelude: Consultants understand how to innovate to overcome complexities, cross boundaries, and create new paradigms.

Management consulting has become the primary source for innovation in the practice of management, forming a bridge between academia, firms, and thought leaders in other fields.

Wikipedia, 2006

Complex adaptive systems (CASs) are ubiquitous. Stock markets, human bodies, forest ecosystems, manufacturing businesses, immune systems, and hospitals are all examples of CASs.

What is a complex adaptive system? Each word is significant. "Complex" implies diversity—a great number of connections between wide varieties of elements. "Adaptive" suggests the capacity to alter or change—the ability to learn from experience. A "system" is a set of connected or independent things.

Brenda Zimmerman, Curt Lindberg, and Paul Pisek, 1998

Medical researchers and clinicians often work in isolation, yet, as pointed out in this book's introduction, innovation requires teamwork, organizational leadership, capital, and exposure to a larger world if it is to make a difference.

This is especially true in today's complex health care world with so much at stake. This is also where consultants come in. They see a wider world than the typical research worker or practicing doctor.

What are the similarities between researchers and clinicians? Researchers and clinicians similarly understand the power of science, curiosity, and independent work, but they may not understand health care collectively is a huge enterprise, calling for diverse talents from other fields outside their own.

- Physicians may not understand they may need expert and impartial outside advice if they are going to produce significant innovations.
- They may not understand that traditional scientific methods do not always work in a complex world.
- Physician thinking may rest on linear thinking, on conceiving of the human body and of health organizations as logical machines.

Modern health care, however, is nonlinear. It is rife with outside influences, office politics, gossip, competing factions striving for wealth and position, internal and external conflicting patterns of behavior, and positioning of the organization to please stakeholders, stockholders, and society at large. Sometimes only a consultant who has roamed through multiple organizations and across multiple boundaries understands how all these variables interact.

The worlds of scientific research and clinical medicine are, well, complex. In a classic book, *Edgeware: Insights from Complexity Science for Health Care Leaders,* these truths for functioning and surviving in a complex world emerge:

- View your world, your organization, and your work through the lens of complexity. You are part of a dynamic, ever-changing system and part of a much larger world. It may take an outside eye to understand.
- Build a good-enough vision, provide minimum specifications, and do not plan every little detail. Look at what others are doing. There may be connections. You may not see them if you are too insular or too focused.
- Balance data and intuition, planning, acting, safety, and risk, giving due honor to each. Innovate. Look for what connects you, not what separates you.
- Tune to the edge of your world. Look for connections inside and outside the organizations. Don't try to control information, force agreement, and ignore contentious groups. People are political animals. You have to work your way through the hierarchy.
- Learn to uncover and work with paradox and tension. They are a natural part of being human—and of finding innovative niches.
- Let your direction arise from the circumstances. You don't have to be certain— to be "sure" before you proceed with anything. Ready, fire, aim.
- Listen to the shadow system—gossip, rumors, and hallway conversations. This shadow system is important. It moves organizations. It creates insights, connections, and innovations.

- Grow complex systems by chunking. Start small. Complex systems emerge out of simple things that work well independently.
- Cooperate and compete at the same time. It's not one or another. (Zimmerman, Lindberg, & Pisket, 1998)

In other words, do not work in isolation. Understand you are part of something bigger. If your enterprise is big enough, on the average, good things, often random things, but big things, will happen. Also understand you need innovations—new ways of looking at things—if you and your organization are to remain vital and sustain freshness and growth.

One problem with researchers and physicians and hospitals is that because of past public support and generous funding, both have succeeded on their own relatively isolated terms within their own cocoons and have been relatively immune to economics of the outside world. As costs rise, taxpayers resist paying more, and competition for dollars and support intensifies, the old isolationism is fading.

Enter the Businesspeople

As medicine has become commercialized and has been taken over by large organizations, more businesslike thinking has entered health care, research activities, and clinical practice. Businesspeople understand complexity. In health care, the dynamics of capitalization, the law of large numbers, and "economies of scale" become important. Businesspeople understand they must be big enough if good things and sustainable innovations crossing organization and societal barriers are to have impact. Consultants understand this too.

Researchers and clinicians, often isolated and preoccupied with their one-on-one relationships with experiments and patients and with little training in business, may not grasp the magnitude of the health care enterprise—nor do they have the organizational structure, traditions, or capital resources to call upon such management consulting firms as McKinsey and Company, Booz Allen Hamilton, Boston Consulting Group, or Bain & Company for help. Outside consultants sometimes see what internal stakeholders do not see: that health care is a huge and potentially lucrative enterprise if properly capitalized and organized on the basis of economies of scale.

In the 1990s, the practice management industry, led by such organizations as PhyCor and Medpartners, and other specialty management companies, rushed in to fill the corporate void. However, because of resistance by hospitals and physicians, these physician management firms lost money, physicians lost confidence in them, and the stock market abandoned them. The industry virtually disappeared in the late 1990s.

Of course, a few health care organizations like Kaiser Permanente, the Mayo Clinic, academic institutions, and large hospital-based health care systems were big enough and corporate enough to make it on their own without outside corporate help or advice. Most doctors, however, still did not quite grasp this reality. Collectively, health care is the biggest single economic sector of the U.S. economy and the fastest growing (Kolata, 2006b).

A few doctors understood what was going on, and they left their clinical careers to become physician executives. They helped found an organization called the American College of Physician Executives, which now has about 12,000 members. Compare this to the number of consultants hired by the major management consulting firms: just one firm—Booz Allen Hamilton, for example—has 17,000 consultants, not all devoted to health care, but a significant number nonetheless. There are many large health care consultant companies and a number of national health care law firms as well, all anxious to offer their consulting services.

Large Corporations Will Shape Physicians' Futures

Large health care corporations with capital, market reach, and ability to generate billions of dollars will shape physician practices in the future. This should not come as a surprise. Society has entrusted the huge social task of health care to corporations, with their concentrations of money and power. As Peter F. Drucker (1968) observed nearly 40 years ago, society entrusts large social tasks, like health care, to large organizations.

Corporate power came into sharper focus with the 2005 World Health Care Congress, held in Washington, D.C. Sponsors included the *Wall Street Journal, Accenture*, Booz Allen Hamilton, CIGNA, the UnitedHealth Group, and AstraZeneca. Attending were 136 senior executives from large health care corporations. Independent practicing physicians simply weren't there in 2005.

Either physicians weren't invited to the congress or they couldn't afford to be away from their offices. Besides, many of them wouldn't have been comfortable in this corporate meeting. Eighty-one percent of independent clinicians belong to practices of nine or less, lack expertise to market, have insufficient funds to build information infrastructures, and don't have the time to be at the negotiating table (AHRQ, 2005).

You could argue physician associations should perform these functions. Unfortunately, professional associations are not effective business organizations. Lack of effective business organizations among primary care clinicians leaves little room for leverage or expansion, as noted in a 2006 *Journal of the American Medical Association* article:

> The absence of a professional organization for all primary care professionals, linking family medicine, internal medicine, and pediatrics, and advance practice nursing renders coherent primary care workforce planning substantially more difficult. (Rosenblatt, Andrilla, Curtin, & Hart, 2006)

Innovation Talking and Action Points

Large organizations have capital and other resources, including skilled managers and support personnel, to make large-scale innovations. Physicians with backgrounds in both clinical practice and the marketplace are positioned to be major contributors to these new innovations.

Many attribute the incredible success of the UnitedHealth Group to the clinical experience and insights of Dr. William McGuire, a former pulmonologist. Through his knowledge of small practices and his subsequent experiences in building in HMOs (which profit by knowing the needs of and marketing to large populations), McGuire knew the limitations of small numbers, the law of large numbers, the importance of public capital, and the opportunities of the economies of scale in health care.

Innovation management has become a discipline among management consultants. It is now understood sustainable growth requires constant and incremental innovation. Health care now consumes 16 percent of the GNP, and exploding health costs make systematic innovation imperative. Because of the scope and intricacies of health care, outside impartial and objective advice is needed. For hospitals, which alone account for about 4 percent of the GNP, calling upon outside consultants is a tradition.

That is why, of course, the management consulting industry and practice-management consultants market their services to hospitals and to large physician groups. There—to use the Willie Sutton expression of why he robbed banks—is where the money is.

Management consultants recognize, in Peter Drucker's language, "systematic innovation consists of the purposeful and organized search for changes, and in the systematic analysis of the opportunities such changes might offer for economic or social innovation" (Drucker, 1985). According to Drucker, in *Innovation and Entrepeneurship,* there are seven sources for innovative exploitation of change:

1. *The unexpected*—the unexpected success, the unexpected failure, the unexpected outside event
2. *The incongruity* between reality as it actually is and reality as it is assumed to be or as it ought to be
3. *Innovation as a process need*
4. *Changes in industry structure or market structure* catching everybody unawares
5. *Demographics* (population changes)
6. *Changes in perception, mood, or meaning*
7. *New knowledge,* both scientific and nonscientific

These are the changes health care organizations and health care stakeholders have to exploit through innovation if they are to succeed. In addition, these are changes management consultants often understand better than the stakeholders because of their broad view of society and industry.

Case Study

Research Meets Practice: A Nationwide Cancer Information Network Could Use Cross-Boundary Knowledge to Promote a Broader Base of Breakthroughs

By Robin Portman, Kevin Vigilante, and Brenda Ecken, consultants for Booz Allen Hamilton

Robin Portman is a vice president of Booz Allen Hamilton in Rockville, Maryland. Portman leads health-related programs for strategic planning, program management and evaluation, and technology systems integration and delivery in support of research programs.

Kevin Vigilante is a physician and a principal of Booz Allen Hamilton in Rockville, Maryland. Dr. Vigilante leads health-related programs related to biomedical informatics, preparedness, health safety and quality, and strategic planning.

Brenda Ecken, a senior associate with Booz Allen Hamilton in Rockville, Maryland, has more than 20 years of health care experience. She specializes in leveraging technology within the health care industry for improved performance, reduced costs, and improved market penetration.

This case study is from *Strategy and Business,* a Booz Allen Hamilton publication.

In Seattle and Baltimore, two university-based cancer research teams competed for years. Isolated from each other, the teams spent countless hours creating similar software tools intended to mine a variety of genomes for clues to cancer.

Now they've each had a breakthrough: The two teams separately discovered the same gene. However, they've given the gene slightly different names, and they correlate it with different functions—one team associates it with the efficacy of a cancer drug; the other sees it as a marker for certain types of brain cancer. Linking these two observations would provide valuable insights for the drug-development process, but barriers to communication, both technical and cultural, prevent that crucial connection from being made.

Another story is unfolding in a small suburb outside Buffalo, New York. A cancer patient named William B visits his oncologist to treat the stage 4 glioma that has invaded the left side of his brain. Mr. B asks his Buffalo-based doctor if he is aware of any experimental drugs or research programs that might help him.

The physician, already 2 hours behind schedule with 20 more patients to see before running back to the hospital, stares back at Mr. B blankly, says he will look into it, and scribbles a reminder in the paper chart. Of course, he never follows up—so Mr. B never learns about the clinical trials at an academic medical center in Cleveland, where a doctor—we'll call her Dr. Kelly—is struggling to recruit a sufficient number of glioma patients to test the efficacy of a new investigational drug.

Unfortunately, these two stories represent the rule, rather than the exception, in biomedical research.

In the first case, expensive redundancy drives up the cost of taxpayer-funded basic research while information silos undermine the potential for scientific collaboration.

In the second case, a patient is denied treatment that might have been beneficial while inefficiencies in recruiting research subjects drive up the cost of a clinical trial designed to test a promising new compound.

The second story also illustrates a particularly compelling challenge: how to build stronger links between medical research and medical practice. Doctors and their patients desperately need information on the latest therapeutic breakthroughs and clinical trials, but "bench scientists"(scientists who work in the laboratory) and research physicians who run clinical trials rarely interact with community physicians—yet the care that a patient receives represents the end of a long value chain to which each of these individuals, and many others, make important contributions.

Finally, both stories help explain the current stagnation in new drug research. The pharmaceutical industry and the National Institutes of Health have each more than doubled their investments in research and development over the last decade. However, despite this dramatic increase in spending, the number of new chemical compounds submitted to the U.S. Food and Drug Administration annually has declined from approximately 45 in 1996 to approximately 25 in 2003, according to a March 2004 FDA report titled *Innovation/Stagnation: Challenge and Opportunity on the Critical Path to New Medical Products.* The shortfall in biomedical research won't be cured by infusions of cash; we've tried that. What is required is a fundamental change in the way research is conducted.

Collaboration and Communities

The National Cancer Institute (NCI), the lead federal agency for cancer research, is confronting these challenges through a paradigm-changing program called the Cancer Biomedical Informatics Grid, or caBIG. Launched by the NCI's Center for Bioinformatics in 2003, caBIG aspires to create an informatics network that connects cancer researchers (and eventually all researchers) nationwide: a World Wide Web of cancer research.

Using common standards and an open-source approach (one that encourages participants to join in designing and expanding the system), caBIG links data, research tools, scientists, and organizations in a virtual research environment. The goal is to create a voluntary forum in which the sharing of data produces research synergies and speeds the process of discovery. The most significant challenges are not technical, but cultural. For scientists to achieve the vision, former competitors will need to collaborate.

Today, research teams sequester precious data as they race to publish their findings in peer-reviewed journals. Those who publish first, and most often, are rewarded with grants, promotions, and tenure. Although competition certainly encourages productivity, the stagnation in discovery of new chemical compounds suggests that the benefits of isolated research do not outweigh the costs. Therefore, in addition to making information sharing technically feasible, the caBIG designers are seeking to prompt a dramatic cultural change in the cancer research community to make collaboration more likely. This will not occur through goodwill alone; incentives such as grant awards, academic promotion, and tenure are needed to break down the information silos that separated those researchers in Seattle and Baltimore.

Now consider the case of William B, the patient in the second story, who is grappling with brain cancer—and a communication breakdown as well, though he doesn't know it. The inability to match Mr. B in Buffalo with Dr. Kelly in Cleveland is both tragic and expensive. Currently, it costs an average of more than $900 million to bring a new drug to market, with an average clinical trial budget of $162 million.

Approximately 16 percent of the clinical trial budget goes to patient enrollment: finding people like Mr. B whose diseases qualify them for participation in the experiments. Pharmaceutical company executives have ranked patient enrollment as the process with the greatest opportunity for improvement in their clinical research enterprise. This perspective is supported by the Center Watch's State of the Clinical Trials Industry report for 2005, which estimates that more than half of the delays in clinical trials can be attributed to patient-recruitment problems.

Why is it so hard to find patients for trials? Because physicians don't have the information they need for referrals. Only one third of patients learn about clinical trials from their primary-care or specialty-care physicians.

That's hardly surprising, given the results of another Center Watch study (March 2004) in which 58 percent of physicians said they don't refer their patients because they lack information on the treatment or trial, followed by 30 percent who said they didn't have enough time to learn about and evaluate the trial, and 28 percent who said they were unsure where to refer their patients.

Intelligent Health Care Records

Imagine a different scenario for Mr. B. Instead of a paper chart, his physician uses an "intelligent" electronic health record (EHR) that links to a research infrastructure network such as caBIG. Smart applications scan Mr. B's health data and note that he is 53 years old, that his liver and kidney functions are normal, and that his CAT scan reveals a brain mass measuring 4 centimeters in diameter.

The biopsy report in the EHR confirms the diagnosis of glioma. The computer then scans a list of current clinical trials in NCI's databases, whittles it down to those relevant to glioma, and further examines inclusion and exclusion criteria for those trials—factors such as tumor size, duration of previous treatment, age, and kidney and liver function. The EHR recognizes that Mr. B may be eligible for at least three clinical trials that are still recruiting patients, including Dr. Kelly's.

A message appears on the computer screen in Mr. B's physician's office, stating Mr. B may be eligible for clinical trials at one or more NCI-designated cancer research centers. Mr. B's physician clicks on one of the links and a user-friendly recruitment process has begun.

Except for one or two trips to Cleveland, Mr. B receives his care and experimental medications from his current oncologist near Buffalo. Reports regarding tumor response and side effects of the treatment are automatically extracted from the EHR and sent to Dr. Kelly and the study nurse coordinator in Cleveland for review. Not only have Mr. B and Dr. Kelly been matched at low cost and almost without friction, but the trial is being monitored remotely without the need for paper files.

The benefits of building this type of intelligence into the health care records system are obvious. Patients get access to the newest treatments; researchers can conduct trials more efficiently; and those who pay for these trials—largely the pharmaceutical industry and the taxpayers supporting NIH—can expect better results at a lower cost. In addition, the available pool of cancer patients for trial recruitment is richer and more easily identified.

Linking community oncologists with the research enterprise will enable them to become true customers of research, giving them ready access to the rapidly expanding body of medical understanding that can improve their practice.

It has been well documented that disparities exist between new research evidence, particularly those involving effective medical interventions and the general state of clinical practice. Outdated therapies persist despite new findings; advances in medical knowledge and treatment capabilities can take years to reach patients.

To be sure, physicians are supposed to base their practice on the evidence of new research studies, as published in the academic peer-reviewed literature. However, there are thousands of journals publishing many thousands of articles each year. It is almost impossible for busy clinicians to keep up with the abundance of new information coming from the scientific community.

Physicians are often influenced more by the practice habits of local colleagues in their social networks than by the evidence-based literature. Therefore, although evidence-based medicine is the foundation of sound judgment and quality care, there are significant challenges to infusing this evidence into clinical practice.

If practitioners were linked with research networks and cutting-edge evidence, patients (and their insurers) could be reassured that they were receiving the most appropriate care for their medical condition. Evidence-based medicine would also reduce variability in practice and contribute to improvements in the quality of care in other ways. Physicians are more likely to refer patients to clinical trials when research results will be readily shared with the referring physicians. All of this is technically feasible, and yet, like so many other forms of innovative infrastructure, a research web connecting laboratories to community physicians remains a vision for the future.

However, progress toward this goal is accelerating. In 2004, President George W. Bush called for the widespread adoption of EHRs by 2014. He also appointed Dr. David Brailer as the national coordinator for health information technology in an effort to jump-start the vision. Dr. Brailer modified existing conceptual frameworks to describe two important concepts that would facilitate the achievement of the president's goals: a national health information network (NHIN) and regional health information organizations (RHIOs).

The NHIN can be thought of as a national infrastructure designed to support connectivity and information flow among health care organizations, professionals, and citizens across the country. RHIOs are the local governance structures that foster EHR adoption and interoperability in communities.

Currently, RHIOs tend to focus on connecting community doctors, hospitals, labs, and pharmacies in the service of everyday care. Their role in supporting research is often overlooked.

However, it wouldn't take much to extend the RHIO concept to include the creation of "research RHIOs." These local organizations could focus on connecting the network of community caregivers with the network of cancer researchers, using caBIG as their medium. (Of course, these projects would have to be careful to safeguard the privacy of patients and would need to comply with privacy rules mandated by the U.S. government's 1996 Health Information Portability and Accountability Act.)

Personalized Medicine

Although decreasing friction in research and clinical information flow is important today, it will become even more important as care becomes increasingly customized to an individual's genetic characteristics. Today we create drugs for populations that are differentiated mostly by the disease or condition they happen to have—arthritis, hypertension, elevated cholesterol, non-Hodgkin's lymphoma.

For often unclear reasons, drugs work better for some than others and produce side effects that vary from person to person. This variability is probably due in some cases to subtle differences in genetic characteristics of the individuals taking these drugs, and, in the case of cancer patients, genetic differences of the cancer tissue. As research reveals the underlying genetic differences that drive the different responses to the same drugs, compounds that are tailored to the genetic characteristics of individuals will be created.

This will improve drug efficacy and safety while creating challenges in clinical trial recruitment. In the future, the fictional oncologist, Dr. Kelly, may not be looking merely for glioma patients with normal liver and kidney function. She may be looking for glioma patients with certain genetic characteristics. Instead of choosing from the universe of existing glioma patients, which is already a relatively small population, she will be looking for a subset, say the 20 percent of glioma patients with certain genetic characteristics that correlate with a higher response rate to the drug she is testing.

In this environment, it will be vital to use national networks to identify patients for clinical trials. Without such networks, the costs of recruitment will continue to climb and will become increasingly disproportionate to the size of the market for which a given drug is relevant. In some cases, the costs of development will become prohibitive and the drug will not be produced. In other cases, the cost of the drug will be significantly higher than it otherwise would have been and will create added financial stress for organizations already buckling under the pressures of health care costs. The promise of personalized medicine will not be fully realized until information networks link researchers with community caregivers and the patients they serve.

Weak Ties, Strong Science

In the process of linking scientists and practitioners through an informatics network, not only is the transfer of information being facilitated, but vital social ties between individuals and social systems that previously had no reliable links are being created. Such "weak links" (or casual and informal social ties and connections) are easily fostered by electronic networks and have been shown to be effective in exposing people to types of information they are unlikely to encounter in their usual social environments. For example, sociologist Mark Granovetter studied job referrals in the early 1970s and found that attractive opportunities were unlikely to come from close friends and coworkers, who travel in the same social circles. By linking researchers in different "ivory tower institutions" with one another, and then linking them with community-based medical caregivers "in the trenches," this new network facilitates a web of weak social ties.

This should be the broader objective of any new research-oriented electronic network: to enable the sharing of information and knowledge across different disciplines and thus create a more robust network in the research and practitioner communities. Although the Internet has provided a way for highly motivated actors to forge weak social ties with one another, there can be time and effort barriers that make it difficult for beleaguered physicians like Mr. B's doctor to identify researchers doing highly specialized clinical trials.

In other cases, as with the research teams in Seattle and Baltimore, information systems that speak different scientific dialects prevent scientists in different social networks from sharing information with one another. Bringing these communities together in the service of science and patients promises to provide synergies in both domains that could not have otherwise been achieved.

Mr. B was looking for a simple answer to a simple question: How can science help me live longer? His doctor probably knew that somewhere in the large social system of medical researchers, someone could answer that question, but, unfortunately, he was not aware of a mechanism to find that person. Properly constructed information tools and connections could have provided that answer and linked the researcher with the practitioner. Such episodes of interdisciplinary social linkage can be life-changing for people like Mr. B, and over the long term can accelerate the pace of basic scientific discovery.

Chapter 19

Employers' Push to Release Medicare Claims Data

Prelude: When managers know what you're talking about, they can express it in numbers. That is why Medicare claims data is so fundamental in judging health cost, quality, and outcomes.

In God we trust. All others use data. If there is any credo for statisticians, it is that. Critical to the Deming method is the need to base decisions as much as possible on accurate and timely data, not on wishes, or hunches, or "experience."

Mary Walton, 1986

Using Medicare Claims Data to Judge and Pay for Health Care

Other than Medicare itself, one of the more profound innovations over the last three decades has been the use of Medicare data to judge practice variation, outcomes, and performance. Medicare claims data is also the instrument through which it pays hospitals. Medicare pays America's 5,000 hospitals approximately $125 billion a year—or $25 million per hospital. Using a contract with the 3M Corporation, which has a sophisticated software program analyzing Medicare claims, Medicare plans cuts of:

- 33 percent for cardiac stents to $7,590
- 23 percent for implanting cardiac pacemakers to $22,000
- 10 percent for hip and knee replacements to $14,500
- 35 percent for clot-busting drugs for strokes to $11,758
  (Pear, 2006)

If the corporate world has a mantra, it is "Data! Data! Data!" Data are:

- impersonal, objective, and nonpolitical—although practitioners challenge this by saying medicine is an art, as well as a science
- a road map for disease management, festooned with mile markers by which one can judge continuing performance improvement
- a carrot to entice hospitals and physicians to practice quality and to be paid for achieving it
- a stick for flogging nonperformers and noncompliers; lend themselves to computer tracking, aggregation, and integration
- a management platform for restructuring, managing, comparing, and controlling costs at the individual disease, individual physician, and group levels
- an unsurpassed "drill down" tool for fleshing out details (i.e., computer software can be used to dig deeper into details of cost and outcomes of health care events)
- an ideal vehicle for studying statistical variation, the bedrock for improving quality

In health care, the corporate mantra has a government-attached tag line—Medicare. This data, growing by one billion transactions each year, is bigger and better than any private data source. Medicare data's very size overcomes data critics' objections that data from any private source is too small to judge performance of individual doctors.

Medicare "Biggers" Its Database

The huge growth of Medicare data can be described by a verse in a Doctor Seuss story about the Lorax, a mythical creature who cuts down trees, which happen to be the source of pulp for printing reams of Medicare data.

> *I meant no harm. I most truly did not.*
> *But I had to grow bigger. So bigger I got.*
> *I biggered my factory. I biggered my roads.*
> *I biggered my wagons. I biggered the loads*
> *of the Thneeds I shipped out. I was shipping them forth*
> *to the South! To the East! To the West! To the North!*
> *I went right on biggering . . . selling more Thneeds.*
> *And I biggered my money, which everyone needs.*

In 1973, John Wennberg and Alan Gittelson at Dartmouth published a paper describing how they used Medicare data to calculate medical procedure and episode variations in different sectors of the country. Ever since, Medicare data have been considered the *sine qua non* for studying and judging health costs and outcomes.

Wennberg, still active at Dartmouth as well as Harvard, considers the wide variations of medical services across regions and academic center as "unwarranted."

The variation data, he and his Dartmouth colleagues conclude, do not correlate with better outcomes data. He has proved, without statistical doubt, "more is not better" (Fisher, 2003).

Small wonder, then, the Business Roundtable, a health care coalition of national business leaders based in Washington, D.C., stung by roaring health inflation and representing 1,600 major employers covering more than 25 million people, is demanding the White House release all Medicare data (Halvorson & Isham, 2004). George W. Bush administration officials say they cannot do so because of a 1979 court ruling in which a federal district judge blocked disclosure of Medicare payment information on individual doctors as an invasion of privacy.

Critics have countered by saying the ruling is no longer relevant because doctors now practice in professional corporations rather than as individuals. Furthermore, Peter V. Lee, CEO of the Pacific Group on Health, says the privacy argument does not hold water because the data can be stripped of patient identity information. Privacy aside, Lee's reasoning goes:

> *To measure performance accurately, you need big numbers; the best source of big numbers is Medicare. One employer may have 12 patients seen by a particular doctor. Medicare may have 100 patients treated by the same doctor. If you combine the information, you get a much better picture of the doctor's performance.* (Halvorson & Isham, 2004)

Not only can you get a much better picture of the doctor, but you can get a much clearer and bigger picture of the costs and outcomes in the environment in which the doctor practices. You can "aggregate" (the buzzword of health care statisticians, which means bringing different data sets together) the following:

- Costs and outcomes of doctors
- Diseases they treat
- Hospitals they use
- Drugs they prescribe
- Providers to whom they refer

Given these practice patterns and disease-episode information, as a payer, you can begin to pick and choose among efficient and high-performing doctors and hospitals.

Researchers have found startling variations, as much as five- to twentyfold, in the amounts and costs of care by different doctors treating patients with the same disease and same severity of illness (Jerry Reed, personal communication, 2006). Wennberg praises the Business Roundtable for their "splendid effort" in pressuring the White House to release Medicare data, but cautions against "a simplistic effort to measure efficiency. It's very difficult to get reliable data on cost and quality at the individual physician level" (Pear, 2006b). This resonates with what many physicians feel: Data alone can be an unrealistic "straitjacket," because it does not take into account diverse circumstances and infinite variables at the patient–doctor level.

Government's Clash with Its Own Consumer Rhetoric

The government's reluctance to release Medicare data flies in the face of President Bush's repeated insistence that doctors should post prices and outcomes to "empower consumers" and those doctors should "make all information about prices and quality readily available to all Americans" (Weintrub, personal communication, 2006). It is difficult to do this when the prices vary by health plan and by Medicare zip code, and when the doctors themselves do not have the individual quality information in hand. It is true, of course, to again quote President Bush, "You can't make good health decisions unless there's transparency in the marketplace." What President Bush is saying is consumers cannot determine the value of prices unless prices are known in advance.

However, it isn't easy.

Transparency a Hard Sell

Transparency, generally defined as knowing prices and other data on quality and outcomes in advance, is a hard sell to doctors and hospitals, who fear data-based unfair profiling, unrealistic report cards, deep pay cuts, and devastating lawsuits. Lawyers and doctors affiliated with Harvard University say the lawsuit fear is overblown at present (Kirkpatrick, 2006).

In a 2005 *Journal of the American Medical Association* article, Aaron Kesselheim, Timothy Ferris, and David Studdert studied the probable impact of physician clinic performance assessment (PCPA) on medical legal claims and concluded:

> As long at PCPA measures aggregate episodes of care, aggregation will severely limit the prospects of their use as evidence in malpractice litigation. On the other hand if future initiatives move towards substantially greater specificity in format and content, PCPA data may reach the level of specificity required to gain admission in a wider range of circumstances. (Kesselheim, Ferris, & Studdert, 2005)

In other words, don't count out Medicare data in the future as a tool for punitive litigation. Releasing Medicare information might help insurance companies and employers deal with which doctors to use. Properly scrubbed and evaluated, it might help patients choose if health costs continue to escalate and the consumer-driven movement gains real traction.

Innovation Talking and Action Points

According to Drucker, one of the fundamental sources of innovation is "incongruities." An *incongruity* is a discrepancy, a dissonance, between what is real and what ought to be and what everybody assumes it to be. An incongruity speaks of a fundamental fault in the system. In the case of using data to judge quality and outcomes, there is a fault between too few data and enough data to make a reasoned statistical judgment.

Practicing doctors often object to statistical judgments, which are far from certain. With cancer, for example, there may be a statistical aggregated prediction of when a person will die, but patients die individually. Doctors say judgments of their quality must balance judgment with intuition and common sense, not things we usually attribute to government or payer bureaucracies. Unfortunately, data may be the only realistic tool bureaucracies have to make judgments on performance.

Will the use of Medicare data to judge performance influence what hospitals and doctors do and charge? So far, the answer seems to be: not much. According to an article in the *Wall Street Journal*, the chances a Medicare patient will be admitted to an intensive care unit vary by a factor of five times and the cost of care is more than twice as high in major academic medical centers (Winslow, 2006). Reasons given in the article are familiar.

- Robert Dickler, senior vice president of health care affairs at the Association of American Medical Colleges, which represents more than 400 teaching hospitals, says simply, "Medicine tends to be practiced differently in different parts of the country."
- Dr. Max Cohen, chief medical officer at the New York Medical Center, referring to days spent in the hospital during the last six months of life, says, "There are very distinct patient and family preferences, and major differences in the culture of different patient populations."

Dickler and Cohen are right. Medicare data will never be homogeneous across the country. Medical cultures vary too much in different regions. Providers will not change their ways just because the government says they must do things in certain ways. Those giving care respond to local cultures and preferences, rather than to some distant Medicare drummer.

Keep in mind it was over 30 years ago that Wennberg expressed concern over practice variations and showed more care is not better care in terms of statistical outcomes. Not much has happened since to change how hospitals and doctors behave economically. Medicare data generated by the Dartmouth Medical School's Center for Evaluating Clinical Methods showed that the New York University (NYU) averaged $79,280 for NYU patients while it was only $37,271 for Mayo patients for the last 2 years of life. Regional differences have had no effect on local spending patterns. These institutions respond to their own financial needs, not to Medicare data.

This response is not likely to change in future, except perhaps at the margins. One of these marginal changes may occur when consumers investigate and compare charges at Web sites such as www.medicarecompare.gov or www.dartmouthatlas.org, which will list costs and intensity of care for hospitals in their community or region. In theory, Medicare can homogenize payments across regions, but that is unlikely. In most cases, it is unreasonable given the differences in care expectations in different institutions.

Case Study 1

Health Care in a New Light
By Brian Klepper, PhD

Brian Klepper is founder and president of the Center for Practical Health Reform, a broad-based nonpartisan effort to reestablish stability and sustainability in U.S. health care. An active author and speaker, Dr. Klepper regularly writes commentary for popular and industry publications and presents to major health care and employer groups on practical policy and market-based approaches that can meaningfully affect the health care crisis.

••

Hospitals [and surgeons], if they wish to be sure of improvement . . . must analyze their results, to find their strong and weak points, [and] must compare their results with those of [their peers]. . . . [They should] make this information publicly known so that the future patients might make informed decisions.

Dr. Ernest Codman, Massachusetts General Hospital, 1914

If the feudal knight was the clearest embodiment of society in the early Middle Ages, and the "bourgeois" under Capitalism, the educated person will represent society in the post-capitalist society in which knowledge has become the central resource.

Peter Drucker, 1993

Perfect Information—a term used in economics to describe a state of complete knowledge about the actions of other players that is instantaneously updated as new information arises.

Wikipedia, 2006

This book was published at an auspicious moment in health care's history, nearly 100 years after Dr. Codman's famous advice, and just as health care "transparency" efforts finally are proliferating around the nation. "Transparency" refers to clear information in advance about pricing, value, quality, and outcomes. It's not a moment too soon. U.S. health care is becoming a case study in the excesses and economic disruptions that can occur when a market-based system lacks transparency, and a culture of opportunism takes root—and yet, just in the nick of time, transparency has become all the vogue.

A Crisis of Health Care Cost

Today, U.S. health care continues its long, accelerating descent into deep crisis. Unrelenting cost growth is pricing increasing percentages of mainstream purchasers out of the market for care and coverage. According to Dr. Brian Gould, between 2000–2005, the inflation of health care premiums, where costs converge from the continuum of care, grew a spectacular 5.5 times general inflation, 4.0 times workers' earnings, and 2.3 times the growth of business income.

Employers, who fully or partly subsidize the coverage of more than half of all Americans, are retreating. The U.S. Bureau of Labor Statistics reported that, by 2003, only 45 percent of private sector workers had health benefits, down from 77 percent just 13 years earlier. That number was eroding by 4.5 percent per year, double the annual erosion rate experienced during the 1990s. Employers who still offer health benefits have cut back with narrower coverages. They have also shifted more financial burden to their employees by requiring higher contributions to premiums and significantly higher out-of-pocket expenses. In real terms, premiums are higher for less coverage, so actual inflation rates are even higher than the numbers just cited.

The human toll of this crisis is harrowing and well publicized. Hospital emergency departments are overwhelmed by un- and underinsured people seeking primary care. Patients are experiencing unprecedented levels of personal debt and bankruptcy due to an inability to pay health care bills.

However, the economic prospects of the crisis are equally daunting. Demand for health care services continues to grow, but fewer people are buying coverage, which means that fewer dollars are available to pay for health care products and services. Fueled by skyrocketing costs, the intensifying mismatch between demand and resources threatens to destabilize the health care marketplace. Because health care is the nation's largest economic sector—one seventh of the U.S. economy and one eleventh of its job market—instability in this sector could cascade to and disrupt the nation's larger economic stability (Kolata, 2006b).

The Structural Roots of the Cost Explosion

Why has health care's cost explosion been uncontrollable? Because its deepest roots lie in three structural defects. First is a fee-for-service (FFS) reimbursement system (the current paradigm) that pays for procedures without considering quality or appropriateness. This not only encourages unnecessary care, but discourages adjusting practice to obtain the best possible clinical and financial results.

Second is an inability to identify problems and opportunities as they occur because, at least until now, the infrastructure and processes to track pricing and performance were unavailable to most of us. The invisibility of corporate and professional conduct has cultivated an opportunistic culture throughout health care. Without the information that regulates vendors' behaviors in most markets, health care's players have freely pushed ahead, constantly pushing the envelope on both utilization and pricing. Of course, none of this is lost on an entrepreneurial health care industry that knows a good thing when it sees it.

Third, the combination of FFS reimbursement and a lack of transparency has created a well-funded, broadly distributed power structure that, intent on maintaining the status quo, has shaped U.S. health policy for its own purposes for decades.

Taken together, these problems are a recipe for a perfect economic poison. More services translate to more money, so inappropriate and unnecessary procedures have come to dominate every nook and cranny of this country's vast health care continuum, from the supply chain to care delivery to finance. While luminaries such as Dr. Donald Berwick, CEO of the Institute for Health Care Improvement, and Dr. John Wennberg, author of the *Dartmouth Atlas of Health Care,* insist that half of or more health care is wasted, so far we haven't been able to easily see what things actually cost or how effective our practitioners and institutions are.

Leveraging Claims Data for Transparency

Until now, the health system's most powerful counterweights to the health industry—employer and government purchasers—have resisted mounting the efforts that would be required to effect change. Health industry lobbies have, for the most part, effectively neutralized government initiatives that might compromise short-term profitability and employer interests have been focused elsewhere. However, when faced with health care costs that threaten their bottom lines, their employees, and the larger marketplace, new transparency projects are afoot, sponsored by employers and government.

In fact, for several years, most large employers have used sophisticated analytical tools to evaluate their health plan claims data. Nearly all big corporations are self-funded for their health coverage, and so they have every incentive to identify ways to tweak and improve their health plan operations.

Claims analysis tools perform several important functions. Most important, they group all the data associated with each clinical episode, gathering all claims from any part of the continuum (e.g., physician offices, ambulatory centers, hospitals, laboratories, diagnostic centers, and pharmacies) pertinent to a specific patient, condition, and time. These tools also apply one of several commercially developed algorithms to "risk adjust" the claims, based on the severity of the patient's condition. This function permits apples-to-apples comparisons of the performance or experience of physicians, hospitals, or employer groups.

The reports that result allow managers to identify problems and opportunities in their health plan experience. For example, analysts can easily and credibly identify

- Patients with chronic disease who should be managed
- Patients with emerging acute care conditions
- High- and low-performing physicians and hospital services
- Average costs of care for specific conditions, specialties, and providers

While these tools are powerful, they generally have been applied by individual employers, who have analyzed and adjusted their plans in isolation—however, even the largest employers cannot muster the claims data-sample sizes to credibly evaluate all the health care vendors in a region. (Many commercial health plans have large, statistically credible data sets, but have typically considered their data proprietary.) By sharing and analyzing aggregated data, though, employers can.

Even better, if employers choose to publicly report the results, they can have several impacts. In an increasingly high-deductible health plan world, consumers might use that information to make wiser purchasing decisions, identifying better and more economical doctors, hospitals, and diagnostic centers. That said, the jury is still out on whether consumers are inclined to actually use the information available.

Better candidates for using the data are the purchasers from employers and government, who are very likely to avail themselves of information that can help shape improved health plan performance. The evidence to date, however, suggests that the health care industry itself would likely be most responsive to public reporting of pricing and performance information. Nobody wants to be publicly identified as a poor performer.

Transparency: The Best Driver of Market-Based Reform

This new transparency information will precipitate tremendously positive changes in the U.S. health system. Readily available health care pricing and performance data will likely accelerate the transition away from FFS and to pay-for-performance reimbursement, which will tie payment to results. Establishing targets for higher payment should reduce unnecessary and inappropriate utilization (and cost), should improve outcomes, and should encourage physicians and other providers to become more efficient by joining larger practices and investing in better management tools.

Together, these changes can break the cycles that have held U.S. health care captive for years and lay the foundation for a more stable and sustainable health system that truly adheres to market-based principles.

Case Study 2

Giving Medicare a Little Credit
By Richard L. Reece, MD

So far in this book, scant praise has been given to Medicare, more appropriately called the Centers for Medicare and Medicaid Services (CMS), as an innovative force. This may be unfair. Innovation is hard for any large bureaucracy because it has multiple constituencies to please, multiple regulations to meet, and multiple implications of its decisions to consider, and it takes a long time to do what it wants to do.

Still, through multiple partnerships with the private sector, the CMS has embarked on the CMS Roadmap to Quality. For the template of its road map, the CMS is using milestones set forth by the Institute of Medicine in its book *Crossing the Quality Chasm: A New Health System for the 21st Century* (2001). These road markers are to make health care safe, effective, efficient, patient centered, timely, and equitable. These are no small tasks. The CMS's five strategies for improving care are to:

1. Partner with federal and state agencies and health professionals.
2. Publish frequently and openly quality data and information.
3. Pay for performance; improved quality and better outcomes at lower costs.
4. Help doctors and hospitals install a nationwide electronic system.
5. Use federal leverage to drive innovations of information technologies. (Straube, 2006)

The CMS is under no illusion any of this will be easy. To say it will measure and improve quality is one thing; putting these concepts into operation is quite another. The CMS has been frank by saying it may take a decade to do what it wants to do—but there are signs progress is being made: The electronic health record is taking root with surprising speed. Doctors are realizing the combined effect of data display, data retrieval, work-flow improvement, decision support, and predictive modeling makes their work easier, better, and more profitable.

This is happening for five reasons:

1. Constant hammering by authorities on themes of patient safety and preventable medical errors
2. Growing numbers of anecdotal stories of physicians' positive experiences

3. Fear of being left at the gate when the electronic train is pulling out
4. Technology advancements making systems more affordable and more flexible, even for miserly, underautomated solo and small groups
5. The move toward pay-for-performance, requiring an automated system to get paid

Congress is helping the CMS toward its goals by changing the Stark laws to make investment in EHRs easier for hospitals and doctors cooperating in information technologies. Stark laws make joint hospital–physician investments difficult. In addition, the CMS is helping itself by requiring doctors to better identify and document patient conditions, which can only be done electronically. The CMS is also risk adjusting its revenues. Meeting these risk-adjusted payments requires electronic documentation. Another driver is the CMS's and commercial insurers' use of information technologies to aggregate electronic data to discern patterns of economic and practice behavior so that only those practicing cost-effective medicine are rewarded or excluded for payment.

Chapter 20

Health Plans and Banks Move to Ally with Doctors

Prelude: Health plans and banks now seek to win doctors as allies in the use of electronic health records for documentation of cost and quality. New consumers in high-deductible plans with HSAs will be carefully watching their health care dollars and will want this documentation.

In the cast of banks, HSAs will be sold at either independent or health-plan-owned banks, and HSA transactions will be processed at the point of care through smart cards containing financial information about HSA financial status and may be backed by bank credit cards.

If you ask patients, the vast majority want to communicate with their doctors via the Internet. Once physicians become enthusiastic, there will be a tipping point. Given the convenience and efficiency for both patient and physician, I think it will rapidly expand.

Dr. Charles Cutler, Aetna National Medical Director for Quality, 2006

Sometimes a health plan innovation will improve the lot of physicians by uncovering an innovative company that helps physicians install electronic health records. As explained in Chapter 4, Blue Cross Blue Shield of Massachusetts in 2005 provided $50 million to the Massachusetts eHealth Collaborative, a nonprofit organization, to coordinate a medical records experiment in three Massachusetts communities: Newburyport, North Adams, and Brockton. About 450 physicians practiced in these communities, and 170 of 180 picked the electronic health record system of Eclinicalworks because it was cheaper, more doctor friendly, and flexible the competitors' systems for small practices. This was a win-win, for the Blue Cross plan, for doctors, and for patients, for it is generally acknowledged that widely available electronic health records in doctors' offices will improve care.

Electronic health records may make it possible for physicians to be paid faster, to be paid for performance, and to be more productive and profitable in the process. For patients, electronic health records offer prospects for safer, more efficient, and better documented care.

However, that is not the point of this chapter. The point is that innovative health plans can make a difference by subsidizing or facilitating the introduction of electronic health records for physician practices to make them more efficient.

Putting Aside Past Antagonisms

In the past, doctors have often perceived health plans as enemies. In 2001, this enmity culminated in a class-action lawsuit lodged by 19 state medical societies against the national HMO industry (Reece, 2005c). In 2003, Cigna and Aetna settled, and others have agreed to settle, including Health Net, Prudential, WellPoint/Anthem, and Humana.

The terms of the Cigna and Aetna settlement were that the health plans would ensure new transparency standards were enacted in settling claims and would pay to help doctors set up two foundations that would issue grants to help doctors improve their business practices. The Aetna Foundation is called the Physicians Foundation for Health Systems Excellence, and the Cigna foundation goes by the name of the Physicians Foundation for Health Systems Innovation.

However, health plans are not out of the woods with doctors yet. Doctors continue to be rankled by late and partial payments for their services. A *New York Times* article (Freudenheim, 2006d), quoting data from athenahealth.com, a claims-processing company for doctors, says health plans and Medicare continue to delay payment by an average of about 30 to 40 days after the service is delivered (Humana 29.0 days, Aetna 31.6 days, Medicare 34.4 days, Cigna 36.2 days, WellPoint 36.8 days, United-Health 37.4 days, and Champus/Tricare 41.4 days).

Most of the time Medicare and health plans do not pay in full. The percentage of the time plans do not pay in full include Medicare 92.0 percent, UnitedHealth 89.1 percent, Humana 87.7 percent, Aetna 86.7 percent, Cigna 86.6 percent, WellPoint 86.3 percent, and Champus/Tricare 85.1 percent (Freudenheim, 2006d). In other words, overwhelmingly doctors are not paid for what they bill.

For physicians, health plans' slowness in paying claims may add as much as 15 to 20 percent in overhead costs. This high overhead forces doctors to pursue claims or pass along costs to other patients, according to Jack Lewin, a family doctor who is CEO of the California Medical Association, a professional group of 35,000 physicians (Dalzell, 1999). Many California physician groups are going bankrupt. In 1999, Only 44 percent of California's 200 medical groups met the state's solvency requirements, and Lewin asserted, "For HMOs to claim that groups are failing because of mismanagement is the source of unbelievable anger on the part of California physicians."

HMOs are beginning to make peace with doctors after 30 years of alienating them. They are buying them computers and prescribing devices, helping them get automatic payments at the point of care, and paying for "virtual" e-mail visits. These applications help health plans make sure the reasons for claims are justified and also reduce the number of health plan personnel needed to process the claims. In the case of physicians, they can be paid faster with fewer claims rejections.

Some insurers are trying to lure doctors into the digital age by offering free computers. In 2004, WellPoint offered to give free personal digital assistants (PDAs) and free personal computers (PCs) to 19,000 doctors in California, Georgia, and Wisconsin (McGee, 2004). In the future, health plans may offer free electronic health records and personal records to doctors in exchange for participating in networks, meeting quality standards, updating personal records, and prompt payment at the point of care.

The Central Role of Banks in Processing HSAs

In addition to health plans, banks are being drawn into the physician business. With the dawning of the health savings account (HSA) era, banks, those owned by the health plans themselves, by community banks, and by larger national banks, like the HSA Bank in Sheboygan, Wisconsin, may also be central players in bringing electronic solutions to bear. Banks will serve as custodians for HSA funds and will serve as processors of HSA claims for physician offices and hospitals.

Banks have well-established information infrastructures. They can expeditiously process claims and serve as custodians for HSAs and other funds. They can set up HSAs, provide credit lines for HSA holders, and develop card technologies that will make it possible for consumers to pay at the point of care with the swipe of a card. In the future, this secure card may well contain personal health records. The idea of being promptly paid with a card appeals to doctors (Reece, 2005b).

Drivers of Provider-Friendly Health Plan Services

Forces driving physician-friendly services among health plans include:

- Pleasing employers who are shifting health costs to employees and who stand to gain from satisfied employees who experience simpler and more convenient medical services
- Hospitals and doctors may accept discounts in exchange for prompt payment; a bird in the hand at the point of care is worth two in the health plan bush
- Simplified bill paying for members of consumer-driven plans who may become overwhelmed by medical bills that are either impossible to comprehend or impossible to pay in one fell swoop

- The appeal of systematic pay-down plans initiated by the swipe of a credit card at the point of service, particularly for patients with HSAs
- Health plans providing incentives and mechanisms for consumers to pay at the point of care

Expanding on this last point, according to the *Wall Street Journal* (Haines, 2006), physicians' accounts receivable balances average 100 days for the uninsured (with 31 percent uncollectable), 92 days for co-insurance (with 16 percent uncollectable), 80 days for deductible (with 18 percent uncollectable), and 16 days for copayments (with 3 percent uncollectable).

UnitedHealth Group's "OnePay"

Since April 2006, UnitedHealth Group has offered an automated payment plan at the point of care. This plan assured hospitals and doctors that patients will pay, because if they don't, United will get money regularly out of their paychecks, with interest at the prime rate, 7.5 percent (2006 rates).

The new plan, dubbed "OnePay," will pay the patient's bill directly to the hospital or doctor as soon as it processes the claim.

To collect money, United will turn first to money in the HSA, or if patients don't want money extracted from that account, they can use personal funds or have money extracted from their paycheck. United, which has chartered its own bank, Exante, will serve as a lender if employers participate in OnePay; in effect, extending lines of credit to employees to pay health expenses.

Doctors may welcome this new approach because they have learned it is hard to collect once the patient leaves the office or after a procedure has been done. Collecting before a procedure is done or at the office window helps reduce accounts receivable, but patients may regard these tactics as heavy handed. It is more palatable to shift collection responsibilities to the health plan.

Aetna and RelayHealth, Inc.

Starting May 3, 2006, Aetna, Inc., began offering groups and individual members of its plans in six states a variety of online services from primary care offices of RelayHealth, Inc. RelayHealth, based in Emeryville, California, has been in existence since 1999, but in 2002, changed its name from Healthlinx to RelayHealth. From Aetna.com or the Relayhealth.com Web sites, by providing credit card information, consumers can:

- Obtain online doctor consultation via e-mail; expect a return e-mail consultation within hours at a charge of $25 to $30 with an additional copay.

- At no charge, request prescriptions, make appointments, get referrals, and receive lab test results or reports of other procedures. If problems cannot be resolved on-line, the doctor may suggest an office visit.

Aetna is rolling out RelayHealth in California through its health plan, and in Florida, where Blue Cross Blue Shield of Florida has made RelayHealth available to 500,000 of its 3.8 million members.

Some doctors say they like RelayHealth because it replaces advice they've been giving for free for years. Cigna plans to offer RelayHealth in four states next year. Competitors to RelayHealth include Dallas-based Six Corporation, which purchased MYDOCOnline from Aventis Pharmaceuticals, Inc.; Medfusion; and Medem, which provides secure Web sites for doctors and is owned by the American Medical Society and other medical societies.

Innovation Talking and Action Points

Efficient electronic health record systems in doctors' offices, consumer-driven high-deductible health plans linked to HSAs, and consumers demanding value and convenience for their money, with card-swiping devices in doctors' offices and refinement of health plan Web sites, and outsourcing of HSAs to banks will be converging forces driving a future electronic health system.

Electronic health record systems are already common in large physician practices and are catching on fast in smaller practices, as less-expensive, more user-friendly, and less-unwieldy systems are introduced. Banks like United's Exante and the bank being set up by National Blue Cross Blue Shield, and banks set up by organizations like RelayHealth, Six Corporation, and Medem are catalysts for these new HSA developments.

Case Study

eClinicalWorks: Changing the Electronic Health Record Landscape

By Garish Navani, Chief Executive Officer

Founded in 1999, eClinicalWorks is an established, profitable, private clinical information technology company. Several factors, including the popularity of tablet PCs, coming together made this the right time for electronic health records. The five founders of eClinicalWorks, one physician and four IT professionals, saw a gap in the current electronic health records industry that was just waiting to be filled. Comparable to what Southwest Airlines did to its industry, eClinicalWorks planned to do with the medical electronic business, i.e., make cheaper, more convenient, more flexible, and more functional.

From the start, eClinicalWorks knew what business it was in—developing electronic health record solutions for physician practices of all sizes. Offering an award-winning, integrated electronic health record and practice-management solution, the company does not make hardware and has never burned a CD.

Products are distributed and updated electronically over the Internet. There is onsite training, but no shipped boxes. Also, eClinicalWorks offers more functionality than traditional electronic health records, listening to its customer base and tracking its user group Web site. When enhancements can be made, the development team is immediately involved in an upgrade. The turnaround for getting a requirement to development is usually less than a week.

Part of that fast response is that eClinicalWorks does not have a traditional executive structure.

"Our company is team based with team leaders—that's it," said Garish Kumar Navani, president and cofounder of eClinicalWorks. "Like a football team, there are groups specializing in offense, defense, and special teams, all of which have coaches, but there is no hierarchy. We believe that people will realize their full potential as part of a team rather than a rank in a chain of command. Plus, the lack of hierarchy allows us to be flexible to quickly meet customer needs."

eClinicalWorks has extended its nontraditional approach to include how it financed the company. From the beginning, the founders chose to forgo venture capital funding and began eClinicalWorks literally on their own. The lack of investors has given the founders a flexibility and control that few start-ups can claim, allowing them to shape the future as they see fit. The company is still free from debt.

This strategy has paid off. eClinicalWorks currently has more than 2,000 customers across all 50 states. Revenues have grown 100 percent year after year and are projected to reach $40 million for 2006. By looking at the current industry and finding ways to turn it upside down, eClinicalWorks has built a solid business that will be a driving force in the market for many years to come.

Chapter 21

Pay-for-Performance— a Seemingly Inevitable Trend

Prelude: The siren cry of pay-for-performance (P4P) advocates is: "An ounce of performance is worth a pound of quality—and is worth paying for." This expression may hold true in California, but P4P has yet to be shown to work effectively on a broad scale outside of California.

[M]omentum is building to develop a national P4P model as more projects— and more financial rewards—come online in communities across the country.

One successful project that is drawing a lot of attention is the pay-for-performance program developed and run by the California-based Integrated Healthcare Association, which now covers 225 medical groups and individual practice associations whose members care for 6.2 million Californians enrolled in seven different health plans.

With three years of reporting experience and two years of payouts that have sent approximately $90 million in performance bonuses to physicians across the Golden State, the program is now one of the largest and most lucrative in the nation. But is this the model that other regions should seek to emulate? Or do the idiosyncrasies of the California market—one dominated by several large HMOs with delivery networks composed of organized medical groups and IPAs operating under a capitated model—preclude replication in other regions?

Brad Cain, 2006

The pursuit of evidence-based medicine is now at the core of the agenda for improving health care in the United States. All major quality measurement systems use science-based indicators of proper processes of care. All-or-none assessment of process quality represents an impressive advance in the level of ambition, patient-centeredness, and system-mindedness of performance measurement and reporting as assets in the pursuit of better health care.

Thomas Nolan and Donald M. Berwick, 2006

In his 1968 book *The Age of Discontinuity,* Peter F. Drucker opened with:

> *In guerilla country a handcar, light and expendable, rides ahead of the big, lumbering freight train to detonate whatever explosives might have been placed on the track. This book is such a "handcar."*
>
> *For the future is, of course, always "guerilla country" in which the unsuspecting and apparently insignificant detail derails the massive and seemingly inevitable trends of today.*

The "successful" California experience noted at the opening of the chapter with pay-for-performance (P4P) over the last 5 years may be such a handcar. It may explode myths about the workability and practicality of P4P. However, will P4P work elsewhere in the United States where big, integrated delivery networks and dominant HMOs are rare?

P4P Trend Not Inevitable

The P4P trend would seem to be massive and inevitable. A survey of 252 HMOs in 41 metropolitan areas indicated more than half of the HMOs, representing more than 80 percent of persons enrolled, used P4P in their physician contracts. Of the 126 health plans with P4P contracts, nearly 90 percent had programs for physicians, and 38 percent had programs for hospitals (Rosenthal, Landon, Sharon-Lise, Frank, & Epstein, 2006). A survey of health care stakeholders, explained in this book's first chapter, ranks P4P as the number one innovation.

However, a seemingly and apparently insignificant detail could still derail this trend. It is resistance of primary care groups in small groups. These doctors have neither the means, will, nor the time to enter the data or install the computer systems to make P4P a reality Nor are they yet persuaded that P4P bonuses, now being paid in the 5 percent to 10 percent range by California health plans, will improve care (Robinson, 2001).

What works in California, with its dominant HMOs and its huge multispecialty groups, does not necessarily work elsewhere as shown by the capitation experience—nor is the formation of large multispecialty groups being replicated in most parts of the United States. California is unquestionably a unique place; it:

- is home to nearly 35 million Americans
- has a greater nonwhite population than any other state
- attracts immigrants from everywhere
- has a large and growing uninsured population
- has more than 70,000 physicians

If P4P works in such a diverse state, it ought to work elsewhere. Medicare officials and the Robert Wood Johnson Foundation, leaders of most of the nation's health plans, and integration experts like Stephen Shortell look approvingly on the 5-year-old California experience as a model for P4P for the rest of the United States.

As one of the leaders of the California Integrated Health Association's efforts to implement P4P for 6.8 million Californians covered by 225 medical groups and seven large health plans, Shortell, dean of the School of Public Health at the University of California–Berkley, effectively presents the case for P4P. Of the reason for lack of quality in U.S. health care, his message is this:

> *The largest limiting factor is not lack of money or technology or information, but rather the lack of an organizing principle that can link money, people, technology and ideas into a system that is more cost-effective (i.e., more value) than current arrangements.* (Mongan, Mechanic, & Lee, 2006)

Current arrangements include lack of integrated systems with a unified vision and an overarching system that gives incentives for quality clinical care. That overarching system includes P4P.

According to Shortell, the California Integrated Health Association (IHA) plan's P4P goal was to give "a compelling set of incentives to drive breakthrough improvements in clinical quality and patient experience through a common set of measurements, a public scorecard, and health payments" (Mongan, Mechanic, & Lee, 2006). Using this goal, Shortell says the IHA has achieved these measured results:

- Widespread improvements, with 87 percent of clinics improving their ratings by an average of 5.3 percent
- A 65 percent improvement in patient experience
- A 34 percent improvement in IT systems in clinic settings

To make the P4P system work, Shortell says these criteria must be met:

- Building and maintaining trust among physicians and health plans
- Securing physician group participation

- Securing health plan participation
- Collecting and aggregating data in a neutral fashion

As he looks to the future, Shortell sees these necessary steps:

1. Increasing incentives to physicians
2. Developing and expanding measures that incorporate outcome measures, including more specialists
3. Applying risk adjustments to measurement sets
4. Adding efficiency measurements
5. Including Medicare HMO plans

The California P4P initiative is an effort to be admired. But keep in mind the California health system is a different breed: big integrated systems dominate; a few large HMOs hold sway there; and collectively, California physicians are at the lower end of the scale economically compared to the rest of the United States.

Physicians elsewhere may resist the California model. In my mind, whether the California model is translatable to the rest of the country remains an open question. After all, capitation, California-style, did not catch on in most of the rest of the United States, and neither have large multispecialty groups dominated elsewhere. Consequently, the California-inspired P4P movement is not without skeptics. More than one hospital observer has remarked, "I find it unseemly to reward doctors for quality. Isn't that their job?" Dr. David Blumenthal, of the Institute of Health Policy at Massachusetts General Hospital–Partners Health System in Boston, gives a thoughtful evaluation of prospects for P4P in a health policy report:

> *Along with consumer-directed health care, a second strategy to reform the health care system pursued in employer-sponsored insurance is paying for performance, through which employers, working with insurers, agree to reward providers who offer a better quality of care, care at a lower cost, or both. Pay-for-performance arrangements have exploded in number and no systematic list of them exists, but it is clear that they vary widely in what they reward and how they do so. Some arrangements are focused on hospitals, some on groups of physicians, and some even compensate individual physicians on the basis of their performance.*
>
> *At first glance, the pay-for-performance idea has a compelling logic. It corrects a major flaw in the current fee-for-service system, which compensates providers without regard to the quality or efficiency of their services and thus offers them no financial incentive to improve their services. However, paying for performance also has potential downsides. Performance is difficult to measure, and there is concern that what is measurable might drive out what is important. Providers might also avoid sick poor patients whose care may be more difficult to manage than that of healthy rich*

patients, thereby improving the providers' cost or quality statistics. It is also unclear whether employers would be happy if paying for performance resulted in an increase in the quality of care but at a higher expense than in the current system. Systematic studies have just begun to test the effects of pay-for-performance programs. (Blumenthal, 2006)

The pay-for-performance movement is a strong trend.

1. All major payers—the Centers for Medicare and Medicaid Services, other government health agencies, the Bush administration, all private health care measurement organizations, and most other entities in the health plan industry—have deemed it the wave of the future. As Dr. Carolyn Clancy (2006), director of the U.S. Agency for Health Care Research and Quality, put it in a Medscape podcast: "Pay-for-performance: The train has left the station, but where is it taking us?"

2. "Innovative" means to create something new and creative. Paying for performance, common in other industries, is hardly new and creative. It is an idea borrowed from industry—that universal standardization and specification of vendors based on evidence will lead to continuous quality improvement.

3. The idea of universally applying quality indicators, now numbering 469, to all hospitals and medical practices (Asch et al., 2006), inpatient and outpatient, and commanding all hospitals and doctors to enter into computers all relevant quality indicators in overly busy medical practices and in overcrowded hospitals are "all-or-nothing" mode. Paying nonperforming institutions and individuals at a lower rate, thereby characterizing them as of lower quality, may be unworkable.

Physicians Are Not Servants of Payers

It is not that critics are against bonuses for following quality processes or better outcomes; many simply are wishing for a realistic collaboration of payers with physicians. Physicians, after all, are trained knowledge workers. Physicians consider themselves independent, beholden only to themselves and their patients. They do not think of themselves as servants of government, health insurers, or employers.

To impose upon busy practicing doctors, many of them struggling to make ends meet now, the additional work, time, and expense of entering by computer all relevant quality indicators may be impractical. That is why the American Medical Association, the Medical Group Management Association, the American Academy of Family Physicians, and other specialty societies have fought quality mandates and have substituted their own principles.

Best and Most Practical Principles

The best set of realistic principles that puts the matter in proper perspective is articulated by a working group of Massachusetts physicians:

1. **You get what you pay for.**

   Payment should be neutral or better when it comes to value, meaning that payment and quality are inextricably linked together.

2. **Follow the Willie Sutton rule.**

   In any given year, most people have small medical bills, while a few people have very large bills. In 2003, health spending roughly followed the "80–20 rule": 20 percent of the population accounted for 80 percent of expenses.

   Therefore the second principle is that P4P should be focused on where the return on investment will provide the greatest increase in total (largest number of dollars) value (maximum quality/minimum cost) for the smallest number of patients.

3. **Incentives must be completely transparent for all members of the health care team.**

   The health care team can act on the understanding of the link between payment and quality only if the incentives, including risk adjustment, are based on logic that is transparent and open for examination by all health care professionals.

4. **Improve value starting with the hospital framework and then moving in concentric circles into larger episodes of illness.**

   This specifically means starting with adjusting hospital payment for severity of illness beyond Medicare's current diagnostic related groups (DRGs), then moving to correctly identifying potentially preventable hospital complications, and at the same time, moving to the coordination between inpatient and outpatient services by providing financial incentives.

5. **With respect to physicians, start first with their hospital practice.**

   The approach to improving value outlined in Principles 2 and 4 implies that one moves the effort from the health professionals working in the hospital and then to outpatient specialty services providing care to expensive or about-to-be expensive chronically ill individuals. Only after this low-hanging fruit has begun to create savings should one move to engage primary care physicians and practices.

6. **The tools exist today to implement Principles 1–5.**

   Principles 1–5 implicitly entail bundled payments adjusted for severity for each type of health care encounter (ambulatory visits, hospital stays, yearlong episodes of illness, and post acute care). Some recommend aggregating the unit of service beginning with the ambulatory visit, moving to the hospital stay, and then linking those together into a classification tool describing the patient over a year's period of time.

7. **Data and metric integrity is important. If existing data resources are to be used, they need to be up to the task.**

    Claims data elements not currently being used for payment purposes need to be validated in terms of both coding and completeness before being used for P4P. Success is more likely when there already is measurement going on, and where the validity/reliability of the measures has been vetted by experience and accepted by clinicians.

8. **Focus on outcomes as good processes lead to good outcomes.**

    Start this focus on outcomes by aligning payment incentives with specific, measurable goals.

9. **Public reporting is key to increasing value.**

    Public reporting of validated process and outcome metrics is a strong catalyst for providers to improve care and enhance the value of the care provided. Making performance reporting completely transparent to consumers and the entire health professional team assists both consumers and providers seeking to improve.

10. **All providers need to be engaged with feedback on their performance.**

    Financial incentives are necessary but not sufficient. Frequent, clear, and actionable feedback is essential. Central to these efforts is the ability to compare performance to others based on measures whose logic is transparent (does not need to be in the public domain). They also need to be given tools and guidance on how they can improve.

11. **P4P needs to use national metrics but reflect local priorities and choices.**

    P4P needs to incorporate national metrics (e.g., core measures), but priorities and implementation of the program needs to be locally driven.

12. **Benefit design needs to be linked into P4P, making the consumer part of the health care team.**

    It is important provider payment incentives are consistent with benefit design. For example, per diem limitations on mental health coverage will not work with a case-based payment approach. Innovations in clinical practice that are not specified in the benefit are often the best path to enhanced value (improving outcomes while lowering costs). P4P needs to create, encourage, and enable providers to improve performance, and a component of that effort includes the removal of barriers related to benefit design while aiding transparency and consumer choice. (Goldfield et al., 2006)

Innovation Talking and Action Points

To implement P4P, Norbert Goldfield and associates are saying to start with specialists and hospitals because that is where 80 percent of the money savings is. Other things need to be said, too.

- Bonuses in the 5 percent to 10 percent range are not likely to get the attention of doctors who may correctly perceive it will take that much to change practices and set up systems to justify bonuses.
- Open up those "black boxes," that is, software undecipherable to outsiders, containing computer-crunching methodologies for calculating quality and rewarding bonuses for all to see.

At this time, no one knows whether P4P will work, but everyone agrees it is here to stay, and a formidable group of payers and players—Medicare, Medicaid, other government agencies, hospital associations, health plans, and medical associations—are behind it.

All eyes are on California where a consortium of health plans and big medical groups, representing about half of California's 70,000 doctors, has been experimenting and working on the concept for 5 years with promising results. Right now physician bonuses are in the $8,000 to $10,000 range in a state where primary care incomes are in the $100,000 to $150,000 range.

California, Always a Leader in Health System Restructuring

California has always been a leader in restructuring its health system, in the managed care and capitation movements, and in inducing doctors to join large multispecialty organizations. The fact that a greater percentage of doctors work on salary in California, or are dependent in other ways on large organizations, may make P4P a reality quicker there than in the rest of the nation. Furthermore, because the California climate is so idyllic and because many physicians fantasize about living there, doctors make sacrifices to live there at any cost.

Case Study

Pay-for-Performance Case—a Key to Universal Coverage in the United States: Suggestions on Improving Value (Quality/Payment) of Health Care Services in Massachusetts

By Norbert Goldfield, MD

Dr. Norbert Goldfield is medical director for 3M Health Information Systems. In this capacity, he has worked on a number of projects including:

- The development of the outpatient visit-based prospective payment system used by CMS, the refinement of DRGs adjusted for severity/mortality used for quality and payment (proposed by CMS in March 2006 to replace the current inpatient acute hospital payment system) purposes, and the development of risk adjusters for capitation payment/retrospective analyses of episodes of care.
- New methods of measuring quality of care such as a tool to avoid readmissions and a tool to not reimburse hospitals extra for patients incurring avoidable complications during their hospital stay. Many countries throughout the world use these tools for quality-management purposes.

Goldfield has presented many papers on topics ranging from quality of care measurement to history of efforts to enact national health reform. He has published extensively and is editor of the peer-reviewed *Journal of Ambulatory Care Management*. Goldfield is a practicing internist with a subspecialty in adolescent medicine. He works 2 days a week at a community health center and has introduced new coordinated care programs for patients with significant chronic illnesses. He teaches medical sociology at the University of Massachusetts, Amherst.

Goldfield also has helped form several volunteer organizations including Hampshire Health Access (providing access to care for the uninsured in Hampshire County, Massachusetts, where Goldfield lives), the Palestinian Medical Access Partnership (providing major surgeries to Palestinian children living in the West Bank and Gaza), and Healing Across the Divides, an organization that serves to improve the health of both Israelis and Palestinians. He is also on the board of Health Care for All based in Boston.

• •

This study will provide specific suggestions that can be implemented today to reverse current practice and instead pay appropriately for quality care in a transparent manner. All of these measures can be implemented by a state over a period of only a few years, putting continuous downward pressure on the rate of health insurance premiums. Some of these measures, such as readmissions, could be implemented immediately, resulting in significant savings. These suggestions, put into place as incentives, need to be built into every type of health care encounter. These encounters include:

- Ambulatory visits (or very short strings of ambulatory visits)
- Inpatient stays (including readmissions)

- Long-term care including but not limited to home health care, acute long-term care hospitals, and rehab hospitals
- Episodes of illness or yearlong episodes of care for chronic illnesses such as diabetes

The tools described in this article should be useful not just to improve quality in a public manner but also to align reimbursement methods with policy goals.

The measures that comprise the P4P data set could be disclosed to the public at regular and predetermined intervals as part of a community or statewide report card for providers. This would provide patients and advocates with the data they need to find high-quality care at a better price. Such public disclosure leverages the natural synergy between P4P and consumer empowerment.

Transparency is key to success. All parties (state and federal government, consumer advocates, patients, providers) need to be able to understand, if they so choose, the underpinnings of any payment incentives. If the payment system is not transparent and is loaded with so many bells and whistles such that no one can understand the impact of the incentive, it will be ineffective at modifying the behavior of health professionals, payers, and/or patients. Therefore, the first step is to improve transparency.

Once a more transparent reimbursement system is achieved, one should focus, in order of importance/ease of implementation, on:

- hospitalization-based P4P together with the period immediately after hospitalization (e.g., readmissions) and before hospitalization (ambulatory care sensitive conditions). The hospital-based P4P should be implemented first because it will result in the greatest improvement in quality and provide the greatest monetary savings. The hospital field alone can take up to 2 years to implement. Expensive services are also provided on an outpatient basis; but are more difficult to control. These outpatient services may include:
  - pharmaceuticals and durable medical equipment
  - mental health services
  - postacute care services such as home health and skilled nursing facilities
  - entire yearlong episodes of care (such as a yearlong episode of diabetes)

The following are specific suggestions.

1. Hospital services: P4P for hospital services. I suggest implementation in the sequence provided. That is
   - Pay on the basis of prospective (a set or predetermined) payment for hospital services that is adjusted for the complexity or the severity of illness of the patient. One can then reliably measure inpatient mortality rates using, for example, Agency for Health Reseach and Quality metrics.
   - Provide incentives to hospitals/medical groups to decrease hospital readmissions. The payment incentives need to be designed to encourage hospitals and medical groups to collaborate. Significant savings are possible.
   - Provide hospital/physician incentives to avoid potentially preventable complications that occur during the hospital stay.
   - Provide incentives to hospital outpatient departments/medical groups/emergency rooms to avoid hospitalizations for conditions that when optimally treated should almost never result in a hospitalization (severity adjusted, ambulatory care sensitive conditions).

2. Outpatient visits

- ED visits and admissions to the hospital following an outpatient procedure
- Pay on the basis of prospective payment for, at a minimum, expensive outpatient services (visits ranging from CT scans to outpatient operations) that are adjusted for the complexity of the encounter
- Precertification for expensive outpatient procedures

3. Reformed payment for pharmaceutical/DME services
   - Use a formulary without all the barriers that currently exist for needed medications
   - Academic detailing
   - Oregon approach to drug pricing involving a combination of evidence-based lists of approved medication together with aggressive price limits on allowable payments to manufacturers
   - Approaches from other countries that take other approaches to combining evidence-based lists of effective medication together with negotiation strategies with pharmaceutical companies. Governments in other countries negotiate with pharmaceutical companies for drug pricing. Other than the Veterans Administration system, this isn't the case in the United States.

4. Reformed payment for mental health services
   - Provide financial incentives to encourage coordination of mental health services. The key issue that is missing from all other managed mental health services is that there is little understanding of the types of services needed by mental health patients. Inadequate risk adjustment has enabled risk selection on the part of managed mental health organizations.

5. Reformed payment for long-term care (LTC) including skilled nursing facilities, home health care, rehabilitation services, and other forms of postacute care.
   - Prospective payment for LTC using a single classification system across all LTC settings. This would allow incentives to be built in to favor home care while using the same classification system and would require careful monitoring.
   - Nursing home disease management in an effort to avoid unnecessary hospitalizations.

6. Paying for disease management/episodes of illness
   - Paying disease management entities/medical groups/managed care companies in a transparent, risk basis adjusted for the value of the care they are delivering/insuring.
   - Encourage severity-adjusted package payment for episodes of illness and/or capitation wherever politically feasible.
   - Encourage provider groups predominantly serving chronically ill enrollees to work together (from a financial, not just organizational, point of view) to apply for waivers from the federal government allowing them to pool resources.

Part Five

Constraining Costs and Expanding Markets

Unsustainable trends will not be sustained.

James C. Robinson, 2004

This is really a landmark innovation for our state because this proves at this stage that we can get health insurance for all our citizens without raising taxes and without a government takeover. The old single-payer canard is gone.

Massachusetts Governor Mitt Romney, 2006

Chapter 22

Imaging: The Blessing of Technology, the Curse of Cost

Prelude: Technologies of computer imaging machines are evolving so fast that doctors cannot keep pace. The pace of technological change coupled with financial incentives to physicians to order more images along with public perception that frequent scans represent the standard of care is resulting in billions of wasted health care dollars. This waste can be reduced through clinician educational and consultative programs and more effective use of data showing clinical yields of various imaging equipment.

Highmark put an imaging pre-authorization program in place in 1999, but abandoned it in 2001. Since then, the insurer has experienced a dramatic increase in both its number of imaging facilities and advanced imaging costs— growing 20 percent annually for three consecutive years. In 2003, employer groups paid the price for those increases with a rise in premiums equaling 20 and 30 percent.

C. Lyn Fitzgerald, 2004

This chapter has been co-written with Brian Baker. This was necessary because imaging technology is a highly technical field requiring special knowledge. With more than 23 years of diagnostic imaging and health care technology experience, Baker has dedicated himself to solving some of health care's challenges from new and sometimes different perspectives. As a strategist and serial entrepreneur, he has held senior-level positions at some of the most recognizable health care technology companies including Philips and General Electric. Today, Baker is vice president for Regents Health Resources, Inc., a Brentwood, Tennessee, based health care consulting company specializing in development and consulting services for the diagnostic imaging industry.

The Beginning

The evening of November 8, 1895, Wilhelm Conrad Roentgen discovered an unknown phenomenon that had the unusual ability to make objects appear transparent. When subjected to the path of this phenomenon with a screen covered with barium platinocyanide, from as far away as 6 feet, objects became transparent. The image of his wife's hand was the first "Roentenogram" or "X-ray" ("X" because the nature of these "rays" were unknown) ever produced (see Nobelprize.org). Within a year, the first angiographies (moving X-ray pictures) were being produced, intent on disease discovery. Ironically, a short 28 years later, the Nobel Prize–winning physicist died from carcinoma of the intestine.

However, modern diagnostic imaging had begun.

Excitement over this new technology was tempered by its apparent but unexplainable side effects. Objections began to surface, but the revolutionary and superior nature of the new technologies overrode these objections.

In April 1972, G.N. Hounsfield, senior scientist for EMI Ltd. of England, and Dr. James Ambrose, a London radiologist, sprung an innovative technological wonder when they presented their work on the computerized tomographic (CT) scan before the British Institute of Radiology.

Hounsfield foresaw CT scanners would start a radiological revolution:

> It is possible that this new technique may open up a new chapter in X-ray diagnosis. Previously, various tissues could only be distinguished from one another if they differed appreciably in density. In this procedure absolute values of the absorption coefficient of the tissue are obtained. The increased sensitivity of computerized X-ray section scanning enables tissues of similar density to be separated, and a picture of the soft tissue structure within the cranium is built up. (Hounsfield, Ambrose, Perry, & Bridges, 1973)

In 1977, after 7 years of work (and using information gathered from countless physicists dating back to the late 1930s), Raymond Damadian completed the first MRI (magnetic resonance imaging) scanner, calling it "Indomitable." In 1978, he founded the Fonar Corporation, which manufactured the first commercial magnetic resonance imaging scanner in 1980. Fonar went public in 1981 (Weed, 2004).

In 1983, Toshiba obtained approval from the ministry of health and welfare in Japan for the first commercial magnetic resonance imaging system. FDA approval was granted to Fonar in 1984 for the first magnetic resonance imaging commercial scanner in the United States. Starting in 1992, Fonar was paid for patent infringement from all the major multinational corporations; however, the main "goal" for the magnetic resonance imaging, the reason it was originally pursued by Damadian, has yet to be achieved. That reason? The separation of benign from malignant tissue (differentiation).

Almost immediately, political objections arose to the widespread use of this new computerized tomography imaging technology. Health, Education, and Welfare Secretary Joseph Califano declared, "There are enough CAT scanners in Southern California for the entire western United States" (Califano, 1977). (The terms CT scan and CAT scan are used interchangeably to indicate computerized tomography scanning.) Not to be outdone, Dr. Howard Hiatt, dean for the Harvard School of Public Health, compared the use of CT scanners to overgrazed medical commons in which too many were foraging for too little. He said a national center for technological assessment and suppression of new technologies should be established and argued:

> *There is no doubt that the scanners provide additional diagnostic information, and frequently with less discomfort and hazard to the patient, however, it is not clear that the diagnostic information very often leads to a better outcome for the patient. Until this important information is available from careful studies, would we not be better served limiting the use of such expensive technology?* (Hiatt, 1976)

Califano and Hiatt overestimated the power of federal regulations and underestimated the thirst of doctors and the public for this clearly superior technology. Neurosurgeons immediately embraced computerized tomography scans. Their enthusiasm soon spread to orthopedic surgeons, who soon after saw the potential of magnetic resonance for joint, bone, and soft-tissue imaging.

Most recently, oncologists have welcomed PET (positron emission tomography) scans to check for subtle cancer spread. Computerized tomography and magnetic resonance scanning have become the modus operandi for evaluating all manner of physiological anomalies.

In 2001, 225 internists, when asked to evaluate the relative importance of 30 medical technologies, rated computerized tomography and magnetic resonance imaging scans as the number one innovation of the last decade (Fuchs & Sox, 2001). Today, the utilization of imaging exams is growing between 9 percent and 11 percent annually.

The Accepted Standard of Care

Physicians and the public alike accept and demand imaging as the standard of care. The public may regard scans not only as being of diagnostic but of therapeutic value. A story I heard recently from a friend shows the public's attitude and acceptance of the new technologies:

"You know, I've had four CT scans and two in the last 6 months to check on my back, and I feel a lot better."

Scans have become a leading cost component in the practice of modern medicine. Several other factors are at work:

- Entrepreneurs, radiologists, and specialists have been quick to set up screening and imaging centers, with and apart from hospitals, and "partner" with referring physicians (Hiatt, 1976).
- Some primary care physicians—suffering from lower Medicare and managed care reimbursements, rising costs, and lower incomes—have banded together to set up their own imaging centers (Ruff, 2006).
- The aging boomer generation expects complete access to new and innovative technologies.
- New technologies are offering more options for, and better ways to, image the patient.

Small wonder, given these combined forces, that imaging has become one of the largest single aspects of health care costs in the United States, currently valued at $80 billion and growing 16 percent per year (Kuhn, 2006). Health plans have sought to check this inflation through utilization review, and Medicare, through the Deficit Reduction Act (DRA), has lowered certain reimbursements, expecting to save $2.8 billion over 5 years (Griggs, 2006). Debate is currently under way that will define the future of the DRA and its final effects. However it turns out, something must be done to reduce the rising utilization and costs of imaging services and their impact on overall health care spending.

Trends, Innovation, and Symptomatic Solutions

For a host of reasons, the diagnostic imaging industry with its use of computerized tomography scans, magnetic resonance images, positron emission tomography scans, nuclear medicine, ultrasound, and others is seen by many payers as being out of control. The rising utilization and subsequent costs have caused Highmark Health Plan in Pennsylvania and Tufts Health Plan in Boston to issue preauthorization decrees and other standards to try and restrict imaging use. In the case of Highmark, the utilization requirements include requiring:

- Diagnostic imaging services to be offered for a minimum of 40 hours per week on business days, including one evening per week until 8:00, and at least two Saturdays per month for a minimum of 4 hours per day
- Centers to be staffed on-site by a Highmark-credentialed radiologist with advanced cardiac life support (ACLS) certification
- A minimum of five modalities at each provider location offering computerized tomography scans, magnetic resonance imaging, and fluoroscopy
- PET (positron emission tomography) technology to be provided in a hospital setting only (Fitzgerald, 2005)

In addition, providers now must notify Highmark when ordering magnetic resonance imaging, computerized tomography, or positron emission tomography. The insurer wants to use data gathered through the notification process to identify appropriate and inappropriate utilization trends of these high-end imaging modalities. While these rules on the surface might seem reasonable, they only address the symptoms of the disease— rising costs.

With every cost problem of this magnitude, there beckons an opportunity to restructure the industry, to educate physicians on proper use of new technologies, and to define and refine the indications for imaging technology use. Some industry groups have conservatively estimated that 30 percent of the $80 billion worth of annual imaging exams is unnecessary or inappropriate (Baker, personal communication).

Unfortunately, technology has advanced so rapidly that the imaging industry and imaging professional societies have not been able to adequately keep physicians abreast of the options and proper utilization. This education issue along with litigious proliferation has caused many caregivers to get a second opinion themselves. How do they get that second opinion? They cannot find such an opinion because it does not currently exist in a convenient format. So physicians often order multiple exams on different imaging technologies to "cover" themselves. Even with this additional data, a confident diagnosis determination is still problematic to achieve for the referring physician. The real solution lies in standardized (accessible) protocols that recommend technology usage according to the clinical indication and then associate it with local technology availability. Furthermore, each physician will need the tools to understand and delineate each technology's capability for an indication.

In other words, the capabilities of technologies or vendors within a given modality are not equal in their ability to image. However, clinicians are unaware of these subtle differences and therefore overutilize the technology or order exams on technology that is incapable of producing diagnostic results for the indication. Caregivers must be given the tools to quickly and easily understand the technology differences and their application to clinical indications.

Technology's Financial Impact

As providers continue to adopt emerging technology solutions like computer-aided diagnosis (CAD) software, electronic health recores, robotic surgery, and sophisticated information technology programs, and everyone moves closer to a paperless all-digital world, solutions will need to be developed to manage the financial impact. Meanwhile, the industry wrestles with the cost of it all. Numerous surveys have shown more than half of all hospital IT budgets have increased dramatically in the last 5 years.

Ask almost any hospital CEO what the most capital-intensive department is in their facility and they may say imaging services and its associated support infrastructure, but radiologists may not agree (Beinfield & Gazeel, 2005).

Historically, when building or remodeling a health care facility, somewhere between 25 percent and 35 percent of the entire capital needed for the project is spent on medical equipment and its support needs (Firestone, personal communication, 2006). Today and more so tomorrow, this will only increase with information technologies; electronic health records and the like in the digital hospital will mandate these technologies and the associated costs.

In the past, a medical office could buy routine X-ray equipment for about $100,000. With today's advancing technology, that same office now has the option to buy a digital X-ray room for $350,000. It's more complex, requires more staff, and a more expensive service contract, but it does not need film. Instead it needs _____ (insert a portion of your IT budget) PACS (Picture Archiving and Communication System) to transmit and/or print its digital images.

So, where is the value to this new technology?

On the surface, the new system looks more complex and expensive with little or no return. In this example, although both systems accomplish the same goal, a diagnostic X-ray represents a paradigm shift in the way things are done. The new paradigm demands greater speed, high-quality images, exposes patient to greater radiation doses, and requires more sophisticated and expensive technician help.

One digital X-ray room, with good planning and infrastructure support, can potentially produce the same volume of exams as two or three analog X-ray rooms. In addition, it provides information for many other clinical data systems along with customer satisfaction benefits through reduced time to exam, lower repeat exams, almost instant quality assurance, and faster results to the referring physician.

When the office manager begins to consider the positive deeper ramifications this new "more expensive" technology can have on the larger picture, there are many benefits to this new technology, including earlier, more precise diagnoses, and higher cure rates due to early detection.

Preemptive Medical Imaging: Smaller Slices, Greater Yield

By Brian Baker, Vice President, Regents Health Resources, Nashville, Tennessee

As noted in the introduction to this chapter, Brian is experienced in evaluating costs and impact of imaging technologies. Prior to joining Regents, Brian started and ran a division of the nation's largest health care construction company, Turner Construction, as the general manager within logistics for Medical & Research Solutions Group. Their charter was to strategically plan, implement, and procure the health care technology within Turner's health care building projects for selected clients. Brian gained his diverse experience by working with some of today's most recognizable health care companies such as GE Medical Systems and Philips Medical Systems in various roles of increasing responsibility. His clinical environment experience includes Hospital Corporation of America, where he helped implement a national Biomedical Service program that reduced service and maintenance costs for HCA, along with his role as vice president for a surgery center development company. Brian has completed numerous technology training programs focused on diagnostic imaging while also receiving Six Sigma training at GE.

• •

Less than 5 years ago, because of limitations in technology, it was not possible to accurately measure small changes in a lesion's growth to make a diagnosis for symptomatic lung patients. As clinicians know, it's difficult to distinguish between benign and malignant lung tumors on imaging characteristics alone. Growth rates are the most reliable sign (other than a biopsy) that a nodule is cancerous.

As the 16-slice scanners were just coming to market, one small company purchased rights to artificial intelligence (AI) imaging software used in military applications, realizing the potential application of this AI when combined with the improved resolution capabilities offered by new CT scanners.

After a couple years of work by some very gifted scientists, this small company had what they thought were some usable algorithms for lung nodule imaging in 16-slice CT applications for segmentation, computer-aided detection, and computer-aided diagnosis. In the next step, they purchased a new 16-slice scanner and started the clinical experiments applying these algorithms to computerized tomography data sets and then comparing their outcomes to actual clinical diagnoses to refine the software.

The goal was to see if this software would really show anything new in the way anomalies were classified. As they were installing and configuring the software, they started looking for asymptomatic volunteers to image.

As just mentioned, until recently, it has not been possible to accurately measure small changes in relatively small nodule sizes with imaging technology. A doubling in volume from 3 mm to 6 mm or more was needed in order to make a diagnosis with previous CT technology. In addition, the tools to measure the imaging data sets typically available were not accurate or advanced enough and many times would not allow reproducible measurements on the same data sets. The new AI-CAD software had been designed to measure extremely small changes in volume provided a clear data set was provided by the now more accurate computerized tomography.

Early in the imaging of asymptomatic volunteers, a patient was identified by the medical director to have a small area of interest, a lung nodule. It was classified as only a couple of millimeters in size and marked for follow-up. In the past, it was not uncommon for several months to pass before a follow-up exam was performed due to technology limitations for visualization and measurement.

As part of this experimental phase, the patient was asked to return in less than a month—certainly a much shorter follow-up exam time than past protocols dictated. On his return visit and reexamination, this new, more accurate technology revealed a noticeable change in nodule volume: rapid growth. The volunteer was immediately sent for biopsy where it was determined as stage 1 lung cancer and it was immediately removed: asymptomatic and curable. Certainly the ability to detect tumors when they still remain small enough for their removal and therefore curative is of benefit.

Now, some would argue that the most ubiquitous X-ray exam, the chest X-ray, can offer the same early detection result. However, as radiologists are aware, lung nodule characterization on a simple chest X-ray even with CAD applied is limited to 5 mm or larger. Today's computerized tomography technology can image to 2 mm routinely with slice thickness selections of less than 1 mm. Several studies have shown CAD-software technology, when applied as a secondary read, provides double-digit percentage increases in the radiologist's accuracy in detection of pulmonary nodules, which may be the reason imaging technology is growing much better in detecting early lung cancers (Kolata, 2006c). With lung cancer still the leading cancer killer in the United States, what do you think the new CT and CAD technology is worth clinically and financially for the health care system? Is this preemptive medicine? The goal is becoming more visible through the fog.

As demonstrated earlier in this chapter, an industry often questions the efficacy, application, utility, value, and benefits of new technology. This is mostly because those in the health fields don't completely understand it, how to use it, or its potential benefits. Even considering limitations, cost, and dangers of modern imaging technology, the medical field is on the cusp of achieving what Damadian and other scientists were pursuing with the magnetic resonance imaging back in the 1970s: differentiation of disease process from normal tissue with imaging techniques.

Combine differentiation with early detection and the industry is closing in on real preemptive medicine. Although CAD software has a long way to go in its development, the future looks promising for imaging technologies and their abilities to produce amazing data. So many technologies, like functional imaging, hold the promise for new clinical discoveries. Utilization is not forecast to decline any time soon, nor is the cost of new technology predicted to decline.

What the industry must do to leverage the real utility and value of new technologies is continually rethink operational paradigms, considering not only the higher cost of new technology but also the advantages new technology provides within the context of the larger health care picture.

Clinicians must be supported in the adoption of the new technology by developing operational and educational tools that enable sound clinical diagnoses through a complete knowledge of the technology and its clinical application, thereby reducing unnecessary and inappropriate usage.

Chapter 23

Flattening Supply Chain Costs

Prelude: The bane of hospital chief financial officers: the supply chain cost drain. Supply chain costs for managing and acquiring medical equipment—such as coronary stents, joint replacements, information technologies, and various other items—are the single fastest growing costs for hospitals.

"Supply Chain Management" encompasses the planning and management of all activities involved in sourcing and procurement, conversion, and all logistics management activities.

Importantly, it also includes coordination and collaboration with channel partners, which can be suppliers, intermediaries, third-party service providers, and customers. In essence, Supply Chain Management integrates supply and demand management within and across companies.

Council of Supply Chain Management Professionals, 2004

Supply-chaining is a method of collaborating horizontally—among suppliers, retailers, and customers—to create value. Supply-chaining is both enabled by the flattening of the world and a hugely important flattener itself because the adoption of common standards between companies (so that every link of every supply chain can interface with the next), the more the efficiencies of one company get adopted by the others, and the more they encourage global collaboration.

Thomas L. Friedman, 2005

In 2002, the *New York Times* ran a series of articles on questionable business practices of group purchasing organizations (GPOs) within the hospital industry. It was alleged that GPOs have conflicts of interests (e.g., they controlled the stock of Internet-based company purchasing supplies) and the magnitude of their commissions and discounts were unknown to hospitals that used their services (Bogdanich, 2006). The U.S. Senate investigated these allegations in hearings (Walsh & Meier, 2002).

There may be yet another link in the hospital supply chain. In 2006, Attorney General Richard Blumenthal of Connecticut built upon the Senate findings by issuing more that 100 subpoenas to hospital CEOs belonging to the Healthcare Research and Development Institute. Members of the institute are paid to give advice to companies like Eli Lilly, Johnson & Johnson, Becton Dickson, and Morgan Stanley. These companies sell either supplies or financial advice to hospitals. Blumenthal was investigating whether the organization allows vendors to buy access to hospital leaders who are in a position to influence what supplies or services their institutions purchase. Blumethal said, "At the very least it suggests insider dealings—an insidious, incestuous, insider system" (Bogdanich, 2006).

In 2003, most of the journalistic fire and the Senate investigation focused on Premier, Inc., and Novation, Inc., the two largest group purchasing organizations, which account for about two thirds of the nation's hospital supply business. Congressional hearings were held in 2002 and CEOs of major GPOs testified (Bogdanich, 2006). In the course of the hearings, it became apparent hospital supply costs, delivering through the *supply chain,* a mix of manufacturers, distributors, marketers, e-procurement firms, GPOs, and providers, constituted the fastest growing segment of health care costs, second only to employee costs. Supply costs were critical to hospitals, whose margins averaged less than 4 percent. (Average hospital margins, 2006). Hospitals needed greater margins to maintain access to capital and to fund capital improvements, implement IT systems, and invest in high-tech equipment.

To remain competitive and to hold onto specialists, hospitals felt obligated to participate in the "medical arms race," a race that was expensive. Imaging costs, for example, are outstripped all other health costs (Iglehart, 2006).

According to the VHA, Inc., one of the nation's largest hospital systems, supply costs break down into these categories:

- Surgery: 20 to 22 percent
- Pharmacy: 16 to 18 percent
- Dietary: 7 to 8 percent
- Cardiac: 6 to 8 percent
- Laboratory: 5 to 8 percent
- Radiology: 5 to 6 percent
- Other (state room, central supply, and sterile processing): 20 to 40 percent

Physicians' loyalty to certain product brands makes supply chain cost reduction difficult. The ultimate solutions, said one hospital CEO, resided in having doctors use the same product, measuring outcomes, sharing data with doctors, and focusing on quality rather than costs. In other words, focus on quality data rather than brand.

The *New York Times* series and the congressional hearings caused a furor in the GPO industry. Some hospitals dropped contracts with Premier and Novation, others turned to e-procurement firms, and still others upgraded the position of hospital purchasing office. Together, GPOs started a collaborative effort called the Health Care Group Purchasing Industry Initiative. At the Web site, www.healthcaregpoii.com, one will find this definition of purpose.

> *The initiative is a voluntary association of health care GPOs created in 2005 to encourage and sustain best ethical and business conduct practices in the GPO industry. The Initiative's founding members are Amerinet, Broadlane, Child Health Corporation of America, Consorta, GNYHA Ventures, Inc., Healthtrust Purchasing Group, MedAssets, Novation and Premier Inc. These companies include most of the largest group purchasing organizations in the United States, estimated to represent more than 80 percent of the volume purchased through GPOs.*

This set of six core ethical principles is also located on their Web site.

1. Have and adhere to a written code of business conduct. The code establishes the high ethical values expected for all within the Signatory's organization.
2. Train all within the organization as to their personal responsibilities under the code.
3. Work toward the twin goals of high quality health care and cost effectiveness.
4. Work toward an open and competitive purchasing process free of conflicts of interest and any undue influences.
5. Have the responsibility to each other to share their best practices in implementing the Principles; each Signatory shall participate in an annual Best Practices Forum.
6. Be accountable to the public.

What the impact of this initiative and principles will be is unclear at the time, but there is no doubt that the importance of the health care supply chain has been highlighted and that some actions will be taken to standardize and rationalize the workings of the supply chain. That will require knowledge of how other industries control supply chain costs.

Flattening Supply Chains

In his now-famous book, *The World Is Flat* (2005), Thomas Friedman talks about the global supply chain. He wrote of Wal-Mart and how its elaborate inventory- and supply-chain management system gave it an enormous competitive advantage because it could set standards and cut costs of manufacturer suppliers.

Friedman also told the story of the building of his Dell Inspiron 600m notebook that he ordered on April 2, 2004. Dell's total supply chain, including suppliers or suppliers and manufacturers, involved 400 companies in North America, Europe, and primarily Asia, with 30 key players supplying the parts for Friedman's computer (Friedman, 2005). The completed computer arrived in Bethesda, Maryland, on April 19, 2004, where Friedman signed for it. Friedman's point was the Internet-connected companies made all of this possible at a decreasing cost each year.

Why is this not possible in the country's hospital market, with the 4,800 hospitals supplied by 150 health care suppliers, all belonging to an organization known as the Health Industry Group Purchasing Association (HIGPA)? Probably because hospitals consider themselves independent, have different purchasing system, and most do not have executives assigned to supply chain management.

This may change. The cost to hospitals is still running about 35 percent to 40 percent of their budgets and is rising at a rate of 15 percent to 20 percent each year. The CEOs of the nine largest GPOs insist they are negotiating as large a discount as they can from manufacturers (Firestone, personal communication, 2006). However, commissions extracted from the hospitals and discounts for manufacturers, for the most part, remain a trade secret. There are cries from reformers for more transparency and greater accountability on the part of the GPOs.

An organization, the Center for Practical Health Reform, held a Health Care Supply Summit in March of 2004 to consider approaches to increase transparency, establish standards, improve operating procedures, remove conflicts of interest, and preempt government regulations. Not much came out of their efforts (except to form study committees), but it was clear the supply chain industry was threatened by the prospects of government regulation and dangers of making trade secrets known to their competitors within the industry.

By April 3, 2006, HIGPA successfully headed off government regulation by adopting a code of conduct for self-regulation, requiring compliance by all 150 supply chain members, and by telling Congress that government regulation would increase costs by at least $30 billion.

Neither the federal government nor HIGPA has the top-down business structure or leverage or motivation of a Wal-Mart or a Dell; however, the ultimate power of transparency and the "flattening power" of an interconnecting management system will prevail. Transparency may not come from the supply chain but from government itself.

In Florida, under Governor Jeb Bush's leadership, state government has launched a Web site, FloridaCompareCare.gov, that provides detailed quality and cost comparisons of the state's hospitals and ambulatory surgery centers for certain procedures. It will not be long before government begins to cut down on the cost of supplies as a contributor of unrelenting rises in hospital costs and begins to attempt to standardize the costs and standards of supplies.

Innovation Talking and Action Points

One of the major sources of innovation is a change in perception. With computer systems, one can quickly perceive that anything is possible—like managing the inventory of a Wal-Mart, putting together a Dell computer with inventories from 30 different countries, or managing inventories of hospitals from 150 different supply chain companies.

Case Study

2006—The Year of Transformation for the Health Care Supply Chain
By Greg Firestone, CEO of NCI, Tampa, Florida

After college, Greg Firestone worked in the food manufacturing industry for 10 years. In 1989, he went to work for Richard Allen Medical, which sold instruments to hospital operating rooms. To gain access to group purchasing organizations, Richard Allen retained a firm called NCI, a consulting and education firm. Firestone went to work for NCI in 1995, bought out the owner in 1999, moved the company from southern California to Tampa, and converted it into a health education company for purchases.

Today NCI is a leading health care information, communication, and education company specializing in supply chain, IT, and professional education. By encouraging close associations with health industry stakeholders, Firestone hopes to advance common interests, the exchange of views, and the settling of differences between different constituency communities. He believes this collaboration and consensus are predicate to high-quality, affordable health care for all Americans.

• •

If you have been contemplating when to "truly begin" the process of transforming your supply chain, clearly, the time is now.

During 2005, we saw GPO business models changing radically. Many providers are beginning to better manage the exorbitant cost of high-technology products. While these changes are encouraging, from my perspective, we are only scratching the surface. Successfully managing the supply chain is no longer as simple as inventory management and demand fulfillment. It's really the combination and integration of strategy, financial, revenue, operations, and clinical performance management.

Unfortunately, this requires specialized knowledge and know-how, commonly lacking among health care providers. Currently, as we all know, few hospitals and integrated delivery networks employ a senior-level executive with the necessary qualifications to effectively manage their supply chains. Attaining/retaining financial viability in the current environment depends on a chief resource officer's attributes, with experience implementing total quality management (TQM) systems.

The cost of supply chain inefficiencies is staggering. According to accepted industry estimates, as much as 35 percent of total supply chain costs result from inefficiencies. This has been known for some time, yet many providers have chosen to pursue the business-as-usual approach. In my opinion, this is no longer an option.

We're all aware of the number of health care providers—from every type of provider network—that are in critical financial trouble; many have already filed for bankruptcy. In contrast, we have also read about those providers that have recognized significant cost savings by merely "cutting the fat." Consider the following examples provided by health care systems that have already instituted strategic supply chain initiatives:

- Swedish Health Care Services of Seattle, Washington, undertook a strategic supply chain initiative in 1998 when it was a two-hospital system. Since that time, Swedish added its third hospital (2000) and was still able to cut its total supplies expense as percentage of net revenues 4.5 percent, from 21.0 percent to 16.5 percent. With net revenues for 2005 at $1.0 billion, that's a savings of $45.0 million. Allen Caudle, Swedish's vice president—supply chain management, estimates Swedish's annual expense reduction to be approximately $30.0 million (Carey, B., 2006).
- In 2002, the management of the Health Alliance of Greater Cincinnati decided to make supply chain management a core competency. A two-state, seven-hospital system, the health alliance was spending $269 million of its $1.3 billion in annual patient revenues on supply-chain items (Market competition, 2004). Dorman Fawley, chief operating officer, says the health alliance showed an audited expense reduction of $34.3 million over the 4-year period ending December 31, 2005.

Five steps are required to achieve this magnitude of success. In priority order, they are:

1. Developing an operating plan with defined performance metrics
2. Optimizing employee knowledge of supply chain management practices
3. Driving toward a financially, administratively and clinically integrated supply chain
4. Focusing on total supply spend to improve financial management
5. Assuring continuous improvement in relation to economic, health, and satisfaction outcomes of care

The path to rigorous supply chain management and financial health in health care is not unknown, only infrequently traveled. My colleagues and I at NCI have written a 14,000-word white paper explaining the importance of the health care supply chain. Its title is "Profit-Driving Opportunities in Health Care Supply Chain Integration," and it discusses the strategic implications of the supply chain evolution in health care and the value-creation imperatives for today's health care stakeholders.

Executive Summary of NCI White Paper

Why is supply chain integration important? Supply chain integration connects the supply chain management (SCM) and enterprise performance management (EPM) systems of material suppliers, medical product manufacturers, healthcare distributors, providers and other end-users.

It offers the healthcare industry a chance to reduce costs, improve revenue, enhance profitability, and deliver greater value to the marketplace.

The healthcare industry is challenged to offer a greater number of individuals access to quality care at a reasonable cost. Business process synchronization across organizations helps to integrate healthcare information, technology, financing and delivery systems to achieve greater efficiencies. These efficiencies allow more individuals to receive the healthcare products and services they need, at a lower total cost.

At no time in history have enabling technologies and societal needs converged to the degree they have in healthcare today. The open architecture of the Internet and the benefits of wireless communications come at a time when our society finds itself unable to properly care for all acutely, chronically and terminally ill individuals and unable to support wellness in our populations.

Technology-leveraged supply chain integration offers an unparalleled opportunity to better manage the health of populations of healthcare beneficiaries at the least possible cost. It also offers our healthcare organizations greater financial security at a time when that security is threatened.

The healthcare supply chain is very poorly evolved. The industry is easily a decade behind the supply chain status of the more advanced retail, electronic and automotive markets. Inefficient movement of goods, redundant processes and excess inventory plague the industry.

The Balanced Budget Act (BBA), the Health Insurance Portability and Accountability Act (HIPAA), Ambulatory Payment Groups (APGs), potential malpractice litigation aimed at Managed Care Organizations (MCOs) and a variety of other short-term impediments to profitability have put unparalleled cost pressures on healthcare players. The industry critically needs solutions that save money and still support quality healthcare.

Supply chain integration helps achieve these needed savings through the efficient movement of goods, information and funds to and from source and end-user. It establishes an information technology infrastructure that links healthcare participants and aligns their performance goals with improving the health of covered populations of beneficiaries at the lowest possible cost.

The resulting virtual healthcare organizations (VHOs) are better informed about what types of healthcare interventions are appropriate, when particular products or services are needed and how best to provide them. These VHOs are better positioned than non-integrated healthcare participants to innovate and generate wealth and value in business and medicine.

Chapter 24

Skinning the Universal Coverage Cat the Massachusetts Way

Prelude: Politicians in the Commonwealth of Massachusetts have decided universal coverage can be achieved through political consensus and compromise. It is not yet known whether this model can be implemented in the Bay State or expanded beyond its borders.

Our health care system is a mess. The number of uninsured Americans is approaching 50 million. The costs of health insurance are too high, and they are rising rapidly. Polls repeatedly show that a majority of Democrats, Republicans, and Independents favor universal health insurance. The trouble is that we cannot agree on a solution.

Stuart H. Altman and Michael Doonan, 2006

The Innovative Path to Universal Coverage

The Massachusetts Universal Health Coverage bill, which passed in April 2006, is unquestionably innovative in these ways:

- It mandates every citizen who can afford health insurance must buy it or pay an income tax penalty.
- It converts $500 million in the states' free health pool to help low-income citizens buy an insurance policy.
- It creates a way for businesses and individuals to save on insurance by using pretax dollars. (Belluck, 2006)

Other details and highlights of the bill are:

- All residents will be required to have health insurance.
- All employers are required to offer insurance or contribute up to $295 a year for each uninsured employee.
- Fines will be levied against residents or businesses that do not comply—except individuals unable to find "affordable" policies, or businesses with 10 or fewer employees.
- Something called the Connector will link individuals or companies with under 50 employees to a choice of affordable private health plans paid out of pretax dollars. The Commonwealth Connector is a new agency that serves as clearinghouse to help both workers and small companies buy insurance. The Connector allows individuals to maintain coverage from job to job and even between jobs. It also cuts down the administrative costs that make it so expensive for insurance companies to market to small businesses and their workers.
- Health insurance obtained through the Connector will be portable when the enrollee changes jobs.
- Subsidized premiums will be offered on a sliding scale for enrollees with incomes up to 300 percent of the federal poverty level. (Rowland, 2006a).

Three big questions swirling around the bill are:

1. Is the bill a trend for other states, or just another turn to the left in a very liberal state, which like another liberal state, Vermont, is the first to offer universal coverage? Probably not. Massachusetts is unique—it has relatively few uninsured (about half the national average of 15 percent), already spends $500 to hospitals to cover the uninsured, and employers in other states are likely to resist mandates to pay for the uninsured.
2. Will it contain costs, and or simply spin out of control and plunge the state deeply into debt? No one knows at this point, although the Medicare and Medicaid experiences over the past 40 years indicate costs are vastly underestimated. In 1965, Medicare spending was projected to cost no more than $9 billion, but now is over $250 billion.
3. Will it work in a vacuum in which other states do not have such a bill and the United States lacks universal coverage? Americans are mobile. Census figures show that each year some 20 percent of Americans move. The IRS reports that five million people file from new states each year (Nancy DuVerge Smith, personal communication, 2006).

There are doubters as well about the trend-setting potential of the Massachusetts plan. Some note universal coverage initiatives in other states—Maine, Vermont, Minnesota, and Illinois—have either yet to be followed up upon by other states or have yet to bear fruit. Others say it is difficult to put universal coverage into play in a vacuum (i.e., without national reform).

In Massachusetts, the political left says the poor cannot afford individual mandates, and the right has claimed these mandates invade privacy. Conservative commentators in other states question the workability of a $295 per employee levy, saying it may work in liberal Massachusetts but not in their backyards. Romney vetoed the $295 levy, but was overridden by the legislature. Some on the left are furious a Republican governor has taken credit for the Massachusetts universal coverage bill. The left is also unhappy that Massachusetts must ask for a waiver from the federal government to proceed with its plan to cover Medicaid recipients and other plans to cover 460,000 other uninsured Massachusetts residents.

Even Dr. David Himmelstein who founded a physician group for a single-payer system, questions whether the Massachusetts approach will work. The law, he says, "Will force you to purchase either something you can't afford or something you can afford but which will be nearly useless in the actual coverage it offers" (Barry, 2006).

Tenncare, an ambitious health care Medicaid experiment introduced in the 1990s to cover the uninsured, failed for multiple reasons: Tennessee's doctors did not support it, it lacked financial controls, and it ended up devouring one third of the state's budget (Hurley, 2006).

Brendan Miniter, assistant editor of the *Wall Street Journal OpinionJournal.com,* doubts Massachusetts can force Medicaid patients to pay their bills and questions if Massachusetts will save money with Medicaid reform (Miniter, 2006).

He refers to Tennessee's Tenncare as an example of why Medicaid reform, even with the best of intentions, does not work. Tenncare was introduced in the 1990s to cover everyone who couldn't afford or didn't qualify for health insurance.

Tenncare ended up eating up one third of Tennessee's budget. Romney insists Massachusetts will not make Tennessee's mistake, because the Bay State's plan doesn't not try to expand Medicaid, but to reform insurance.

However, by and large, editorial writers and pundits have been enthusiastic about Romney's assertions. They say the clue to wider coverage lies in insurance reform rather than expanding Medicare.

Romney is given credit for effectively crossing party lines and satisfying partisan on the left and right. Says Stuart Altman of Brandeis University, "Every once in a while, a political person or event comes up and kicks this thing [universal coverage] into the mainstream. The Massachusetts plan could become a catalyst and galvanizing event at the national level and could be a catalyst for other states" (Rowland, 2006a).

Even some conservatives give guarded praise. Robert E. Moffitt, director of the health policy center for the conservative nonprofit Heritage Foundation, notes its innovativeness, "The idea of creating a consumer-driven insurance market is different. Nobody in American has ever done anything like it" (Rowland, 2006a).

Innovation Talking and Action Points

The most impressive thing about the Massachusetts achievement is the bringing together of diverse points of view in a complex political system to reach consensus. But will the political center hold? There is a lesson to be learned here, and it comes from one of the principles and insights of complexity science. It is this: "Build a good enough vision and provide minimal specifications rather than trying to plan out every little detail" (Miniter, 2006). A democracy is based on compromise and consensus, and it seems to me that Massachusetts, while having a Republican governor and a heavily Democratic legislature, showed compromise and consensus are possible on a very controversial issue—universal coverage.

Case Study

Finding a Way to Achieve Universal Coverage
By Governor Mitt Romney

March 11, 2006, *Wall Street Journal*

BOSTON—Only weeks after I was elected governor, Tom Stemberg, the founder and former CEO of Staples, stopped by my office. He told me, "If you really want to help people, find a way to get everyone health insurance." I replied that would mean raising taxes and a Clinton-style government takeover of health care. He insisted: "You can find a way."

I believe that we have. Every uninsured citizen in Massachusetts will soon have affordable health insurance and the costs of health care will be reduced. And we will need no new taxes, no employer mandate and no government takeover to make this happen.

When I took up Tom's challenge, I assembled a team from business, academia and government and asked them first to find out who was uninsured, and why. What they found was surprising. Some 20% of the state's uninsured population qualified for Medicaid but had never signed up. So we built and installed an Internet portal for our hospitals and clinics: When uninsured individuals show up for treatment, we enter their data online. If they qualify for Medicaid, they're enrolled.

Another 40% of the uninsured were earning enough to buy insurance but had chosen not to do so. Why? Because it is expensive, and because they know that if they become seriously ill, they will get free or subsidized treatment at the hospital. By law, emergency care cannot be withheld. Why pay for something you can get free?

Of course, while it may be free for them, everyone else ends up paying the bill, either in higher insurance premiums or taxes. The solution we came up with was to make private health insurance much more affordable. Insurance reforms now permit policies with higher deductibles, higher copayments, coinsurance, provider networks and fewer mandated benefits like in vitro fertilization—and our insurers have committed to offer products nearly 50% less expensive. With private insurance finally affordable, I proposed that everyone must either purchase a product of their choice or demonstrate that they can pay for their own health care. It's a personal responsibility principle.

Some of my libertarian friends balk at what looks like an individual mandate. But remember, someone has to pay for the health care that must, by law, be provided: Either the individual pays or the taxpayers pay. A free ride on government is not libertarian.

Another group of uninsured citizens in Massachusetts consisted of working people who make too much to qualify for Medicaid, but not enough to afford health-care insurance. Here the answer is to provide a subsidy so they can purchase a private policy. The premium is based on ability to pay: One pays a higher amount, along a sliding scale, as one's income is higher. The big question we faced, however, was where the money for the subsidy would come from. We didn't want higher taxes; but we did have about $1 billion already in the system through a long-established uninsured-care fund that partially reimburses hospitals for free care. The fund is raised through an annual assessment on insurance providers and hospitals, plus contributions from the state and federal governments.

To determine if the $1 billion would be enough, Jonathan Gruber of MIT built an econometric model of the population, and with input from insurers, my in-house team crunched the numbers. Again, the result surprised us: We needed far less than the $1 billion for the subsidies. One reason is that this population is healthier than we had imagined. Instead of single parents, most were young single males, educated and in good health. And again, because health insurance will now be affordable and subsidized, we insist that everyone purchase health insurance from one of our private insurance companies.

And so, all Massachusetts citizens will have health insurance. It's a goal Democrats and Republicans share, and it has been achieved by a bipartisan effort, through market reforms.

We have received some helpful enhancements. The Heritage Foundation helped craft a mechanism, a "connector," allowing citizens to purchase health insurance with pre-tax dollars, even if their employer makes no contribution. The connector enables pre-tax payments, simplifies payroll deduction, permits prorated employer contributions for part-time employees, reduces insurer marketing costs, and makes it efficient for policies to be entirely portable. Because small businesses may use the connector, it gives them even greater bargaining power than large companies. Finally, health insurance is on a level playing field.

Two other features of the plan reduce the rate of health-care inflation. Medical transparency provisions will allow consumers to compare the quality, track record and cost of hospitals and providers; given deductibles and coinsurance, these consumers will have the incentive and the information for market forces to influence behavior. Also, electronic health records are in the works, which will reduce medical errors and lower costs.

My Democratic counterparts have added an annual $295 per-person fee charged to employers that do not contribute toward insurance premiums for any of their employees. The fee is unnecessary and probably counterproductive, and so I will take corrective action.

How much of our health-care plan applies to other states? A lot. Instead of thinking that the best way to cover the uninsured is by expanding Medicaid, they can instead reform insurance.

Will it work? I'm optimistic, but time will tell. A great deal will depend on the people who implement the program. Legislative adjustments will surely be needed along the way. One great thing about federalism is that states can innovate, demonstrate and incorporate ideas from one another. Other states will learn from our experience and improve on what we've done. That's the way we'll make health care work for everyone.

P.S. to Case Study

Even the most ardent proponents of universal coverage are cautious about the so-called "Romney Plan" succeeding in the long run in the Massachusetts or in the United States as whole. Here, for example, are comments from two faculty members of Brandeis University:

> Massachusetts has now sent a new message to the rest of the country; providing health care to the uninsured is possible. This move will embolden leaders in other states. One day, Washington may follow suit. (Altman & Doonan, 2006)

Here is what the national correspondent for the *New England Journal of Medicine* says about the Massachusetts plan:

> The Massachusetts health care reforms are ambitious and complex. State officials anticipate that adjustments will be needed along the way. Perhaps the most important assumption, however, is that the costs and economic burden will be acceptable in the long term. When the economy slows, state tax revenues decline.

> Simultaneously, Medicaid spending accelerates and the number of people who enrolled in Medicaid or uninsured increases. For the reforms to succeed, Massachusetts will have to sustain them through the economic hard times, when they will be needed most. (Steinbrook, 2006b)

Massachusetts voters do not often reflect U.S. voters' opinions, as evidenced in recent presidential elections of Richard Nixon over George McGovern, George H.W. Bush over Michael Dukakis, and George W. Bush over John Kerry—yet with the Massachusetts universal coverage bill, they may be right that they can "lead the nation" and absorb the burden of covering the uninsured without raising taxes. Now that would be political innovation worth bragging about.

Behind all this speculation one huge question remains: What does each state do about Medicaid when the going gets tough?

Nationally three entitlement programs—Social Security, Medicare, and Medicaid—eat up 52 percent of the federal budget. Medicaid, which covers 52 million Americans, is the single biggest and fastest growing component of most state budgets (Review and outlook, 2005).

What to do?

According to Tom Coburn, MD, senator from Oklahoma, and Regina Herzlinger, PhD, professor of business at Harvard Business School, senior fellow at the Manhattan Institute, the answer may be Personal Health Accounts (PHAs), a Medicaid variation of Health Savings Accounts (Coburn & Herzlinger, 2006).

In a recent *Wall Street Journal* article, Coburn and Herzlinger (2006a) noted three states—Florida, South Carolina, and Oklahoma—had already moved decisively to provide Medicaid recipients with PHAs (Personal Health Accounts). PHAs allow recipients to chose whatever services, doctors, and other providers they want. Enrollees, in effect, can shop for care. If PHAs were to spread to other states, including Massachusetts, Coburn and Herzlinger claim these accounts could revolutionize Medicaid, just as Wisconsin revolutionized welfare in the early 1990s. Something must be done, they said, to fix Medicaid, which is out of control, grew 9.1 percent in 2004 alone, and is already gobbling up over 20 percent of many states' budgets.

Part Six

Consumer Innovations

The consumer voice has advanced from a whisper to a holler.

David Nash, 2000

Health Savings Accounts: Wall Street, Health Plan Web Sites, and Preventive Services

Prelude: Health Savings Accounts have far-reaching implications for Wall Street investors, health consumers, physicians, hospitals, health plans, banks, and chronically ill patients. Because of the extent of these implications, this chapter is longer than other chapters, consisting of three parts, each part followed by appropriate case studies.

Part 1: Wall Street and Health Savings Accounts

When it comes to medical benefits, millions of Americans already have a health insurer. Soon, many will also have a debit card and a bank tied to their medical plan.

Banks, credit unions and money management firms are now quietly positioning themselves to become central players in the business of health care, offering 401(k)-type accounts to cover future medical expenses.

Eric Dash, 2006

A Health Savings Account (HSA) is a combination of a high-deductible insurance plan coupled with a safe tax-free savings account used to pay for qualified health care expenses. Large employers—Wal-Mart, Guidant, Microsoft, Fujitse, General

Motors, DaimlerChrysler, and Nokia—already offer HSAs to employees. Eight percent of companies with 10,000 to 20,000 employees now provide HSA benefits as compared to 1 percent in 2004. Three million Americans have HSA-qualifying high-deductible plans (Dash, 2006).

HSA Financial Management

Banks, credit institutions, financial firms, and money managers are rushing into HSAs. Soon, millions of Americans will have a bank tied to their medical plan. The Bank of America, J.P. Morgan Chase, and Wells Fargo have joined the HSA chase. UnitedHealth Group owns a Utah bank, Exante, and National Blue Cross Blue Shield Association is establishing a bank covering 94 million Americans.

Experts predict 15 to 25 million Americans will own HSAs by 2010 when the average individual's account balance will grow to $3,500 from today's $1,500. Ballooning balances may mean $75 billion in new money to manage (Dash, 2006). Banks may generate lucrative fees by offering consumers mutual funds and other investment vehicles as account balances grow.

Why are Wall Street and the banking industry rushing into the consumer-driven/ HSA industry? The reason is because Wall Street and the banks smell big opportunities, not only in managing funds, generating related investment business, and processing claims, but in simply being part of the next big move in the health care industry. Wall Street and the stock market are involved because they advise and invest in banks and health sector organizations.

Riding the HSA Wave?

As a health care participant, how do you ride the consumer-driven HSA wave? How do you innovate to the meet the new challenges? According to Cambridge, Massachusetts–based Forrester Research, 5.9 million people have enrolled in consumer health plans. Scott Spiker, president and CEO of Chicago-based Destiny Health, says 4.1 percent of Americans are now in plans in the private marketplace and that this will grow to 7.8 percent by the end of December 2006 (Betbeze, 2006). The actual HSA membership was probably just over 4 percent by the end of 2006 (Claxton et al., 2005).

What to Do?

St. Luke's Health System, a 10-hospital system in Kansas City, Missouri, is responding by setting up a system to make shopping easier for HSA holders and consumer plan members. St. Luke's is repricing inpatient obstetrical care, outpatient tests, outpatient procedures, and CT and MRI scans—anything likely to concern price-conscious consumers. It is not an easy process. St. Luke's calculates the price by finding out what the consumer's plan is, checking out the contract, and calculating the coinsurance (Butcher, 2005).

Consumers Want to Know in Advance What Things Will Cost

However laborious it is to discover, the first-time consumer wants to know in advance what something is likely to cost. This may be obvious in the retail world, but for the health care world, knowing in advance what products or services cost is revolutionary. This type of innovation will almost certainly spread to other hospitals.

In the meantime, the health plan industry is doing its own innovations. Humana, Aetna, UnitedHealth Group, and others are spending millions building transparent consumer-support tools. Some of these tools allow shoppers to compare hospital and physician prices and outcomes.

Entrepreneurs are also at work. Steve Case, AOL founder and now head of Revolution Health, is pouring $500 million into various segments of the consumer health industry; WebMD, the informational Internet-based health care Web site, is betting on the rapid growth of HSA-linked personal health records to spur consumer use of its online services (Yang & Cappell, 2005).

Case Study 1

Health Savings Accounts from a Physician's Point of View

By Dr. William West, founder of First HSA, Inc.

Seven years ago, Dr. William West, an obstetrician and gynecologist in private practice in Reading, Pennsylvania, co-founded First HSA, Inc., a nationwide health administration company. He and his partner started First MSA (Medical Savings Accounts) in 1999 and changed the name to First HSA when the Health Savings Account legislation was passed on January 1, 2004. First HSA provides the custodial services and accounts management for a Health Savings Account.

The company is now the eighth largest HSA administration company in the country, is doubling its business each year, and is actively partnering with third-party administrators and other insurance companies to foster the HSA movement.

• •

Those health care expenses in HSAs include expenses that count toward the deductible of the insurance plan and can also include other qualified health care expenses including home care, vision care, chiropractic care, and other things that may not actually count toward the deductible.

Our HSA offers an FDIC-insured checking account that provides unlimited checkbook and debit card access to the fund. We provide monthly statements that detail their account activity, deposits, transactions, interest earned, and ending balance. We provide competitive interest rates on the fund that start at 1.4 percent and that go up to 4.5 percent based on the balance. In addition, there's 2-hour telephone banking, free Internet access, live customer service from 8:30 in the morning until 6 in the evening, a periodic newsletter, and investment options when they reach a certain threshold they can invest in mutual funds.

We believe the current health care market is unsustainable. Businesses, employers, and individuals cannot afford current double-digit increases in insurance premiums. That's what we will see in the current HMO/PPO marketplace because there is no cost containment. HMOs were built on "Economic-Negative 101": high utilization at low cost. In other words, HMOs offered broad benefits with low premiums—an impossible promise.

At first, managed care worked because of limitation of access, restriction of referrals, and utilization review, and ratcheting down of payments to providers and hospitals. Eventually there was a backlash because the providers couldn't go any lower, and now you're seeing the double-digit increases with the indemnity model.

Health Savings Accounts reconnect the patient and provider by revealing the true costs of health care services. What we have seen so far is a 20 percent to 50 percent decrease in cost utilization. This is because of consumerism—people being alert to true costs. Consumers now shop for health care services, they increasingly use generic drugs, and they ask questions about the necessity or need of additional testing.

Although critics say there is the threat of decreased use of preventive care, we have seen the opposite. Use of preventive services is greater than or equal to use of preventive services in the current HMO/PPO model. HSAs with high deductibles will be the dominant market force by 2010 to 2012. Furthermore, almost half the employers offering these plans did not offer coverage before and 30 percent of those signing up were previously uninsured. The reason is the 20 percent to 40 percent decrease in premiums compared to traditional HMOs and PPOs.

In Pennsylvania, the premium for a healthy family in 2006 was $1,600. People don't see the value of that high a premium when they're healthy. So what are they doing? They are either self-insuring or going without insurance.

My wife and I have five children; we have a $5,000 deductible and we are covered for $300 a month. We put $420 in our HSA so our total cost is $720—not $1600. In our practice, we have 22 employees, and we went 100 percent HSA. Because of the savings from our old PPO, we were able to fund 90 percent of the deductible of the out-of-pocket risk for our employees, which was less than in the traditional PPO plan. We see small businesses across the country completely replacing HMOs and PPOs with HSAs.

Larger companies are offering HSAs in combination with other plans. I have concerns with that policy because of adverse selection. People with diabetes and other chronic illnesses are better off with HSAs, but they tend to stick with traditional plans because they understand them.

However, because they are paying with pretax versus post-tax dollars, people with chronic disease actually save money. The HSA legislation allows high-deductible plans to pay for first-dollar coverage of things like immunizations, mammograms, and Pap smears so the money does not come out of the HSA. The same goes for wellness and disease-management programs. In fact, some high-deductible plans will pay for Lipitor because it is "preventive" in the sense it will prevent a heart attack.

One of the problems physicians face across the country are mounting accounts receivable. That is happening, not because of HSAs, because PPOs and HMOs alike have raised their deductibles. "Real-time" adjudication systems are developing that allow us to know exactly what patients owe before they leave the office, but they are still in their infancy. The technology is there, but insurance companies have not built the systems to answer questions in real time.

When that happens, when questions can be answered and payments can be made at the swipe of a card, HSAs and high-deductible plans will take off. Doctors may be paid less per service, but they will be paid promptly rather than waiting months to be paid.

Only two companies, Humana and Blue Cross Blue Shield of South Carolina, have real-time adjudication systems—but the technology for prompt adjudication is coming fast, probably within 1 or 2 years. If it doesn't come, there will be a backlash, and doctors may drop health plans and begin to negotiate on their own.

Another thing that may develop fast is patient discounts at the point of service. Look at Lasix and ophthalmologist, Botox and dermatologists, facelifts and plastic surgeons. Take third parties out of the equation and prices drop and quality improves.

In any event, we firmly believe high-deductible plans with HSAs will grow exponentially and will become dominant within 5 years. People will be better off, consumers and doctors will know what things cost, and costs will be contained.

Case Study 2

HSAs: A New Paradigm in Payment and Collections

By Dr. Neil Baum

Neil H. Baum, MD, is an urologist in private practice in New Orleans. He is the author of *Marketing Your Clinical Practice—Ethically, Effectively, and Economically* (Jones and Bartlett, 2004). Baum is considered an expert on practice marketing, information technology applications in medical practices, and taking steps to ensure patient satisfaction. This case study appeared in the June 1, 2006, issue of *Urology Times*.

Most of us have survived managed care and capitation, or getting paid for not treating patients under the concept of covered lives. Unfortunately, the government and insurers are not content until they have modified the American health care delivery system. So what's new on the horizon? It is health savings accounts (HSAs) and consumer-driven health care.

What is an HSA? It consists of a contribution made by an employer to an employee's tax-free savings account. The HSA combines an insurance policy with high deductibles of $1,000 to $5,000 (compared with the current $300 to $400 per year deductible paid by the employer) to help people pay pre-deductible expenses.

As a result, the responsibility for the payment of health care services shifts from the employer to the employee or the patient. Any money not spent by the patient will be allowed to accumulate tax free, and employees can take the account with them if they decide to change jobs, making the health care plan very portable.

Because this concept has already achieved critical mass—nearly three million Americans are currently signed up for HSAs—we need to understand what this will mean to our practices and what we can do to prepare for it.

For this article, I have interviewed Anthony Crillo, a health care consultant and an expert in HSAs, to spell out what they will mean to you and me. After reading this article, you will have a much better understanding of the new paradigm and what you can do to make your practice HSA friendly.

Payment at the Time of Service

One outcome of HSAs is that patients should be more financially prudent with their health care decision-making processes. Early research on HSAs suggest that people who pay more of their own costs up front are more aware of what they spend and make choices based on cost as well as quality.

This new paradigm is based on the theory that patients can make good choices regarding the selection of their health care and will look for services that are most reasonably priced and that offer the most quality. The presumption is that this method of paying for health care by cost-conscious consumers will control spiraling health care costs. If the proponents are correct, the result will be lower costs paid by both employers and employees.

Under the HSA model, physicians will find it imperative to collect fees for their services from their patients. Historically, patients have had low or relatively low co-payments that were easy to collect or that didn't make a huge difference if one or two slipped through the collection cracks. The remainder of the bill was of no consequence to the patient because it was paid by the insurance company. Our payment from the insurance company was based on a negotiation between our practice and what the insurer was willing to compensate us for our service on a "take-it-or-leave-it" basis.

With the new paradigm, doctors will have to collect for their services at the time of the service or they are not likely to receive their deserved compensation. We all know how hard it is to collect from patients, so the new mantra will be, "Get paid now or don't get paid at all!"

According to Crillo, you will go broke if you bill patients weeks after you deliver the service. The acronym to know is PATHOS, or payment at the time of service. The origin of this term as applied to health care is a mystery. In literature, "pathos" means "suffering." Perhaps those who apply PATHOS to payment for services feel doctors suffer financially when payment is delaying, and accounts receivable pile up.

Fortunately, getting paid by patients using an HSA may be easier because they will have a debit card by which fees can be deducted from an account created for them by their employer.

Doctors also will need to alter their revenue cycle. One significant challenge is to accurately identify the contracted rate at the time of service so practices can collect the right amount from the patient without having to later bill, credit, or provide a refund. While it sounds easy, there is some infrastructure that needs to be put in place so this can happen.

For example, if you are seeing a patient with a recurrent bladder tumor and you conduct a cystoscopy in the office using a laser to remove a small bladder lesion, then you need to know what the fee for that service is and collect this fee from the patient at that time.

An even better technique is to collect the fee for the service *before* the procedure. This will work if you know exactly what you are going to do and if you know what the expected fee is. Examples include procedures such as vasectomy, minimally invasive therapy for BPH, or neonatal circumcision.

This new system requires educating your patients and staff about how it works. Some, but not all, HSA patients will be knowledgeable about the system and will be prepared to pay at the time of the service or provide their debit card so that your fee is paid when you deliver the service. I recommend that letters be sent to all of your HSA patients explaining the new method of payment.

The new system places a new level of responsibility on your employee who handles collections, as well. Your receptionist and scheduler also must be prepared to inform patients of what is expected at the time of their visit.

What Is Involved?

Accommodating the HSA paradigm will require training in customer service techniques for all of your employees who deal with collections. Remember that they will become public relations ambassadors for the practice.

Adopt a collection agency mentality and you may find patients leaving. Those best at this are credit card companies. Contact some of the leading companies and find out who conducts training and get in touch with them to learn best practices.

The practice must be prepared to accept HSA debit cards. You also should set up a system to provide patients with online access to view their bills and patient balances.

Throughout this process, it is important to create loyalty through outstanding service. My staff and I try to provide excellent service by seeing patients on time; calling them with their lab reports or imaging studies (especially if they are normal); calling or faxing their pharmacy with their prescriptions; and calling patients at home after outpatient procedures such as a vasectomy or a minimally invasive procedure for BPH.

There is going to be price transparency in the new paradigm. In the past, we rarely discussed the price of urologic care with our patients. They really weren't concerned, as they weren't responsible for the fee for the care they received. With HSAs, high deductibles, and higher co-pays, patients are going to be more interested in fees for our services.

We need to know what the costs are and share that information with our patients. We are going to have to compete on price, which means we will need to know what our competitors are charging. Ultimately, we will have to demonstrate the value of what our patients receive.

It may even mean that we have to offer house calls if a patient has a problem with a catheter and they don't have anyone to take them to the emergency room. Airline passengers will travel an hour or more to save $100 on airfare, and patients will travel greater distances to find a practice that offers value and cost savings.

The Bottom Line

Obtaining and maintaining patients will no longer be about signing the right contracts. We are going to have to find techniques to become more efficient so that we can spend more time with patients. We will have to identify what aggravates our patients, such as waiting for physicians, and solve that problem by seeing them in a timely fashion. If we fail to adjust to the new paradigm, patients will keep doctors waiting as they beat a path to someone else's door.

Part 2: Health Plan Web Sites for Consumers

Prelude: Transparency: the currency of consumer-driven care. If all health care transactions were transparent, that is, readily available up front and consumers were paying more out of pocket, costs would likely fall.

The growing effort to enlist consumers in reducing health-care costs has been stymied by the fact that most people just don't know what medical care costs. Private and government health coverage has helped shield them from bills.

And even with newer consumer-driven plans that employ Health Savings Accounts, which give people more of a financial stake in the issue, pricing information can be hard to come by.

Now, a major national health insurer is making an effort to change that. Starting tomorrow Aetna, Inc. plans to make available online the exact prices it has negotiated with Cincinnati-area doctors for hundreds of medical procedures and tests.

The initiative, which Aetna hopes to take eventually to other parts of the country, aims to give patients the tools to comparison shop and make savvier decisions with their health-care dollars. Aetna is the first major health insurer to publicly disclose the fees it negotiates with physicians. Some in the health-care industry say the move is likely to push more insurers to follow suit, which in turn would give a significant boost to consumer-driven health plans.

Vanessa Fuhrman, 2005

Medical groups are just beginning to feel consumer-driven health care's impact. Patients are asking for generic drug substitutes, bringing information for discussion gleaned from the Internet, and becoming more selective because of high copays and high deductibles. Medical groups may be just seeing the tip of the consumer iceberg.

According to *New York Times* reporter Milt Freudenheim (2006d), WebMD signed contracts with Aetna, Cigna, and WellPoint, and with big employers Bank of America, Cisco Systems, Dell Computer, IBM, Pfizer, Shell Oil, and the state of North Carolina to provide private Web sites. The purpose? To help these large managed care plans and their corporate clients track medical records, look up disease information, and compare cost and ratings of doctors and hospitals.

Already Aetna is experimenting in Ohio with comparing physician quality ratings and costs (Fuhrman, 2005). Furthermore, WebMD is holding talks with big banks and financial giants like Fidelity to help sell and manage HSAs. GE is also in on the act. GE recently purchased IDX, which already provides EHRs to tens of thousands of doctors' offices. EHRs will be essential to compete and provide for health consumers' needs.

Big medical groups recognize this. Jefferson University physicians contracted with Allscripts to provide EHRs to its 480 physicians and 700 residents in 75 different locations. Corporate Web sites will be a potent factor in promoting the growth of HSAs and EHRs (*Jefferson University physicians*, 2006).

Innovation Talking and Action Points

For consumer-driven health plans, using their Web sites to help consumers compare prices is a major innovation. Many of the 5,000 Ohio doctors affected by Aetna's price comparison strategy reacted negatively with doctors citing differences in their circumstances, overheads, and clientele. Practicing doctors say no single set of prices fit all practices, which depend on a number of factors. Aetna says prices vary from doctor to doctor for a range of reasons, including prestige, scarcity or surplus of doctors in a given specialty, or whether the doctor belongs to a small practice or large medical group—all factors affecting price negotiations.

The negotiated fees typically are discounted from list prices doctors charge uninsured patients and are available only to Aetna and plan members. The listings, which don't include behavioral-health specialists or dentists, can be viewed by any Aetna member in the country. "To create a more functional health-care market, we needed more transparency," says Ron Williams, Aetna president. The Cincinnati pilot project has yet to spread to the rest of the country but is a sign of the times, and it may lead to doctors listing their fees in their offices and posting them on their own Web sites.

The transparency movement is picking up momentum (Rubenstein, 2006). So far, information indicates prices for simple services are fairly consistent, but hospital costs vary widely. In Wisconsin, for example, hospital knee replacement fees vary from $16,900 to $34,500. Insurers, some states, and Medicare are launching a number of comparison-shopping initiatives.

- As already mentioned, Aetna started a pilot project in Cincinnati, comparing hundreds of negotiated rates with local doctors. By the end of 2006, the program had spread to Cleveland and Columbus, Ohio; Pittsburgh, Pennsylvania; Las Vegas, Nevada; Kansas City, Kansas; and Washington, D.C., as well as southern Florida and the states of Missouri and Connecticut.

- In early 2006, UnitedHealth Group said it had negotiated rates with dentists for nearly 600 procedures, plus expected out-of-pocket expenses for enrollees in dental plans.

- Cigna in April 2006 revealed cost ranges and average out-of-pocket costs in New Hampshire and Wichita, Kansas, for MRIs, CT scans, and PET scans.

- Certain states offer sites with hospital charge information (see www.floridacompare.gov and http://hospitalpricing.sd.gov).

- Some state hospital associations are providing sites with hospital charge information. See www.nhpricepoint.org and www.wipricepoint.org for examples.

- Medicare in June 2006 posted ranges of what it pays hospitals for 30 common procedures and treatments (see www.cms.hhs.gov/HealthcareConinit/01 Overview.asp).

- Drug-cost information at specific pharmacies is available from companies such as Lumenous, Cigna, and UnitedHealth. For instance, see www.myfloirarx.com and www.destinationrx.com.

Case Study 3

Aetna Price Transparency

By Betsy Sell, spokeswoman for Aetna

Betsy Sell is spokeswoman for Aetna, in its Ohio physician transparency project and its expansion to other states. Ms. Sell is located in Cincinnati.

Imagine a world without price tags. You can buy that big screen TV that you've had your eye on, but you won't know the price until your credit card bill comes in the mail. Sounds ridiculous but that's exactly the world the average American lives in when he or she seeks medical care. As reported in the *Wall Street Journal* in February and June of 2005, knowing the cost of a doctor's visit has long been a missing piece of the health care decision-making process. More recently, 84 percent of Americans agreed that hospitals, doctors, and pharmacies should publish their prices for all goods and services.

The Price Transparency Trend in Health Care

Enter an emerging health care trend known within the industry as price transparency. Through price transparency, consumers know what they can expect to pay at the physician's office *before* visiting the physician. While this approach sounds sensible, no health insurer had ever been able to provide this level of detail to its members. The reasons for this were varied: contractual issues, complexities in the rates physicians agree to accept from insurers, and concerns about consumers shopping for health care on price alone.

That all changed in August of 2005, when Aetna announced that we would be the *first* health plan to provide consumers with online access to the discounted rates for the most common office-based procedures provided by primary care and specialist physicians.

Price Transparency in Cincinnati

Aetna's price transparency initiative responded to a call for help. The employer and broker communities asked us for our help in educating consumers about the actual costs of medical care. Despite the fact that we already offered our members a wide variety of information on health issues, health care quality, and average pricing within specific geographies, the increase in adoption of consumer-directed plans necessitated more detailed information. After considering a variety of options, we determined that the time was right to offer physician-specific price information. The question was: How do we do it in a way that was meaningful to consumers and respectful to the medical community?

One of the keys to successful implementation was testing the program on a limited pilot basis, allowing us to solicit feedback and expand and enhance the initiative over time. The greater Cincinnati market—including Dayton and Springfield, Ohio; northern Kentucky; and southeast Indiana—was chosen as the test market for a variety of reasons including the opportunity to test the initiative in three states with three different regulatory environments.

Collaboration would also be key. As the pricing tool was built, our medical directors and network professionals in the Cincinnati market began meeting with large physician groups and organized medicine. We also conducted more than 20 focus groups with physicians and office staff. Feedback from these meetings and focus groups—including changes in the terminology used with members, intense member education, and intense physician communication—was incorporated into the program.

The Launch

On August 18, 2005, Aetna launched price transparency. The initiative was well-publicized in the media, receiving significant attention in the *Wall Street Journal, ABC World News Tonight,* and *National Public Radio*. These media stories helped educate consumers about not only Aetna's efforts, but the trend toward transparent pricing in health care.

With the launch of our pilot, consumers could research what they could expect to pay at the doctor's office *before* going in for a visit. Available via the Aetna Navigator password-protected member Web site (www.aetna.com), the tool includes rates for 5,000 physicians and physician groups. To access pricing, members search for a physician within the "DocFind" physician search engine. Upon selecting a physician, members choose "View Rates for Aetna Members." The rates are provided for office visits, diagnostic tests, minor procedures, and other services. In all, rates are offered for up to 25 services by specialty and, considering the variations in services among specialties, the tool contains rates for 600 services in all.

The Results

Since the launch of price transparency in Cincinnati, between 600 and 1,000 consumers a month have visited the price information site. Increased usage happens at two specific times—as consumers choose their new benefits for the year ahead (typically in the fall) and as consumers begin to use their new benefits (typically in January). While it's too early to say whether consumer behaviors have changed in Cincinnati, we believe that simply raising awareness about the costs of care is one more step in creating a marketplace for consumers as health care decision makers.

Beyond consumers, we have spent months soliciting feedback from physicians, employers, and policy makers. Physician research was conducted in Ohio; Connecticut; Washington, D.C.; and Florida. Overall, physicians have provided constructive comments on improvements to the program, employers have been keenly interested in our plans to expand the program to their employees, and policy makers have asked to learn more about our experiences. In addition, Aetna's move toward price transparency has been hailed by the media as a "watershed in the evolution of a health care policy in the U.S."

Next Steps

Recently, Aetna announced that we would be expanding our health transparency initiatives to include price transparency in all or parts of 11 states and the District of Columbia and price, clinical quality, and efficiency transparency in all or parts of 7 states and the District of Columbia. With these enhancements, clinical quality and efficiency information will be available for more than 14,800 specialist physicians, and specific pricing will be available for more than 70,000 physicians. In addition, we will be expanding the pricing tool to include up to 30 procedures per physician with the addition of major procedures to the list of available services.

In a testament to the collaborative nature of the program, its expansion came in direct response to feedback from physicians, who were very clear that their patients needed enough information to make decisions based on overall value, not simply price alone. Aetna will continue to work with employers, providers, and legislators to push the envelope on health care transparency. We expect to expand the program to additional markets and enhance it with new information over time.

Part 3: Health Savings Accounts, Preventive Safe Harbors, and Chronically Ill Workers

In my twenty-five years of medical practice, I have seen hundreds—perhaps thousands—of people die needlessly. And I cannot begin to count the thousands of patients I have seen suffering through illnesses that could have been prevented.

As much as I love the practice of medicine, I must confess that I'm growing a bit weary of patching up problems that never should have happened in the first place.

Nine of the ten leading causes of death in the United States are preventable. Only one of ten, diabetes, is an inherited disease; the others are affected much more by what we do than by who we are. And since diabetes itself can often be controlled by diet, weight loss, and exercise, it is fair to say that changes in the American lifestyle could help control all of the ten leading American death styles.

Dr. Harvey B. Simon, 1992

HSAs: Just for the Young, Healthy, and Wealthy?

- Are Health Savings Accounts (HSAs) just for the young, wealthy, and healthy?
- Do HSAs punish older chronically ill workers?
- Will HSA shortfalls generate a new wave of personal bankruptcies?
- Will HSAs cause their holders to delay care to avoid dipping into their deductibles?
- Will HSAs reduce costs—or just burden hospitals and doctors with more unpaid bills?

Since HSAs were made widely available with the passage of the Medicare Modernization Act in December 2003, these contentious and unresolved questions have swirled around HSAs. The jury remains out, and it's still early in the HSA game, but so far none of these dreaded things have come to pass.

The overriding fear is healthier, wealthier, and younger workers will choose HSAs because of tax benefits and lower premium costs, thus destabilizing the risk structure and leaving lower-income, older, and sicker workers with higher premiums. A second, less-frequently articulated fear is that hospitals and physicians will pile up unpaid debts that will bring them to their knees.

It is still is too early to tell whether these fears are well founded, but it is safe to say employers and health plans have seized upon a subsequent preventive safe-harbor ruling to help manage and control costs of chronically ill workers.

Preventive Safe-Harbor Services Included in HSAs

High-deductible plans cover most routine preventive services for free. These are the so-called preventive safe-harbor services. On March 30, 2004, 4 months after Congress passed the Medicare Modernization Act, which included a provision making HSAs widely available, the U.S. Treasury Department and the IRS released this statement:

> *Preventive care HSAs can only be established by eligible individuals, who must have coverage by a high deductible health plan (HDHP).*
>
> *Generally, an HDHP cannot provide benefits before the deductible is satisfied, but there is an exception for benefits for preventive care. The guidance issued today provides a safe harbor list of benefits that can be provided by an HDHP, generally clarifying that traditional preventive care benefits— such as annual physicals, immunizations and screening services—are preventive care for purposes of HSAs, as well as routine prenatal and well-child care, tobacco cessation programs and obesity weight-loss programs.*
>
> *The guidance also clarifies that preventive care generally does not include treatment of existing conditions. Comments are requested regarding whether other benefits should qualify as preventive care, including payments of certain drug costs benefits provided by employee assistance programs, mental health programs, or wellness programs. The safe harbor provides employers and plans with the flexibility in designing health benefits, allowing them to provide preventive care benefits that reduce health costs and encourage early identification of health conditions that may require medical attention.*

Preventive safe-harbor services covered by HSAs include:

- periodic health evaluations
- routine prenatal
- well-child care

- immunizations
- tobacco cessation programs
- obesity weight-loss programs
- screening services (Pap smears, mammograms, and bone-density measurements)

How have employers and health plans reacted to this preventive safe-harbor ruling? For the most part, they have reacted rationally and innovatively. U.S. industry knows six key issues:

1. Half of health care costs stem from just six diseases: diabetes, heart disease, hypertension, mood disorders, asthma, and chronic obstructive lung disease.
2. Chronically ill workers generate the most costs.
3. The most effective way to manage these costs is to identify early those with chronic illness or who are likely to develop chronic illnesses.
4. Workers with chronic disease have been reluctant to tell employers of their problems for fear of losing their jobs or of being excluded from traditional managed care plans.
5. Healthy employees are productive employees.
6. The availability of "free" preventive safe harbor benefits (i.e., that do not come out of the HSA accounts) makes HSAs more palatable to employees.

Once employees recognize preventive services are "free," they are more likely to disclose their illness. This is important for employees who are choosing to fully replace HMOs and PPOs with high-deductible/HSA–linked accounts. Individuals with emerging or existing chronic disease detected early can be managed in a more timely and less-costly fashion than those with "hidden" diseases who develop a full-blown crisis.

Sell HSAs as Mutual Benefit to Employer and Employees

Critics of HSAs say high-deductible/HSA plans are nothing but sophisticated cost shifting that will punish sick employees, cause them to delay seeking treatment, burden them with debt, interfere with traditional entitlements, and do nothing to reduce costs.

This may be—but all the evidence is not in. It is doubtful if any amount of evidence will impress policy critics who viscerally disapprove of a consumer-based, market-driven system calling for behavioral modifications and personal and financial responsibility. Those who think of health care as an entitlement believe everyone, by government fiat, is entitled to health care, no matter their lifestyle. Overcoming this laissez-faire entitlement mentality will never be completely accomplished.

However, for employers, desperate to stem costs and maintain competitiveness, these high-deductible/HSA plans offer a window of opportunity. Adding preventive safe-harbor benefits adds to the salability of HSAs to employees and to discussing the advantages of HSAs to employers and employees.

HSA Advantages for Employers and Employees

For the employers, the benefits are that the employee-owned funds:

1. Promote increased involvement in health care decisions for employees to spend their health care dollars more wisely by encouraging them to "shop around" based on quality of care
2. Provide both employers and employees with tax benefits
3. Allow "matching" contribution options by employers and employees
4. Permit the business to remain competitive
5. Promise to enhance worker wellness and productivity

For the employees, the benefits are:

1. Increased consumer choice
2. Funds roll over from year to year, eliminating the use-it-or-lose-it philosophy
3. Tax benefits on the contributions, earnings, and distributions
4. Increased take-home pay
5. Long-term investment opportunity
6. Portability

UnitedHealth Group Joins Hunt for Early Management of Chronic Illnesses

The UnitedHealth Group, the managed care market leader in selling HSA accounts to businesses of all sizes, has joined the hunt to help consumers and employees in the companies the group covers to better understand, manage, and live with chronic illnesses.

The new program, called Rewards for Action, combines personal education with preventive screening and other means of promoting health. The program focuses on diabetes, asthma, heart disease, and hypertension. Rewards for Action encourages employees to actively manage their conditions, partly by strengthening patient–physician relationships.

By deploying relevant personal information, interactive tools, financial incentives, and customized management programs, employees can adjust their lifestyles to improve their health. According to UnitedHealth, 7 percent of people with chronic disease generate 70 percent of health costs. This disproportional cost of chronic diseases may be because employees don't recognize and manage their care early, because they don't make the necessary lifestyle changes, or because only 55 percent (as documented in RAND Company studies) of individuals with chronic disease receive recommended care.

Innovation Talking and Action Points

HSAs and their preventive safe-harbor feature may represent a fundamental innovation for employers and their employees. Depending on your ideology, innovations may be good or bad, succeed or fail. It may be that HSAs will fail to cut costs. It may be a Massachusetts-type solution, combining HSAs with state subsidies and insurance reform will prevail—or it may be that the United States may eventually go for a universal coverage system.

Case Study 4

A Connecticut Manufacturer's HSA Experience
By Jeffrey J. Hogan, Regional Manager, Rogers Benefit Group

Jeff Hogan is the New England regional manager for Rogers Benefit Group (RBG), Inc., a Minneapolis-based privately held insurance marketing and benefits firm. RBG was established in 1947, operates 71 offices nationally, and handles more than $2 billion in annual benefits premium. Hogan manages a regional office in Farmington, Connecticut, that covers Connecticut, Rhode Island, Massachusetts, Maine, New Hampshire, New York, and New Jersey.

Hogan specializes in designing consumer-driven strategies for middle-market companies and has consulted for PHOs and insurance carriers regarding these strategies around the country. He has also recently lectured on advanced CDC implementation techniques and the technical architecture of CDC products. Hogan has provided expert witness services on health insurance issues and strategies.

In 2006, Hogan served in his hometown, Farmington, as the vice chair of the town council and chaired the town's strategic planning implementation committee. He is an avid outdoorsman and in 2005 was the immediate past director of the Appalachian Mountain Club's Mountain Leadership School. This school teaches people outdoor leadership skills. He lectures on wilderness leadership, wilderness medicine, and accident scene management.

• •

Three years ago, a manufacturer in Connecticut faced a dilemma: a 29 percent increase in its base health insurance premium rates. The firm was under tremendous overseas and domestic competitive pressure to hold down costs. A new CEO grasped for a cogent, integrated strategy to control health insurance costs. Dramatically, he implemented an HSA plan for his employees and fully funded the deductibles for all employees with the hope that he would soon manufacture educated health care consumers. His success in achieving this goal makes him the hero of our story.

For the last 15 to 20 years, countless employers have ceded their health plan buying decision to health resource managers and departments. Managed care plans have been sold as commodities with little price or feature differentiation. Owners and CEOs became detached from the buying decision. Over the same period of time, as in the case of this manufacturer, utilization increased unabated and employees indiscriminately used their copay plans without the knowledge of the cost or quality of services and without a real concern for cost.

Consumer-directed health plans have revolutionized the marketplace. Early indications show substantial behavior modification occurring in groups that have adopted intelligent, incremental strategies for properly implementing and monitoring the results of these plans. The unique design of these plans, providing for cost transparency and 100 percent preventative coverage, encourages a new relationship between the user and the plan.

The manufacturer described herein is representative of other fully insured groups on the eastern seaboard. Bottom-line, first-year utilization demonstrated dramatic behavior modification changes within the group on prescription drug utilization, on preventative benefits utilization, and on front-end pick up and management of disease process.

Most employers are aware that 6 percent to 10 percent of their employee population represents 40 percent to 70 percent of their claims. Many employers, including this manufacturer's CEO, committed to a strategy that gives incentives to the 6 percent to 10 percent of their population with disease process to seek health plan resources and contract provisions that help them to manage and control their disease process. Many of the aspects of their respective strategies were quite simple.

HSA plans allow for a preventative safe harbor that permits health plans to pay for a host of preventive services for free. Physical exams, routine immunizations, Pap smears, mammography, bone-density testing—even routine eye and hearing examinations—are often covered. Many large health plans are trying to out-do one another by offering richer preventative services and interpreting the safe harbor in a way that makes them more marketable.

In this case, the CEO invested in a multiyear strategy that promised to:

1. reduce predictable annual premium increases
2. educate his employees on price and quality issues associated with health care and to modify their existing behavior
3. over a number of years create educated employees who appreciate and like their health plan

To operationalize the strategy, the CEO demanded that his agent:

1. secure a carrier that provided an integrated HSA product serviced by superior technology for customer service access and access to online tools to inform employees on price and/or quality
2. provide rich education and collateral materials to his employees during and after open enrollment that would inform them about all of the many programs available to them through the plan including free preventative care, smoking cessation and wellness programs, vision/hearing care, case management for disease management and other concierge services that would incent them to modify their behavior
3. provide quarterly reports back to him that demonstrated the behavioral changes of his employees including reports on how many and how often employees accessed online tools, online customer service, and reports detailing average fund balances in HSA accounts
4. provide a mechanism up front for employees to self-refer themselves to case managers equipped to handle their disease process and, potentially, to offer additional free services to them via the plan's preventive safe harbor
5. provide a facility, via a lunchroom kiosk for employees without home computer access, to access all of the health plan's online functionality while still at work
6. give credit for the group's educational efforts via a prenegotiated renewal methodology that gives credit to the group for positive behavior modification

The manufacturer enacted mandatory enrollment meetings with his employees in small groups. His strategy was portrayed to the employees via a simple financial incentive sheet that explained the financial logic and the mechanisms of the program. Health plan personnel were on hand to explain technology tools, Rx calculator tools, concierge and disease management, and customer service features to the employees in a personalized setting.

Amazingly, in the first year, the group renewed with an 8 percent increase and in 2006 renewed with a 4 percent increase. The group's Rx claims went from 25 percent of gross claims to 12 percent in the first year! Case management proactively handles about 6 percent of the group's population who self-advocated for their disease process. Preventative utilization increased dramatically in the second year (the first year had no comparative data).

Bottom line, once the employer advocated for employee responsibility and provided hard financial resources to force intelligent consumerism from above, the group saw dramatic positive behavior modification within their employee population. Once employees carried cash forward within their HSA accounts, they became invested in the strategy and became desirous of more and better information about their care, services, providers, and alternatives.

The revolutionary thing that occurred within this group and others embracing intelligent CDC strategies relates to the fact that their biggest users of care—persons with disease process—were given the means and the opportunity to get extra preventative services and concierge care management from the inception of their plan.

Previously, managed care required a year of claims data to "discover" persons with disease process via an analysis of Rx claims (hardly an efficient process). The other revolutionary thing about new CDC products is that health plans can provide real-time feedback to employers related to preventative use, case management usage, and other important items.

Health plans are becoming more effective at recognizing the power of incentives and active programs that promote good health and positive behavior modification. They are also discovering that employers are more inclined to stay with plans that partner with them to reduce costs.

Chapter 26

Alternative and Complementary Medicine Enters the Mainstream

Prelude: Why medicine considered complementary may deserve data entry. Alternative medicine continues to grow in popularity among Americans, yet there remains no systematic way for pricing its services.

In their quest for effective health care, they do not feel bound by the traditions of traditional American medicine. Their near obsession with prevention and wellness has taken this generation well beyond the perimeters of mainstream clinical practice.

It has not been doctors and hospitals, but consumers themselves who have brought alternative medicine—including acupuncture, biofeedback, and homeopathy—closer to the modern mainstream.

Health-conscious consumers, including a surprising number of older people, have promoted a huge range of diet, wellness, and self-care options. They buy billions of dollars worth of over-the-counter medications, home test kits, antioxidant vitamins, and dietary supplements. They have given rise to a publishing industry of newsletters, magazines, and lay-oriented medical books. Virtually all of this has been done without any encouragement from the established health care system.

Daniel Perry, 1997

There is much that we can learn from complementary medicine to make our patients feel better while our science attempts to make them get better. However, to encourage the terminally ill to spend the last few precious months of life chasing the false promise of a cure is as cruel as it is intellectually dishonest.

Michael Baum, 1996

269

While the medical establishment questions whether alternative medicine is worthwhile, patients embrace it. According to a *New York Times* article, consumers spend $27 billion a year on alternative medicine. Nearly half of adults used alternative therapy in 2004, up from 42 percent a decade before (Carey, B., 2006).

Venturing Outside the Mainstream

Millions of patients venture outside mainstream medicine. They're taking herbs for colds and depression, getting spines manipulated, having pain sites needled, ingesting dietary supplements to build cartilage in their knees, swallowing palmetto extracts to shrink prostates, buying up anything containing antioxidants, desperately seeking cancer cures, enduring caffeine enemas to flush out toxins, and undergoing intravenous therapies to leach out calcium from atherosclerotic plaques to unclog their arteries.

The National Center for Complementary and Alternative Medicine of the National Institutes of Health (NIH) defines alternative and complementary medicine this way:

> *Complementary and alternative medicine [CAM] ... is a group of diverse medical and health care systems, practices, and products that are not presently considered to be part of conventional medicine. While some scientific evidence exists regarding some CAM therapies, for most there are key questions that are yet to be answered through well-designed scientific studies—questions such as whether these therapies are safe and whether they work for the diseases or medical conditions for which they are used.* (National Center for Complementary and Alternative Medicine, 2006)

Why Patients Like Alternative Medicine

Patients like alternative practitioners because they spend time with patients, promise results, and don't "poison" them with expensive dangerous drugs (Carey, B., 2006). Besides, patients don't have to haggle with insurers or worry about drug or surgical side effects. Herbs, supplements, and acupuncture needles appeal psychologically because they are either "natural" or rooted in long-standing traditions of Eastern medicine. Dr. Neil Baum, a well-known medical marketing expert, advises doctors to ask patients about alternative therapies, show neutrality and understanding, and form relationships and develop referral relationships with legitimate alternative practitioners (Baum, 2004a).

Alternative Medicine Untouched By Health Reform

Alternative medicine is virtually untouched by health reform, yet health plans pay for 40 percent of acupuncture procedures and 80 percent of chiropractic care; consumers visit alternative practitioners 1½ times more frequently than traditional doctors (Molina, 2006, personal communication). The public is clamoring for additional coverage. What is lacking is appropriate coding for alternative medicine procedures and rational measurement systems for determining the effectiveness of alternative medicine.

The medical establishment (i.e., medical schools, doctors, health systems, and even the National Institutes of Health) is buckling under the weight of public opinion toward alternative medicine. For instance:

- Many medical schools now offer courses in alternative medicine. According to the Rosenthal Center for Complementary and Alternative Medicine at Columbia University, the 125 U.S. medical schools offer a total of 130 courses on alternative medicine. (Rosenthal Center, 2006, personal communication)
- Some doctors are conducting "integrative practices" and selling food supplements and herbs. The selling of supplements has created ethical controversies. (Howland, 1999)
- A number of academic centers and community hospitals have set up integrative centers. Here is the stated mission of the Duke University Integrative Center, "Integrative Medicine is based on a partnership between patient and practitioner, within which the best of conventional, complementary and alternative medicine practices can be explored in a whole person approach to health care and healing."
- Even the prestigious National Institutes of Health runs a division of alternative and complementary medicine.

Proponents and Opponents Unswayed by Each Other

Alternative medicine versus scientific medicine is one of those debates in which neither side is swayed by the other's arguments. In 2006, a number of articles in the scientific literature using double-blind techniques to remove bias have shown palmetto for prostate overgrowth, glucosamine and chondroitin for arthritis, echinacea for the common cold, and St. John's Wort are ineffective. About the only thing conventional medicine will admit is that chiropractic medicine has some benefits for back pain, the same effect for acupuncture for migraines, and the placebo effect is powerful in relieving symptoms and making people feel better (if you think something is going to make you feel better, it will) (Norderberg, 2000).

Loyalists of alternative products are unimpressed by scientific studies discrediting their beliefs, saying they will keep accepting alternative nostrums, undergoing its procedures, and downing its pills as long as they make them feel better (Carey, B., 2006). The debate is unlikely to reach any definitive conclusion.

Innovation Talking and Action Points

Many doctors will object to describing alternative medicine as an "innovation." It has been around for thousands of years, but health food chains and alternative medicine entrepreneurs see it as a profound innovation that fills a gap by satisfying those displeased with traditional medicine. In addition, they see a vast number of the population who fear side effects of traditional drugs, who feel capable of caring for themselves, who are tired of the hassles and barriers posed by insurance companies, and who are susceptible to messages that vitamins, supplements, herbs, and other "natural remedies" have magical preventive and restorative powers.

Some academic centers took the concept of integrative medicine very seriously when it started to gain a foothold in these centers in 1990s. In 1993, Duke University Medical Center formed a mind-body interest group. By 1998, Duke had funding that helped launch the Duke Center for Integrative Medicine in 2000. Duke became a founding member of the Consortium of Academic Health Centers for Integrative Medicine. Services offered at the Duke center include preventive and diagnostic screenings, nutritional counseling, physical therapy, massage, acupuncture, hypnotherapy, yoga, and stress management. The center's aim is to merge safe and demonstrably effective complementary medicine with conventional care—the best of both types of medicine. These services are offered by conventionally trained doctors and nurses and other paraprofessionals. According to Dr. Tracy Gaudiest, director of the center, which now has its own $11 million 27,000-square-foot facility,

> We're incredibly fortunate at Duke to have a number of critical factors come together. The 26-acre Center for Living campus is idyllic. We have the support of the leadership and faculty, and the donor's vision. We have an overall environment at Duke that is one of innovation and entrepreneurship. (Spence, 2006; emphasis added)

ABC Codes for Integrative Health Care

By Cynthia Laura Molina, MBA

In the early 2000s, Molina was CEO of ABC Coding Solutions. In the mid-1990s, she directed the Drucker MBA program at the Claremont Colleges and helped the Drucker School achieve even greater national prominence among management-education programs. Between 1990 and 1995, she was a partner in and served as director of marketing research and vice president of industry and business development for Healthy, a reimbursement strategy, health economics, and industry intelligence firm subsequently acquired by Elsevier and Parexel. She now works with NCI, an industrial education, communication, and consulting firm.

Molina—an expert in industry development, market leadership, and quality systems—explains here why all health care interventions (including complementary and alternative medicine) should be represented by complete, accurate, and precise coding if U.S. health care is ever to significantly advance the economic and health outcomes of care.

∙∙

Our ability to identify what does and doesn't work in health care—and at what relative cost—is dependent on:
1. understanding of what kinds of care are being delivered
2. capturing data on who received that care, when, and with what result
3. analyzing and reporting on practice trends and outcomes in a timely manner

The Importance of Good Data

Good decisions—whether in the clinical or business side of health care—are best supported by good data. The collection of good data is supported by standardizing the way we describe what it is that we want to measure—as well as the way we record and report on what is happening.

U.S. Health System Has a Long Way to Go

Those of us who have sat in a physician's office—completing yet another medical history form by hand—can appreciate that the U.S. health care system has a long way to go in terms of getting computerized. Very often, our mechanics have better and more automated "medical histories" on our cars than our doctors have on us. Lack of computerization extends far beyond the point of patient care—deep into the business side of health care. Insufficient reliance on technology is jeopardizing the quality of care, and it is also costing the industry tens (or, some think, hundreds) of billions of dollars in inefficiencies each year.

If we want to efficiently identify and evaluate the care that is being delivered to consumers, then we need standardized ways of referring to that care; tracking when, where, and by whom the care is delivered; and measuring the outcomes.

Learning from the Grocery Industry

In the grocery industry, widespread use of universal product codes or bar codes has automated the identification of food products and their prices and has improved the so-called *supply chain*—the movement of information, products, and money among manufacturers, distributors, grocery stores, and consumers. Product codes, bar codes, and radio frequency technology have led to more efficient business processes and, ultimately, to greater consumer choice and value for each expended dollar.

Similarly, in the financial services industry, the application of information technology has supported the standardization of financial transactions and credit reporting. This is what gave us greater access to money through ATMs and consumer credit.

Few Data Standards in Health Care

In health care, financial and health-related data standards have not been fully developed. As a result, we don't have the best possible flow of information, health care products and services, and money among key stakeholders. We don't get the greatest possible value for each expended health care dollar because about a third of each dollar is spent on administrative inefficiencies. We also don't get the best possible care because we don't have adequate data collection, analysis, and reporting tools to identify and communicate best practices.

Standardization and Digitization Are Key

This is a challenge that deserves and has received national attention. President George W. Bush and the secretary of the Department of Health and Human Services view the development of health-related data and communication standards (coding and interoperability standards), electronic health records (EHRs), and a national health information network (NHIN) as top priorities. The standardization and digitization of terminology that describes health care and its relative value are key.

The Power of Coding

Despite the high level of attention given to setting standards, even among the industry's top experts, few people realize the power of coding itself. Coding is one of the most powerful economic and political tools available to health industry stakeholders—especially to special-interest groups.

The existence or absence of codes determines whether care is visible or invisible to researchers, administrators, policy makers, and practitioners. Coding is essential for establishing the prevalence, patterns, and outcomes of care; factors that determine whether that care is covered and reimbursed or excluded by insurance companies.

Coding determines whether care is mainstreamed or marginalized and whether particular types of caregivers are financially rewarded or systematically disenfranchised.

Without complete, accurate, and precise codes for all types of care, caregivers and sites of service—those who make decisions about health care accessibility, quality, and cost management—are forced to rely on misleading information in their decision-making processes. Codes are specific and objective; other sources of information, such as product descriptions, are more subjective.

Codes for Integrative Medicine

For example, before ABC codes were developed for integrative health care, the nation's older code sets focused on the practices of 15.3 percent of the nation's caregivers and reflected less than 43 percent of the nation's 2.8 billion outpatient encounters—and even fewer inpatient encounters. Imagine the inefficiencies that would result if only 15.3 percent of food products in grocery stores had bar codes! The gaps in the nation's code sets resulted in missing or sub-standard data on care delivered by 84.7 percent of the nation's caregivers, in more than 1.6 billion outpatient encounters—and the vast majority of inpatient encounters.

Supply Chain Inefficiencies

Needless to say, in the past, these gaps created profound inefficiencies in the health care supply chain and they precluded scientific comparisons of the economic and health out-comes of competing sites of service, caregivers, and approaches to care. The gaps added costs and prevented the systematic identification of the nation's most cost-effective health care practices; that is, inadequate coding made evidence-based care an unachievable end-point. That situation has been changing.

In early 2002, I joined a group of data standards experts at ABC Coding Solutions to help ensure the health-related data standards for research, management, and commerce were more complete, accurate, and precise. The company had been systematically filling gaps in older code sets since 1996, with the goal of ensuring codes were eventually made available to reflect every product and service in health care, including medical procedures, pharmaceutical products, medical devices, biological products, supplies used by hospitals, herbal remedies, nutraceuticals (natural, bioactive chemical compounds that have health promoting, disease preventing, or medicinal properties), unconventional approaches to care, disability and rehabilitation services, and the like.

Codes for Every Type of Care

The company's founder was Melinna Giannini. Melinna believed that codes should reflect every type of care available to U.S. consumers—whether that care was delivered by allied or public health professionals, nurses, complementary and alternative medicine professionals, disability and rehabilitation providers, and/or conventional MDs and DOs. Therefore, she and her associates started by standardizing terminology and coding for complementary and al-ternative medicine (CAM) because this area of health care had been so clearly overlooked and yet was of such growing interest to U.S. consumers. (More than 40 percent of health plans provide some level of insurance reimbursement for acupuncture and more than 80 percent for chiropractic care—and consumers visit unconventional and non-MD practitioners far more frequently than they visit conventional medical doctors.)

Once Melinna and her team developed standardized terminology and coding for uncon-ventional care (and rational measurement systems for determining the relative cost effective-ness of those approaches to care), they went into other underdescribed areas of the U.S. health care system: allied and public health services, nursing services, wellness and holistic medical care, and spiritual care in the military.

Today, ABC Coding Solutions works with a broad range of health care professions to standardize terminology and develop representative codes for unconventional and non-MD care. The company also compiles critical data associated with that care. For example, to sup-port assessments of the legality, medical necessity, cost effectiveness of competing or com-plementary care on a per-intervention, per-practitioner, and per-state basis, ABC Coding Solutions offers tools that electronically link individual codes to expanded definitions of care; relative value units; practitioner identifiers; legal practice guidelines; and training, licensing, credentialing, referral, and supervision requirements.

The company also delivers educational programs, research and analytical projects, and management services that help key health-industry stakeholders apply these data elements to their businesses to better support the financing, administration, and delivery of cost-effective care.

ABC Coding Solutions' data standards and services are important because they help improve the efficiency and effectiveness of health care research, management, and commerce so more Americans get the quality care they need at a price they can afford.

Coding for Complementary Care: Opportunity or Threat for Physicians

Not every stakeholder in the U.S. health care industry is happy to see coding emerge for medical products and services beyond pharmaceuticals and MD-directed care. For example, coding for unconventional and non-MD care could be an opportunity or a threat to an average physician, depending on the motives of that physician. About half of family practice physicians believe that their practices ought to extend beyond conventional medicine and include legitimate complementary and alternative care. Some want to do this for economic reasons and others in the interest of patients.

If doctors are interested in providing patients with the best possible care, these physicians would want to know, for each diagnosis, whether a patient should see them first or see a nurse, nutritionist, chiropractor, physical therapist, pharmacist, behavioral health professional, or some other caregiver. A good physician wants patients to get care based on scientific evidence of which practitioner type does the best job of delivering that care for each diagnosis.

Other physicians may be more financially motivated and may recognize that proper coding for cost-effective CAM services would help health plans recognize the legitimacy of these services and develop favorable reimbursement policies. If these physicians were trained to provide CAM, for example, in the case of medical acupuncturists, the physicians would support coding for CAM. If CAM displaced the kinds of conventional medical care that the physicians typically delivered, these physicians wouldn't want CAM codes to be available.

Back Pain Example

Consider a patient with back pain, for example. Several factors will determine whether the care a doctor delivers to treat that back pain is the most cost-effective care available.

1. All approaches to back pain need to be identified.
2. All caregivers who treat back pain need to be identified.
3. All sites of service for treating back pain need to be identified.
4. All costs associated with each site of service, caregiver, and approach to care need to be identified.
5. All health, health-related, quality-of-life, and patient satisfaction outcomes of care need to be identified.

With this information available, researchers, administrators, policy makers, and practitioners can determine in advance who should be delivering what care to whom at what price. That way, if a patient shows up with back pain, a doctor is able to say (based on patient characteristics and the nature of the pain) which treatment would be best for the patient.

The physician would know whether to prescribe pain pills, refer the patient to a physical or medical massage therapist, refer the patient to an orthopedic surgeon, guide the patient in biofeedback techniques, or so forth. The physician and/or the practitioner of choice would be able to bill the insurance company directly for the delivered care and be more certain that cost-effective care would be favorably covered and reimbursed. Insurance claims would be less likely to be kicked into manual review, rejected, or delayed. Coding provides an efficient way of describing delivered care and the economic and health outcomes of that care.

It doesn't (as some fear) guarantee coverage and reimbursement—just as the assignment of a UPC to a food product doesn't guarantee the product will make it to the grocery store shelves or into consumers' hands. Just as bar codes provide an efficient way for a grocer to choose what to put on the shelves and for consumers to get through checkout lines with whatever products they prefer to buy, codes for health care products and services provide opportunities to make better decisions and gain broad-based efficiencies.

For example, with good codes available, health plans are more likely to pay for care that is medically necessary and cost effective, regardless of whether that care is conventional, complementary, or alternative and regardless of whether the practitioner is a doctor or another health care professional. Even when payment isn't intervention-specific (for example, in an inpatient or DRG setting), coding is important because it helps ensure that hospitals understand care patterns and can better staff their facilities to meet patient needs.

Health industry problems can't be resolved without the ability to measure what's actually happening and whether what's happening works or doesn't work. Without complete, accurate, and precise codes for all care, we don't have a complete set of measurement tools to identify what's actually happening, let alone whether it's working or not working. The first step in solving the cost crisis is to get measurement tools in place so we can understand both the nature of the crisis and potential solutions.

The health industry is far behind other industries in the application of information technology. This results in inefficient health care financing, administration, and delivery. It also results in less-than-optimal health care accessibility, quality, and cost management. The industry needs better tools for automating the flow of information, health care products and services, and money to ensure consumers get cost-effective and evidence-based care when they need it.

Every health industry stakeholder sincerely interested in properly balancing health care accessibility, quality, and cost management stands to benefit from complete, accurate, and precise codes, because codes give:

- researchers better data
- administrators critical insight for management decision making
- policy makers a more complete picture of the clinical, financial, and political landscape
- practitioners a mechanism for record keeping, practice management, and billing
- an opportunity for better care for more people at a lower cost

ABC Coding Solutions is a health IT company that develops and maintains data standards and databases essential to EHRs and a consumer-centric and interoperable national health information network. The company's information products and consulting services help health-promoting organizations and individuals finance, administer, and deliver cost-effective care.

Chapter 27

Managing Customer Relationships

Prelude: Customers—informed every step of the way—will stay with you. That is why health organizations are turning to meticulous management of customer relations through use of telephone banks and Internet technologies.

Customer Relationship Management (CRM) includes the methodologies, strategies, software, and web-based capabilities that help an enterprise organize and manage customer relationships. It is the collection and distribution of all data to all areas of the business. The general purpose of CRM is to enable organizations to better manage their customers through the introduction of reliable systems, processes and procedures for interacting with those customers.

A successful CRM strategy cannot be implemented by simply installing and integrating a software package; a holistic approach is needed. This approach may include training of employees, a modification of business processes based on customers' needs and an adoption of relevant IT systems (including software and maybe hardware) and/or usage of IT services that enable the organization or company to follow its CRM strategy. CRM services can even replace the acquisition of additional hardware or CRM software licences.

Wikipedia, 2006

Personally and Systematically Connecting with Customers

The customer relationship management (CRM) movement involves systematically connecting with patients personally by using telephonic communication and using sophisticated computer systems at every care juncture. Personally helping consumers navigate through a complex, sometimes bewildering health care environment through telephone and Internet technologies is emerging as an important way to satisfy corporate employees and members of health plans. Toward these ends, Connextions, a 10-year-old company located in Orlando, Florida, has a 350,000-square-foot call center with 2,000 nurses and other professionals and a computer bank integrating clinical and financial data.

Among its clients are *Fortune* 500 companies (e.g., Mercedes-Benz), large health plans (UnitedHealth Group), home monitoring and disease-management companies (I Care), and major hospital systems (Cedars Sinai in Los Angeles, Presbyterian Health Systems in Albuquerque), and Florida hospital, a 17-hospital system in Orlando.

The company states that its personally directed information services connect with consumers, patients, and health plan members at every "touch point"; these points at which individuals personally interact include hospitals, doctors' offices workplaces, and homes. This strategy, the company is betting, will cement customer loyalty (www.connextions.com). In essence, managing customer relations is sophisticated telephonic and electronic hand holding.

According to Connextions, Inc., their system features IT aggregation and integration of financial, clinical, and personal data, and frequent calls by trained, protocol-driven nurses versed in clinical problems. There may be something to this high-tech/high-touch personalized service. Hospitals and physicians can announce to their patients that they are bringing care and reducing costs to homebound patients, and they are concerned about all aspects of care. Being personally present at the patient's bedside is impossible for doctors, nurses, and other caregivers, but personal communication can be established remotely through the use of wireless technologies.

Innovation Talking and Action Points

As a management discipline, managing customer relationships has not yet significantly penetrated the hospital and physician worlds, but customer relationships are much on the mind of hospital marketing departments and of physicians themselves as health care moves into a consumer-driven world. Some physicians—for example, plastic surgeons and dermatologists—are employing public relations firms to inform customers. Emphasis on customer relationships will develop as the consumer-driven health industry grows. It may take the form of customer satisfaction surveys and focus groups. Both can be carried out fairly inexpensively. Hospitals frequently use firms like Press Ganey, in South Bend, Indiana, to conduct hospital satisfaction surveys.

Why has managing health care customer relationships become important? Because, with the advent of consumer-directed care and HSAs, relationships are changing because price-sensitive consumers want value in the form of personal service for their money. Formerly, payers treated health care as a wholesale business, and they tended to neglect individual consumers. It was wholesale, not personal, relationships. They saw no reason to go out of their way to please customers. No more. Two factors are driving this change:

1. Rising costs are pushing employers to negotiate consumer-driven/HSA health plans that shift costs from employers to members.
2. More people are willing and able to use the Internet to manage their own health care choices. (Novak, 2006)

As plan members become price conscious, plans are looking at customer management technologies, says Peter R. Kongstvedt, a vice president at Capgemini of Vienna, Virginia. "To relate effectively to members, plans must find ways to guide them through all the choices they'll have to make—on benefits and perhaps even treatment" (Baldwin, 2004). Consumer-driven care, in other words, is fundamentally about choices through every step of a patient's health care journey, including treatment in the physician's office or hospital.

If employers and health plans are to succeed in helping more demanding consumers through the system, they will have to resort to more efficient technologies, targeting individuals rather than groups. Payers will have to move beyond Web sites that simply offer administrative and health information, to answering questions online—How do I change doctors and plans?—to personally tracking the progress of a claim or questions of a customer—When will I be paid? Where is my claim in the payment process? How much money do I have left in my HSA deductible account? As health plan members begin to exercise choices, health plan companies will need a mixture of telephonic and electronic technologies to please customers and maintain their market share.

Case Study

Connextions, Inc.
By Ron Tazioli, Executive Vice President, Chief Development Officer

Connextions was incorporated in 1996 as a division of Magnetix Corporation, a provider of CD, DVD, video, and audio replication services. In response to the growing need for direct communication and marketing solutions, Magnetix began offering fulfillment, direct mail, and Interactive Voice Response (IVR) services to its customer base of publishers and marketing companies. To expand beyond the publishing market, Connextions was established with the opening of a customer service center. Today, Connextions has evolved to become a leader in integrated fulfillment, customer contact, and technology services for blue chip clients.

This case study illustrates how one company has integrated human technologies (their large call center) and data-mining technologies to systematically reach health care consumers employed by a variety of corporations and health plans. What is happening is elemental. As employers shift costs and risks to employees through higher deductibles and co-payments, often in HSA-linked plans, they must also often shift attention to please these employees or risk losing them as health plan customers.

• •

Connextions Health has a long and successful track record delivering innovative and profitable direct-to-consumer sales and member retention solutions for industry leaders within health care. Its customer relationship management solutions have produced industry-leading results and differentiated large health plans in the marketplace.

Connextions Health's CRM efforts have demonstrated that reaching out to new and longstanding plan members alike—at key intervals—to identify potential relationship-harming deficiencies that are subsequently and proactively addressed leads to increased member loyalty. For one of the largest health plan providers in the country with a sizable Medicare Advantage and Part "D" membership, Connextions Health lowered voluntary disenrollment percentages by more than 40 percent, leading to enhanced organic growth rates and lower member acquisition costs.

Member Touch Points

As with most of its clients, the primary means by which Connextions Health reduced rapid and voluntary disenrollment for this plan provider was through timely, personalized member touches. While mailings are a part of this CRM program, Connextions Health found the most important touches were proactive telephone calls to new and existing members.

Calls were made to members at five strategic junctures: just following notification of enrollment, at the effective date, 45 days after the effective date, at the point a disenrollment risk has been identified, and postdisenrollment. Each phone call was both an opportunity to enhance customer loyalty and to gather member intelligence that could be used to guide the next generation of loyalty initiatives. Call center agents were able to harvest such important member information as "Why did you choose this coverage?"

The specific opportunities for calls included:

- Preeffective Date: An opportunity to establish the relationship
- Effective Date: CMS mandated actions and gathering member intelligence
- Initial Use of Benefits: A period shortly after the effective date in which the member likely first uses his or her benefits and may become confused or disappointed as a result
- Predisenrollment: A save opportunity, when prior notification of disenrollment intent is received
- Postdisenrollment: An opportunity for win-back and to gather intelligence about what went wrong

Each of these intervention points has specific activities associated with them. In this particular client's case, they all required scripted telephonic outreach; some also had mailings associated with them. The telephone contacts were designed to elucidate any issues or perceptions that might put a member at risk of disenrolling. The calls also were carefully scripted to gather intelligence on members—intelligence that was used retrospectively to determine what differentiated a loyal member from a member who disenrolled. This information was then used to customize future loyalty interventions toward individual at-risk groups.

The Technology Behind It All: Business Intelligence and Data Mining

Data mining of customer usage trends was a key component in gaining intelligence about consumer behavior for this health plan provider. Connextions Health created a repository where defined data elements gleaned from member interactions were stored. A rollup of this information produced a "picture" of each member that was used to model and predict particular disenrollment risk points. These risk points triggered specific outreach activities targeted at a particular need to ensure member loyalty. Examples of these proactive outreaches included a phone call after a successful resolution of an appeal or a thank you for a referral, attendance at a meeting, or use of a preventive service. Many of these outreach activities were automated into Connextions Health's proprietary ConnexSys platform.

The power of the ConnexSys system lies behind its integration of methodologies and health care services required to proactively aggregate, analyze, and utilize member data. Using this tool, Connextions Health's teams of professionals, data analysts, account managers, and IT specialists craft and execute customized outbound call programs. Member profiles are continually refined and updated as information is added.

What Connextions Health Discovered

Connextions Health identified numerous common flags to mark new plan members who were at elevated risk of disenrolling. These flags were built into ConnexSys to trigger interventions designed to deal with these issues and retain likeminded future members' loyalties. Characteristics of at-risk groups include:

- ***Prior plan is Medicare plus Medicaid or fee for service.*** These members may not be accustomed to restrictions or processes of managed care.
- ***Heard of Medicare Advantage through a sales representative.*** There is potential for misrepresentation or misunderstanding of benefits.

- *Unable or unwilling to identify their prior plan, how they heard of Medicare Advantage, or what attracted them to Medicare Advantage.* This is an indicator of an uninformed or disinterested member.
- *Left prior plan due to care concerns.* These members may have special needs or be particularly sensitive to quality-of-care issues.
- *Left prior plan because moved out of area.* These members are likely new to the region and may lack loyalty to Medicare Advantage or knowledge of competitors.
- *Reports difficulty accessing care.* Such failure is a key factor affecting the choice of a plan.
- *Medicare Advantage failed to meet member expectations.* This is clearly identified dissatisfaction.

The Human Element of CRM

Connextions Health member retention specialists (MRSs) have encountered a number of incidents, which have provided insight into specific problems for this particular health plan provider. One example is a member who complained during a follow-up call that he failed repeatedly to reach his sales representative with two care access issues. The Connextions Health MRS contacted customer service on his behalf and relayed the message back to the member to call the plan provider's toll-free number.

Other problems included members alerting us to their physicians threatening to drop out of the network, ID cards being misspelled, and misrepresentations by third-party distributors.

However, the most common "problem" indicated by members has been the belief that their sales representative lied to them about the benefits provided by the plan. More often than not, the issue was either a misrepresentation or a misunderstanding of prescription drug benefits.

The ability of Connextions Health's agents to clarify these misrepresentations and misunderstandings with timely contacts and by having real-time access to the right information stemmed negative reactions, allowing them to better manage customer relationships for this plan provider.

Chapter 28

Meeting Demands for Knowing Hospital Costs Upfront

Prelude: Listen up, hospitals and medical staffs: Just tell health care payers and consumers upfront what your joint efforts cost and what your outcomes are. They will figure out what to do.

I am announcing today that for the first time, Medicare, Medicaid, the Department of Defense (VA and OPM/FEHBP), and the Office of Personnel Management will compile non-personalized claims information and release the information in sufficient detail that a statistically reliable foundation of transparent price and quality data will be available for each hospital and doctor.

We will start with a few of the most common procedures and expand as quickly as possible.

Michael Leavitt, Secretary of Health and Human Services, 2006

Transparency efforts are among the most powerful (but neutral) tools available to facilitate healthy markets, affecting every part of the health care continuum (supply chain, care delivery, financing), and benefiting all health care purchasers (governments, individuals and businesses).

Alan Levine, Secretary, Florida Agency for Health Care Disease Management, 2006

You may have caught the episode of 60 Minutes in February that devoted an entire segment to health care pricing. It featured consumer advocates, senators and everyday people caught in the quagmire of hospital pricing.

The hospital industry did not come off looking too good. On the heels of that, the government announced and then published the prices it pays for the top 20 medical procedures it reimburses. Like it or not, kicking or screaming, hospitals are going to have to address the issue of price transparency. And not just for some obvious reasons like tax exempt challenges and class action lawsuits. It's simply the right thing to do.

Although the government did not publish specific hospitals' prices in its release, assume that in the future your pricing will be public and be prepared to explain it. Know that the uninsured will be looking closely at what you receive, and they will demand the same. As an unintended consequence, insurers may have more power to come to you and renegotiate.

Start with the premise that price transparency is reality, and let your instincts tell you where you need to go next. Put yourself in the consumer's shoes. Think about what you would want, and then act accordingly.

Anthony Cirillo, 2006

Demands for transparent hospital bills, that is, hospital bills posted and known in advance, continue be a strong trend and will call for innovative measures. In a November 17, 2005, *Healthleaders* article, Lola Butcher said:

> *Welcome to the new "transparency" of the hospital industry, where price information is becoming available to the public for the first time. For hospitals, opening this Pandora's Box of information has repercussions across the enterprise, from marketing to collections. Many hospital administrators dismiss the transparency notion as meaningless to the public and impotent in its ability to force prices downward.*

With HSAs catching on and expecting to reach 15 to 25 million holders by 2111; with 78 million baby boomers joining the comparison shopping hunt; with state legislators passing laws requiring hospitals to post "list prices"; and with hospital systems like Saint Luke's in Kansas City, Missouri (see Chapter 25), already telling consumers what costs to expect, transparent hospital pricing is inevitable.

Answering the consumer will not be easy, which is why most hospitals don't know how to answer when they hear the seemingly simple question, "What's it cost?" Unfortunately, the answer to that hospital price question is: "It depends." It depends on what the ordering doctor has in mind, the amount of discounts the hospital has negotiated with the health plan, what services the consumer anticipates, and what additional tests might be needed for any particular procedure.

Therefore, the Saint Luke's price-line representative seeks to clear up these questions before quoting a price. Next the representative tries to determine charges for the needed procedures, which depends on a person's insurance coverage. Beyond that, however, are specifics of the patient's individual policy and how much of the deductible already has been used in the current year.

Transparency is difficult because:

1. Hospitals are accustomed to offering prices to different vendors based on discounts.

2. Billing department personnel are used to dealing passively with organizational payers, rather than actively with individual consumers.

3. Consumers may want to know the *total price*—hospital charges and physician charges—not just the hospital component. In the long run, the total price estimate may require bundled hospital and doctors' bills. Constructing these bills will entail hospitals negotiating with physicians. This is doable because integrated hospital systems, academic institutions with centers of excellence, and PHOs have a track record of negotiating bundled bills between hospitals and medical staffs.

Innovation Talking and Action Points

To say demands for transparency are a trend is understatement. The calls, indeed the demands, for transparency in costs and outcomes are coming from the federal government, consumer advocates, employers, lawyers representing the uninsured, and the consumers themselves. There have been some innovations in the transparency directions: cash-only physician practices; bundled or aggregated physician and hospital bills known in advance and backed by reinsurance; repricing of elective procedures by hospitals; and price and quality comparisons on consumer-driven health care Web sites—but price and quality transparency policies remain in their infancy.

The main problems in implementing transparency are legendary and manifold: the entitlement syndrome that says health care is a right and therefore price is irrelevant; the lack of knowledge about what things really cost; the asymmetry of information between doctors and patients; the multiplicity, permutations, and combinations of third-party arrangements; and the stresses and emotions and confusions around emergencies and chronic illnesses. However, even though the barriers to innovation seem endless, so too do the opportunities for innovation.

Case Study

Bundled Bills

By David Coombes, MHA

David Coombes, MHA, a graduate of Duke University and the University of Minnesota's graduate program for hospital executives, has had many career opportunities, including serving as chief executive of a university research hospital, serving as a state commissioner of health, setting up a series of ambulatory clinics across the Southeast, conducting a faculty practice for a major academic center, developing the billing practices for transplants and other major surgical procedures at a university center of excellence, inducing a community hospital and its medical staff to create a series of 65 bundled bills for common hospital procedures, and serving as the chief executive of a start-up company that used the Internet to bring the latest worldwide clinical research to the fingertips of clinicians. He now works at a consultant for hospitals and doctors who wish to achieve common billing transparency.

• •

If a trip to the grocery store caused the same kind of payment confusion often associated with a trip to the hospital, checkout lines would wind around the store with customers paying separately in different locations for each product purchased. That trip to the hospital results in the utilization of numerous different services that are distinct business entities themselves: the hospital itself, the medical specialist, the family doctor, the radiologist, the anesthesiologist, and so on. The customer pays each of these entities separately and at different locations.

In one Midwest city with some 15+ payers, one hospital and its medical staff simplified this complex payment mix for medical services by making the methodology more predictable for those who pay and budget for these services. A separate company was created, jointly and equally owned by the medical staff and hospital, for the purpose of offering purchasers of health care services a completely new and different route to pay for the services utilized: a single price, one-bill process. Initially, 65 procedures were identified, repackaged, and repriced for flat-rate, one-bill treatment.

The company sent a single bill to the payer and then internally disbursed the payment receipts among the various professional participants itself; clean, simple and without confusion because the "deal" was prospectively understood by all participants as signatories on enabling documents.

The marketing strategy for this single bill, one-price program is simple. The company goes to a purchaser (HMO, PPO, insurance company, employer, etc.) and says that for "Q" dollars per patient, it will do everything involved in X, Y, Z procedures.

The advantage to the purchaser is cost predictability. Contingency considerations are removed from the purchaser's cost equation. Economic risks are borne by the company that now must carefully figure both the good and bad cases into the single-price charge.

This company is a vehicle to bring the hospital and medical staff together from a business standpoint. It can negotiate contracts, develop and sell its products, and speak as one voice for the entire ownership. It is a marketing, development, and risk-sharing partnership that seeks to increase business for all of its owners while providing value-added health care for residents of its service area.

Having this kind of innovative product (and others) on your shelf, whipping it out at just the strategically correct time, and going to market with it like a cannon shot can leave your competitors well back in the cloud of dust that's created by its introduction. Remember, in business, there's something to be gained by doing it first. This company took its new health care business products to market first, created a huge cloud of dust, and in the end reaped both tangible and intangible benefits from the bold, innovative move.

Chapter 29

Quest for Personal Health Records

Prelude: A personal health record shifts responsibility for keeping their health records to patients. Many regard such as a record as the central document permitting patients to track their own health, streamline their entry into the health system, ensure their personal safety from drug interactions and allergies, and avoid duplication of services.

The Electronic Health Record (EHR) is a secure, real-time, point-of-care, patient-centric information resource for clinicians. The EHR aids clinicians' decision making by providing access to patient health record information where and when they need it and by incorporating evidence-based decision support. The EHR automates and streamlines the clinician's workflow, closing loops in communication and response that result in delays or gaps in care. The EHR also supports the collection of data for uses other than direct clinical care, such as billing, quality management, outcomes reporting, resource planning, and public health disease surveillance and reporting.

Health Information Management Systems Society, 2006

The Digital and Personal World

In his 2005 book *The World is Flat,* Friedman notes that the Internet and information technologies have caused a giant discontinuity in how the health care world does business. The world of payers, insurers, patients, doctors, and hospitals will never be the same again. The world of the health industry is no longer paper based, it's digital. Both text and images can now be transmitted over the Internet. With this digital revolution are opportunities for radical innovation—it "flattens" the information landscape, crossing information chasms that separate health care players. Nowhere is this more evident or visible than with the patient record—the common document used by all health care participants. Digital technologies have suddenly made it possible to "personalize" this document by making it fresh, updated, relevant, and in real time.

The Electronic Personal Health Record: An Innovation for Improving Care

Everybody agrees:

- A personal, continually updated patient record would be a major innovation for improving care.
- The record should contain facts about the patient's health status (allergies, mediations, vital signs, diagnoses, recent procedures, care plan, and reason for admission, transfer, or discharge).
- The record would be an ideal vehicle for exchanging clinical information among doctors, nurses, institutions, and other care entities, thereby avoiding duplication and confusion.
- Such a record would enhance quality, safety, convenience, and continuity of care. That is why the record in some quarters has come to be known as the continuity of care record (CCR), although personal health record (PHR) is the more commonly used term. The personal health record is not the same as the electronic health record; the personal health record (PHR) refers to an electronic record owned by the consumer, whereas the electronic health record (EHR) is a record system in physicians' offices. The PHR and EHR are separate entities, but consumers may choose to include their PHRs in their physicians' EHR.

Personal Health Records

Personal health records (PHRs) should contain information about document identification, patient identity, patient insurance and financial status, health status, and what occurred at the last patient visit. The records are a snapshot in time to be organized the same in each encounter, to be transportable, to be updated by the practitioner at the end of each patient visit, to allow the next practitioner to access the information, and to be prepared for transfer and display on paper or electronically. The next caregiver will not have to guess about health status, drugs, diagnoses, and treatment plan, and will not have to ask repeat questions about health, disease, or insurance status.

Presumably (and this might be a giant presumption), the record will reduce costs, speed up care, not invade patient and doctor privacy, not put the doctor in a bureaucratic or technological straightjacket, and be better for all concerned.

Continuity of Care Record: A Tortuous Process

The continuity of care record, a form of the personal care record, is more difficult to create because all users must agree upon its format. Complications are inevitable if more than one organization is involved. In the case of the CCR, which multiple organizations—ASTM International, the Massachusetts Medical Society (MMS), the Health Information and Systems Society (HIMSS), the American Academy of Family Physicians (AAFP), the American Academy of Pediatrics (AAP), the American Medical Association (AMA), the Patient Safety Institute, and the American Health Care Association—are working on, progress has been painfully slow.

The CCR requires agreement on a standard XML document. XML (Extensible Markup Language) is a W3C initiative allowing information and services to be encoded with structure and semantics that computers and humans can understand. This document must be machine and human readable; printable by Web browsers, PDF readers, and word processors; and capable of being sent by secure e-mail Portable Document Format (PDF is a file format created by Adobe Systems, Inc). PDF uses the PostScript printer description language and is highly portable across computer platforms. HL7 is an acronym for Health Level 7. It is a standard for health care and is the interface standard for communication between various systems employed in the medical community. This terminology is not easy to understand or implement. It requires a consensus and common knowledge among many parties on standard specifications.

iHealthRecord: A Medem Innovation

The PHR developed by Medem, Inc., a company owned by the American Medical Association and other medical societies, is simpler in concept and execution than the continuity of care record. In May of 2005, Medem launched its campaign for a secure, interactive, PHR for every American. The iHealthRecord, considered by some as a breakthrough service in the U.S. health care industry, permits Americans to control their PHR and provides new protections for families. It represents an important first step in fulfilling President George W. Bush's call for a PHR for every American within 10 years and EHRs for every doctor's office.

The iHealthRecord empowers and educates Americans. It electronically connects them closely with physicians. Beyond containing critical personal health data for use by physicians or emergency departments (including current medical conditions, medications, past surgeries, and allergies as well as end-of-life directives), the standards-based iHealthRecord allows physicians to increase medication adherence, enhance continuity of care, and improve patient–physician communication.

The iHealthRecord is the result of a multiyear effort led by Medem, founded by leading U.S. medical societies, including the AMA (Medem.com, 2003). "The AMA is committed to improving patient safety, enhancing health care quality and strengthening the patient-physician bond through the use of appropriate technology," stated Dr. J. James Rohack, chairman of the American Medical Association. "We believe that electronic personal health records are an important service for physicians and patients, and a key element of the national IT infrastructure" (Chin, 2005).

About 15,000 individuals have signed up with iHealthRecord. Fifteen thousand is not a huge number, but the transition to a paperless environment is slow and depends on multiple factors: the comfort of physicians with electronic personal records, overcoming fears of invasion of privacy, resistance of some older physicians to the electronic revolution, and, last but not least, the slow acceptance of electronic health record system installation in small practices, in which most of the nation's physicians practice.

Dell and WebMD Personal Health Record

Meanwhile, Dell, Inc., in collaboration with WebMD health care, is developing its own personal health care record. It will soon be offered to all Dell employees to import pharmacy and medical claims data as well as to provide a personal up-to-date history. This recode will allow Dell employees to securely manage their own data and procedures, conditions, and medications from doctors, hospitals, pharmacies, and other care entities (Dell, 2006).

Medical Records Alert—Another PHR System

Individual entrepreneurs are also getting into the PHR business, with the express aim of simplifying the record even more. A New York City dentist, Dr. Barry Linins, has developed a PHR that can be found on the Internet at www.medrecordsalert.com. Linins believes his system is important because of its simplicity and its ability to transmit images of medical records and even radiology scans. For a $36 fee, patients receive a card containing their password. On the card, patients' physicians can enter the clinical history in the form of a list containing test results, X-ray, CT, MRI scan images, ultrasound reports and images, EKG reports and images, and colonoscopy reports and images. Physicians and nurses, usually initially aided by a medical alerts team, enter the data either digitally or by scanning. Handwritten notes or voice recognition reports can be scanned and digitized. A preexisting electronic record system is helpful but not essential for entry. Once entered by the physician, the record is permanent. The patient owns the record and can access it any time on the Internet using the password, as can the patient's physician, a physician to whom the patient is referred, or an emergency room physician.

Other PHR Systems

U.S. IT entrepreneurs are working hard to develop these systems. At a 2006 Medical Records Institute (MRI) Towards an Electronic Patient Record (TEPR) conference, an impartial jury of judges handed out these awards for PHR systems.

First Honors: CapMed—Personal Health Key

Second Honors: Medical Communications Systems—mMD.Net PHR

Third Honors: Cerner—IQ Health

One of newer companies developing a PHR is MDcryption in Raleigh, North Carolina. One million hurricane victims lost their medical records in 2005. To alleviate this and similar problems, MDcryption has come up with a product called VitalChart, a personal health record carried on a waterproof key chain. The company claims their product "is particularly valuable for frequent travelers, patients managing chronic medical conditions, and anyone in a hazardous occupation or who participates in high-risk sports" (Vitalchart.com).

Innovation Talking and Action Points

Developing a universal interoperable EHR for use throughout the health care system and constructing a PHR for use among physicians and their patients are different applications.

The universal record requires multiple committees from multiple organizations agreeing on a common format, a standardized language, and readability and transmission and acceptance by multiple senders and receivers. A PHR, on the other hand, can be developed more quickly. In the case of iHealthRecords and Medical Records Alert, for example, the patient's physician enters the initial data and updates it. The patient owns and controls the personal health record, and other physicians can only see the record when the patient gives the password, which is on a card patients can carry in their wallet or purse. Other doctors can enter data into the patient's "vault" (another name for the record), but the owner controls who reads it.

The American Health Information Association (AHIA) also has developed a personal health record, MyPHR. It explains MyPHR's use this way:

> *Your personal health information is a valuable resource to you, your family, and the doctors, nurses, and other health care professionals who provide your treatment and care. In most cases, a complete record of all of your personal health information cannot be found in any single location or consistent format; each one of your health care providers (family practitioner, allergist, OB-GYN, etc.) compiles a separate medical record on you. These multiple medical records can lead to an incomplete story about your health.*

Keeping your own personal health record (PHR) allows you to provide doctors with valuable information helping improve the quality of care you receive. A PHR can help reduce or eliminate duplicate tests and allow you to receive faster, safer treatment and care in an emergency. In short, a PHR helps you play a more active role in your health care. (MyPHR.com)

In other words, patients own the record and can dole out the information as they see fit, without each doctor having access to the complete record.

Soon a PHR may be offered by all of the nation's health plans. A coalition including the nation's largest health plans intends to begin offering consumers a Web-based personal health record in a pilot program (Pack, 2006b). The coalition includes members of the Blue Cross Blue Shield Association and America's Health Insurance Plans, potentially representing 200 million Americans. The coalition's plan is significant partly because it could create an insurer-based national health information network as an alternative to regional health information networks. The personal record will follow patients from job to job and from one insurer to the other. Details are sketchy, and of November, 2006, the project was still in development.

Up to now, there have been other scattered discussions of creating basic electronic medical records from claims data. Getting all the nation's big insurers on a common platform could boost electronic record keeping nationally, which many doctors and insurers say would help reduce duplicated medical services and make patients' records quickly available to doctors and others. Insurers have a great influence over health care, and electronic record keeping is crucial to reducing waste and improving the quality of care.

In 2005, the government estimated only 31 percent of hospital emergency departments and 17 percent of doctors' offices used electronic health records (Portman, Vigilante, & Ecken, 2005). Pressure is building for doctors and hospitals to make the switch. Proponents say electronic records can reduce costs and errors and make it easier for providers to follow care of individual patients as they move from one town or job or insurer to another.

Some health plans may allow patients to enter other information such as allergies and family medical histories. Under the industry plan, the PHR would be available free as part of people's ordinary coverage. The medical information would not automatically be shared with physicians, but patients could give permission to release it to their doctors.

PHRs on the Internet

It may be difficult for patients, physicians, hospitals, health plans, and other health care organizations to sort out their PHR options. What PHRs are available? What organizations have developed them? The following Internet-based PHR list may help patients navigate through the PHR maze. The list includes Internet-accessible applications that could enable a patient (or care provider for a patient) to create, review, annotate, or maintain a record of any aspect of their health condition, medications, medical problems, allergies, vaccination history, visit history, or communications with their health care providers. This list does not in any way indicate a level of quality, functionality, or usefulness for these PHRs.

- Accordant's Personal Health Manager
- AllHealth.com's Personal Health Record
- AMA Personal Health History
- CapMed's Personal Health Record
- CareGroup's Personal Health Web Site
- Catholic Healthcare West
- Cerner IQ Health
- Cyberspace Telemedical Office
- Elixis Corporation's YourHealthChart
- eMD.com
- 4Healthylife
- GlobalMedic's eHealth Record
- HealthAtoZ
- HealthCompass
- HealthCPR.com
- Healtheon/WebMD
- I-Beacon.com
- IDX's Channel Health
- Kaiser Permanente Northwest Personal Link
- Lifeconnect.com
- LifeLineMed's Record
- Medem
- Medifile
- Medical Records Alert
- Medical Communication Systems
- Medscape's Daily Diary
- mMD.net PHR
- MyHealthNotes
- MyPatientsCharts.com
- MyPHR
- 98Point6

- Personal Health
- Personal MD
- QuickViewHX
- TheMedicalRecord
- UrgentLink's Online Safety Deposit Box
- WellMed—WellRecord
- Your HealthChart.com
- Your Health Portrait
- (www.informatics-review.com)

The following offer personal, disease-specific health profiles on the Internet. These sites are designed to help patients with specific diseases. Physician Web sites also find these sites are useful in directing their patients with certain diseases to specific information on their condition.

- MyAllergy
- MyAsthma
- MyDiabetes

Case Study

The Medem Story
By Michael McGee, Office Manager, Medem

Many personal health records are available over the Internet. Perhaps the most well developed and well known of these is Medem, Inc. This case study tells the story of Medem and its founder, its history, its personal health record, and what it tells patients about its personal health record.

The following organizations founded Medem in 1999 to develop the premier physician–patient communications network.

- American Medical Association
- American Academy of Ophthalmology
- American Academy of Pediatrics
- American College of Allergy, Asthma and Immunology
- American College of Obstetricians and Gynecologists
- American Psychiatric Association
- American Society of Plastic Surgeons

Along with 47 medical societies, Medem's rapidly expanding network includes a growing number of strategic business partners in the health care industry, including national and regional health plans, physician groups and medical centers, and professional liability carriers. Industry partners include:

- Allscripts
- AmerisourceBergen
- ConnectiCare
- First Data Corporation
- MEDecision
- The Doctors Company
- Whole Health Management

Medem's seed funding was provided by the seven founding medical societies in October of 1999. Medem has secured additional funding from Whitney & Co, Sir John Templeton, and Allscripts.

In the 1980s, Ed Fotsch, a San Francisco emergency room physician, watched uneasily as medical societies suffered an identity and clout crisis as managed care rose to dominance. The societies' impotence in dealing with HMOs, legislators, and big business contributed to Fotsch's unease.

Then, while running a 250-person San Francisco Independent Practice Association (IPA) and later an Internet communications company, Fotsch became acutely aware that physicians possessed no communications infrastructure. In 1999, when he became CEO of Medem, Fotsch set about filling two gaping defects in American medicine:

1. Communication systems linking physicians and patients
2. Computer networks connecting physicians and hospitals

To fill the first hole, Medem developed two core products: free physician Web sites and online consultation services. To plug the second hole, Medem and Cerner, a major hospital data systems supplier, agreed to build systems to allow physicians and hospitals to talk to one another (Medem.com, 2003).

Goal

Fotsch's goal is to unite physicians around the country by encouraging them to employ information technologies to achieve clinical and business efficiencies; make revenue increases through these efficiencies; and speed communication between physicians, patients, and hospitals. The road to the future, he maintains, is paved with concrete uses of information technologies. Together with leading health care partners, Medem has established a physician–patient communications network. It is designed to ease online access to information and care for physicians, their practices and their patients, while saving patients time and money and helping physicians generate revenue and reduce their liability.

Medem believes patients will want access to physician-specific information and be able to look it up on the Web. Medeim desires to promote patient satisfaction as well as office efficiency. Secure Messaging, Medem's name for its module that facilitates e-mail communication with other doctors and patients, operates under the pretense that doctors want to communicate with their patients via e-mail. A recent survey indicates that if there is a reimbursement mechanism in place, physicians are willing to adopt this method. This underscores another very important point . . . finances.

The Medem Network

The Medem network, through the American Medical Association and medical specialty societies, allows online access to information and care for physicians, their practices, and their patients. It saves patients time and money by giving them rapid Internet access to their doctors and helps physicians generate revenue through reimbursed patient e-mail communications and reduces their liability by documenting patient–physician electronic communications. Medem offers the following services to health systems, hospitals, physicians/physician groups, and other health care providers. These services are important because they facilitate patient–physician communication and render care more safely, more effectively, and in a timelier manner.

- iHealthRecord for patients, with automated disease management and medication adherence education programs
- Disease-management and medication-adherence programs, written by medical societies, advocacy groups, government entities, and others for use with patients
- Online consultation—HIPAA- and eRisk-compliant messaging, enabling physicians to increase practice revenue and enhance existing patient relationships by providing a confidential reimbursable consultation interface.
- Access to new insured patients via health plan provider directory links
- Integrated HIPAA- and eRisk-compliant secure messaging for patient–physician communication including appointment requests, Rx refills, and general messaging

Medem's Personal Health Record

The iHealthRecord, Medem's name for its personal health record, includes the following features, which make it a powerful tool for linking patients with physicians and improving health care through the use of transparent documented information available to patients, their families, and their physicians.

- A secure personal health record repository for all health information, stored in one convenient and secure place.
- Secure e-mail and online consultation with the patient's doctor (assuming he or she offers these services).
- Automatic, same-day FDA product warning and recall alerts sent directly to patients, based on the indications and medical devices listed in their iHealthRecord.
- Automatic enrollment in health education programs, written by medical societies and others including the American Heart Association, American Cancer Society, the FDA, and CDC.
- Quarterly online patient reminders to keep the patient's iHealthRecord current.
- The ability to access the iHealthRecord during an emergency.
- Complete control over who has access to the health record.
- Patients decide who can have access to the record and for what period of time.
- The iHealthRecord provides patients with a log of who has accessed their information.
- Accessibility from anywhere and at any time.
- A convenient iHealthRecord wallet card providing emergency contact information and directions on how to access the patient's iHealthRecord.

Medem's PHR contains patient-education programs focusing on medical conditions, treatment, and medication adherence to help patients understand and manage their health.

Nearly 20,000 Americans have already created an iHealthRecord for themselves or for a family member. Each day, new partners such as national health plans, large medical groups, and hospitals launch programs to promote and increase adoption of the iHealthRecord within their patient communities.

The iHealth Alliance, a not-for-profit health care advisory organization established to protect the interests of physicians and patients, oversees the privacy program.

Information cannot be sold or provided to any third parties without the patient's permission.

Although the patient's medical information is available to the patient via the Internet, it is very secure. It can only be accessed with ID and password. Patients control their information and only they can provide access privileges to doctors, family members, or emergency personnel. Patients can see who has visited their iHealthRecord by using the tracking log provided by the record. Patients are notified via e-mail each day that someone accesses their iHealthRecord so they can monitor its use.

The iHealthRecord does not sell patient data nor use advertising. The service is funded by physician and hospital groups, health plans, and other organizations who license and private label the service for their patients, as well as through transaction fees paid when physicians offer online consultations to their patients.

The iHealthRecord is something that patients own and update so it is important for them to keep their record current. To assist them with this, Medem sends out quarterly reminder e-mails.

Medem is building interfaces to electronic medical records in physician offices and hospitals, as well as with health plans, to update their iHealthRecord. Patients decide what updates they will keep and which they don't want to have as part of their record.

Once patients have created their iHealthRecord, they can make any changes they deem necessary—at any time—through the overview page. The overview page contains a summary of patient information, with links that take them directly to any section or any entry. This allows them to make additions, changes, or to remove information quickly and easily.

Most people create their iHealthRecord at their own physician's practice or hospital Web site. In doing so, their physician or hospital will be able to view their record, unless they are denied access. In addition, patients can grant access to any other third parties, including physicians and other health care providers, as well as family members and loved ones. All third parties to whom patients grant access appear on a tracking log in their iHealthRecord until patients remove them. Patients can revoke access privileges to anyone at any time. Patients are encouraged to identify a trusted third party to whom they grant access privileges to their iHealthRecord information. If possible, this person should be the same individual identified as their emergency contact in their iHealthRecord.

Medem also allows (and strongly encourages) patients to print a wallet card that contains their basic information (assuming they provide it), including emergency contact, blood type, and allergies. Medem recommends patients keep a current copy of this wallet card at all times and also share one with their emergency contact. Doing so facilitates access to important information in their health record should the need arise. The iHealthRecord is for patients to keep. It is completely transportable, and stays with them regardless of where they live or work. They can grant access to their iHealthRecord to new doctors even if they move or change jobs.

The record saves time because doctors who offer the iHealthRecord often use it as part of their registration process for appointments. Much of the information they currently fill out on the clipboard each time patients visit their doctor is contained in the iHealthRecord. The iHealthRecord also saves patients time, because they only need to create it once, after which they simply review and print it prior to visiting their doctor. Patients should be aware that the doctor may also upload other forms to his or her practice Web site that patients can download, print, and fill out prior to their appointment—instead of having to fill them out in the waiting room. With the data stored in the iHealthRecord and other forms available from the doctor's Medem Web site, patients can register for an appointment more quickly, easily, and accurately and help doctors put an end to clipboard care.

Patients can print their entire iHealthRecord or just selected parts of it for their files and for their medical chart. Because the iHealthRecord is available via the Internet from anywhere in the world, it is not as important to print the entire record to ensure access. Even so, patients are strongly encouraged to print an iHealthRecord emergency wallet card to keep with them at all times.

Online Consultation

Online consultation (OC) is a secure, clinical e-mail service that allows a physician to provide clinical consultations to patients online.

- Control for physicians to choose which patients they will use OC with.
- The ability to set/adjust individual OC fees in $5 increments.
- Response timeframe is determined and posted by the physician.
- The ability to accept or decline an OC.
- The ability to "no charge" an OC.
- The ability to append medical society articles or other information/Web links to an OC message.
- The ability to enroll a patient in an adherence program directly from an OC message.
- The ability to store an OC response as a "template" for future use.
- The ability to designate a nurse or assistant as the first author of an OC (the physician can simply review, edit, and approve the OC).
- Integrated medical professional liability insurer–approved disclosures, terms of service, and informed consent language for patients.
- Notification to the physician if a patient does not open an OC response.
- Print functionality that allows physicians to print time- and date-stamped OCs for inclusion in a patient's medical chart.
- Integrated and automated credit card–based billing, in which the physician's office simply receives payment without having to generate a bill.
- Billing reconciliation.

Chapter 30

Navigating Uncharted Health Care Consumer Waters

Prelude: Winds and waves are always on the side of the ablest navigators.

This book has been called, after Bowditch's Practical Navigator, The Practical Cogitator. *At any rate, it should be a sort of cerebral Coast Pilot, a compilation of what those who have gone down this way before report to those who might otherwise have to pick their course through these channels and into these harbors with nothing but the lead line.*

Charles P. Curtis and Ferris Greenslet, 1953

With high-deductible/HSA health plans, in which consumers are given a wide array of choices to pick from, a new phenomenon has sprung up—health care navigators. Everywhere you look, you will find navigators—at the job site, health plan Web sites, government agencies, disease Web sites, and hospitals and physician Web sites— even emergency room navigators who exist to guide people through hospital emergency departments.

Most health care consumers find it difficult to navigate the health system to find information about their health plan benefits, why claims are denied or accepted, how to settle disputed claims, what costs of health care services are, and where to find the best doctors and hospitals. The emergence of health care navigators should not be surprising. After all, for the newly hatched health care consumer, health care waters are often storm-tossed and uncharted. These new health care consumer-sailors need navigational aids. For them, the Web may serve as a sort of Global Positioning System (GPS). In the computer world, *navigation* is defined as something facilitating movement from one Web page to the next. Navigation buttons and links

303

to other sites are a common feature of health care Web sites. However, the Web alone is not enough. As good as the Web is as a health GPS and as helpful as navigation cues are, the Web alone is not enough. Human help is needed.

Castle Connolly Healthcare Navigation, Ltd.

In 1991, John K. Castle and Dr. John J. Connolly founded Castle Connolly Medical Ltd. after more than 10 years of working together at the New York Medical College where Castle served as chairman of the Board of Trustees and Connolly as president. Castle Connolly Ltd. has produced numerous editions of *America's Top Doctors*, books listing top medical specialists selected on the basis of peer nomination and selection. In addition, in 1999 they were among the co-founders of Castle Connolly Graduate Medical Ltd., which publishes review manuals of medical residents and fellows.

In 2006, Castle and Connolly launched Castle Connolly Healthcare Navigation, Inc., which serves individuals who have problems resolving medical bills or understanding insurance statements. The organization offers an array of services to help individuals and families cope with today's complex health care/insurance environment. The company uses the terms "navigation" and "navigator" to refer to the process of finding reliable health system information, picking and choosing one's way through complex issues.

This "navigation" requires the services of experienced health care. The staff at Castle Connolly reviews bills and statements and encourages clients to seek their advice when changing coverage during job or retirement transitions. The company often works with individuals and families at a time of crisis during a serious illness.

Because the volume and complexity of claims can be overwhelming, Castle Connolly Healthcare Navigation charges $80 per hour and says it is difficult to predict in advance how long it will take to untangle a billing problem or an insurance dispute. The company may save clients tens of thousands of dollars in appeal solutions, finding errors in bills, or in negotiating settlements, but there is no guarantee this will be the case (Carley, 2006, personal communication).

In general, the company offers these patient advocacy services to free individuals from the burdens and hassles of medical coverage disputes, health projects involving the authorization or denial of a claim, the reviewing or interpreting of coverage, and the staging of workshops on how to navigate the health care system. The individual no longer has to slog through the process of finding answers. The company does the slogging for them.

Castle Connolly Healthcare Navigation offers personalized support services to high-end health care consumers. Their array of services helps individuals and families navigate health care and insurance and to leverage health care resources in this country and abroad. Their services include:

1. Personal assistance by a physician or specially trained nurse to identify and gain access to the nation's top doctors and hospitals whenever necessary.

Physician searches will be performed at client's request as a result of a family move, serious illness, need for a second opinion, or other situation.

2. Castle Connolly Medical Ltd., which is a separate company from Castle Connolly Healthcare Navigation, publishes books on top doctors. These include *America's Top Doctors, America's Top Doctors for Cancer,* and *America's Cosmetic Doctors and Dentists.* Castle Connolly is a national leader in identifying top doctors. It does this through a process of peer nominations and credentials investigations. With its extensive database of top doctors and hospitals and detailed information on their special expertise, Castle Connolly is able to quickly identify the best physicians to deal with any medical problem

3. Guidance and assistance in dealing with health insurance matters.

   - Customized research reports on diseases and health problems with which a family member is diagnosed.
   - 24/7 access to health records, advance directives, and emergency contacts.
   - Worldwide medical travel insurance and assistance. This covers 20 days of medical insurance and evacuation coverage for travel outside of the United States.

Cost of the Core Program

The cost of the core program consists of (1) personal assistance by a doctor or nurse to gain access to the nation's top doctors or hospitals; (2) personal guidance and assistance in dealing with health insurance matters; (3) customized research reports on diseases and health problems; (4) 24/7 access to digital health records and emergency contacts; (5) medical travel insurance and assistance worldwide; (6) preparation of health travel alerts prior to international travel; (7) assisting families with issues and services to support elderly relatives.

The core program, as of November 2006, is priced at $3,800 per family member per year for identifying top doctors, research reports, health records, the worldwide medical travel insurance, a welcome and/or annual interview to discuss the family's health care coverage issues, and up to 5 additional hours per year of services related to health insurance matters.

Innovation often results from a need. In this case, the innovation is the necessity for authoritative guidance through a complicated, frustrating health system.

As physicians who must know and treat scores of different conditions and hundreds of patients, we sometimes forget patients are only interested in one disease—their own. With the Internet, patients may now spend endless hours outside the physician's office researching their disease or talking to kindred spirits in support groups or in Internet chat rooms. This new IT environment, aided and abetted by the various media hammering and yammering about health care topics, has created a new phenomenon: informed but confused health care consumers who want and have resources to find exactly the right specialist in the right institution using the right technologies and the right medications to treat the disease inhabiting their bodies.

Case Study

Finding Your Way Through the Health System

By Maura Carley, President and CEO of Castle Connolly Healthcare Navigation, Ltd.

Maura Carley is president and CEO of Castle Connolly Healthcare Navigation Ltd., which provides medical claims and medical coverage consulting services to individuals, families, and corporations.

Prior to 1999, Carley was the vice president of operations for the northeast region of PhyMatrix, a physician practice management company. She was responsible for managing and providing services to over 200 physicians throughout the New York metropolitan area. Before joining PhyMatrix, Carley worked for Kaiser Permanente, one of the nation's largest health maintenance organizations, as New York regional director.

She began her career in hospital administration as an assistant administrator at Yale–New Haven Hospital and later as vice president, administration, at Stamford Hospital.

Carley received her master's in public health from Yale University in 1978 and is a fellow in the American College of Health Care Executives. She is a certified life, accident, and health consultant.

• •

Health care coverage issues are complex and becoming more complex. The stakes are very high if a consumer ends up being uninsured or underinsured because health care charges can be ruinous. In fact, medical charges are a leading cause of personal bankruptcy in the United States (Himmelstein, Warren, Thorne, & Woolhandler, 2005). The following examples illustrate how skilled health care navigators can assist individuals and families with health care coverage issues.

Mistakes

In today's health care world, a mistake by a provider's office or the insurance company can often have adverse consequences for the consumer. Barbara Miller, not her real name, had a serious cardiac event during her early 60s but felt that she had good coverage. The cardiology group, however, after a number of months turned her account over to a collection agency. The collection agency in turn initiated the process to put a lien on the Miller home as a result of an unpaid medical bill.

The Millers didn't understand why they were being hounded by collectors. They paid dearly for their coverage and were told it should have provided good protection. Nevertheless, after they were threatened with a lien, they sought help. A quick look at the insurer's explanation of benefits statement revealed that a CPT code (the five-digit code medical providers use to bill) had been transcribed in error. As a result, the insurer instead of paying for a sophisticated cardiac procedure had paid for a lab specimen handling fee of less than $100. It is not clear why the claim had been processed manually rather than electronically. An electronic transmission may have helped prevent such an error. The cardiologist's billing staff should have found this error when recording the payment but they did not. When the error was brought to the attention of the insurer, the claim was reprocessed and the problem resolved.

Hospitals, doctors, and other providers also make mistakes that affect their patients. Another client's husband had received care at a hospital in Maryland before his death. His care there had been preauthorized by the insurer. In spite of the preauthorization, numerous denials creating stacks of paper had been issued by the insurer. A careful review showed that every time the patient was treated in a special procedure room, his care had been coded as day surgery. The insurer's computer system looked for a preauthorization for day surgery, which obviously couldn't be found because day surgery had never been requested or planned to be performed. Because so many denials had been issued, the hospital billed the family for the care provided which was tens of thousands of dollars. This situation required intervention with both the medical center and the health plan to resolve on behalf of the patient's family.

Catastrophic Illness and the Out-of-Network Benefit

The out-of-network benefit is commonly misunderstood because the patient and family believe the out-of-pocket maximum is the maximum amount they will have to pay in a year. Instead, it is the maximum amount they will have to pay for deductible and coinsurance amounts. However, when one is out of network, provider charges are not limited. Thus the difference between what the insurer deems reasonable and customary and what the provider charges, which can be vast, is the patient's responsibility and is not applied to the out-of-pocket maximum.

One of the worst situations we encountered was a hospitalization for a 3-week stay where the total hospital charges were $302,000. The insurer initially deemed $155,000 of the charges to be reasonable and customary or usual and customary. As a result, the family was responsible for a deductible, the coinsurance of 30 percent, and the difference between $302,000 and $155,000, an amount that was originally greater than what the insurer's obligation was for disease management.

In a situation like this, one would typically try to determine if the insurance payment is low, the charges high, or both, and then negotiate with both parties. In this situation, for still inexplicable reasons, the insurer paid the entire balance as soon as an appeal was filed with the state's attorney general's office.

Another client was a 1-year-old diagnosed with a brain tumor. He was taken by his parents to an in-network hospital emergency room where the pediatric neurologist insisted on an immediate transfer to a major center where surgery could be performed. The center where the child was transferred was out of network and the child was hospitalized there for 7 months with bills in the hundreds of thousands of dollars. The insurer was processing the claims as though they were out of network. The intervention was an appeal filed with the insurer documenting the in-network pediatric neurologist's transfer from the in-network hospital to the out-of-network hospital. The argument made was that this was not a family who chose to be out of network; rather they were directed to receive care at another facility because the in-network hospital could not provide the level of care required. In the end, the hospital and insurer negotiated regarding payment and the family was not charged for any additional amounts associated with out-of-network services.

Coverage Advice

Many problems with health care coverage issues can be avoided if consumers have good, objective advice about health care coverage issues.

One client came to us because she had divorced and her COBRA was about to expire. She was working at a part-time job that did not offer health care coverage benefits. Unfortunately, she had preexisting conditions and would not qualify for individual coverage in the private health insurance marketplace. Upon discussing the various alternative ways to obtain coverage, she shared that she was a serious artist with works being exhibited in the area and sold via her Web site. She considered this activity more of a passion and hobby than an economic activity. However, on closer examination, this activity was significant enough to be handled as a small business through which the client was able to obtain a guaranteed issue policy as a sole proprietor, consistent with the laws and regulations in her state.

Another client came to us in crisis, a crisis that could have been avoided had such advice been provided prior to our involvement. The client's husband had been an engineer and was laid off in his early 60s; at that time, he chose COBRA. His company subsequently went bankrupt so there was no longer a COBRA option. He and his wife bought individual private insurance policies.

Shortly thereafter, the insurance company that sold them the private policies left the state the couple lived in and canceled all insurance policies. Being close to Medicare age and feeling that he could not afford the state high-risk pool premium, the husband chose to be uninsured. At that point, he likely could have legitimately worked as a consultant and been able to obtain coverage as a sole proprietor but he did not know this was an option.

Unfortunately, months later he developed serious medical problems and subsequently died owing a major six-figure amount to the local hospital and many local doctors. We helped the surviving wife complete an application for charity care at the hospital and negotiated major reductions in the charges with a payment plan extending over several years. Many of the local physicians were kind enough to accept substantial discounts from the widow and others wrote off the entire balance for this couple who had always paid their bills.

Chapter 31

Health Care Retail Outlets

Prelude: A series of clinics located in retail outlets—pharmacy chains, discount stores, and grocery stories—is opening around the country. Most of these retail outlets feature operating hours, are staffed by nurse practitioners, treat minor illness, offer routine immunizations, have prices roughly half of those charged by primary care physicians, and are located near pharmacies where prescriptions can be filled immediately.

Coming soon to a mall near you: health care. Most people go shopping for food, clothes or other items, but thanks to a new trend, they may also be able to purchase health care in Target stores and food stores in Minnesota, Indiana, and elsewhere.

Paul Awarder, associate professor of medicine at Johns Hopkins, says such services may prove quite helpful. "These minute clinics are a way really that are a very good effort in medicine to change things from being very physician centered to very patient centered, and it allows physicians to make good use of their time to monitor things that basically don't require an office visit."

Nurse practitioners who staff the clinics will refer a patient who needs a physician's attention for more complex problems. They also keep a record of repeat visits so that if an infection persists, more in depth evaluation will be recommended. And the visits are paid for by most private insurance plans. So perhaps you'll be seeing such a clinic in your local grocery store soon.

Elizabeth Tracy, 2006

Everyday low prices on strept-throat exams. That is the basic idea behind a retail approach to routine medical care now catching on among consumers and entrepreneurs. At Wal-Mart, CVS and chain stores, walk-in health clinics are springing up as an antidote to the expense and inconvenience of full-service doctors' offices or to the high-cost and impersonal last resort of emergency rooms.

Milt Freudenheim, 2006

Retail clinics, located in retail outlets in malls and elsewhere, offer walk-in care by nurse practitioners for simple illnesses. The three largest retail health chains—MinuteClinic, Rediclinic, and Take Care—plan to accelerate expansion in the next few years (American Academy of Family Physicians, 2006a).

Charles B. Inlander, president of the nonprofit People's Medical Society, a consumer health advocacy group in Allentown, Pennsylvania, explains licensed nurse practitioners usually administer care, fees are affordable (about half for similar services in doctors' offices), hours of operation are convenient (usually 12 hours a day), and services are limited.

Inlander says:

> *Retail clinics are not mini-emergency rooms. They do not fix broken limbs or care for severe injuries, such as concussions or lacerations that require stitches. They provide routine medical services, such as inoculations and treatment for minor skin rashes, flu symptoms and other basic health concerns (and are a good option for people with such needs). Contrary to how it might appear your local drugstore or department store doesn't actually own these medical clinics. The clinics are leased by a handful of companies that provide health-care services.* (Inlander, 2006)

On July 13, 2006, CVS Corporation, Inc., which have 6,100 retail and specialty clinics nationwide, announced it had acquired MinuteClinic, headquartered in Minneapolis, Minnesota, for $170 million. The deal made an already close relationship even closer, and it accelerated MinuteClinic's growth. At the time of acquisition, the company had 83 outlets in 10 states; 66 of those were in CVS stores. MinuteClinic plans to triple in size to 250 locations by the end of 2006 and said its earlier forecast of 450 to 500 locations by the end of 2007 was revised upward (CVS Corporation, 2006).

What does this deal portend for U.S. health care? It means the retail clinic outlet phenomenon has become mainstream. It means consumers can seek care for minor ailments 24 hours a day in health clinics in CVS drugstores and have prescriptions filled on the spot—and it may signal another blow to already beleaguered primary care physicians.

As Jeff Hogan, a Rogers benefit broker who specializes in selling high-deductible health plans linked to HSAs, said, "These clinics use 26 of the 29 payment codes most commonly employed by primary care physicians, and the cost to the consumer is roughly one-half what it would be to doctors' offices" (Hogan, 2006, personal communication). This means retail health clinics can compete with primary care physicians at half the price.

The key to MinuteClinic's success has been a proprietary software package that includes all the protocols necessary to guide nurse practitioners through the diagnosis and treatment of simple maladies such as strep throat, ear and sinus infections, and pink eye, to name a few. The company now commonly charges $49 to $59 for visits, with insurers picking up most of that, and had seen 500,000 patients by the time of acquisition (Academy of Medicine of Cleveland and Northern Ohio, 2006).

Note, however, that this retail clinic movement is not assured success. Remember 20 years ago when walk-in or ambulatory clinics were the rage in strip malls? They had no hours, required no appointments, and had cheaper prices—still many of these chains failed. Doctors criticized them, patients weren't used to being seen in commercial settings, and doctors providing the services were of uneven quality. Still, the current clinics tend to be in more consistent settings such as drugstores, the capital backing is better, the nurses seeing patients use best practice protocols, and patient demographics may be different—with baby boomers who are looking for greater convenience, are more aware of consumer rights, and have households with two providers. In families with two wage earners, the wage earners are usually extremely busy and have little time for long waits at doctors' offices. Still, one wonders if the current iteration of walk-in clinics will prevail over the long run.

Clinicians Chained to Offices

The rapid rise in the number of retail clinics has gotten the attention of the American Medical Association (Jansen, 2006). The AMA is pushing for greater scrutiny of these clinics by requesting doctors to be more involved in setting up protocols for evaluating patients and for nurse practitioners to establish referral systems with physician practices.

Why is the concept of clinics in conveniently located retail outlets (pharmacies, discount stores, and grocery chains) that are open 24 hours a day so powerful and so challenging to primary care doctors?

The primary care physician business model has changed little over the last 50 years. The traditional office is where physicians see patients, make money, maintain ancillary services, and pay office overheads varying from 50 percent to 70 percent. Because these clinicians cannot work 24 hours a day, when patients call their office number before or after hours, they often refer the patient to a nearby hospital emergency room. However, now these patients can get care for their minor illnesses without an appointment, in 15 minutes or so, in their local shopping mall or at a drugstore where they can pick up their prescription as the same time.

Medical associations are aware of this retail phenomenon. Even though they know these clinics represent potential competition, they do not necessarily disapprove of them. Dr. Larry S. Fields, president of the American Association of Family Physicians, says that if these clinics "stick to this limited scope, they may have a small role in providing acute health care to people who are mildly ill when their only other alternative might be an emergency room" (American Academy of Family Physicians, 2006).

As an alternative to walk-in clinics, Dr. Fields's organization is promoting the concept of patients using the physician's office as a home base with the physician serving as a coordinator of care. Unfortunately, this physician business model does not lend itself to serving busy Americans, particularly time-starved baby boomers, who are looking for quick, convenient, and inexpensive care on weekends, off-hours, and, in some cases, 24 hours a day.

The physician office as a home base makes a lot of sense to the doctors involved because primary care physicians can serve as coordinators of care and as trusted advisors for a variety of medical ailments. This is a variation of the old Marcus Welby model, which might be defined as a family physician knowing all the problems and needs of families. However, physician office visits for routine care aren't for everyone. A number of entrepreneurs are challenging the medical home concept by establishing companies that provide care away from medical offices. These include:

- **MinuteClinic:** See the description provided earlier in this chapter.
- **Take Care Health Systems:** Founded in Portland, Oregon, 2005, Take Care offers 16 clinics in various retail stores. The average cost per visit is $48 to $68 and their retail partners include Osco Drug and Rite Aid. The company's expansion plans are to have 1,400 clinics by 2009. Hal Rosenbluth serves as chair.
- **Solantic:** Founded in 2002 in Jacksonville, Florida, with two clinics and retail partners, Wal-Mart. Cost per visit of walk-in urgent care is $55. Services offered include occupational health, X-rays, and a pharmacy lab. The group is located in 12 Florida locations. Chairman is now Richard L. Scott, former CEO of Columbia/HCA Health care.
- **The Little Clinic:** In 2006, these nurse practitioner– and physician assistant–based clinics were open in Publix grocery stores in four Florida markets. Charges were under $50 for treating routine infections and their prescribing capabilities.
- **RediClinic:** Founded in Tomball, Texas, in 2005; 1 year later, the company had 11 clinics and an average cost per visit of $45. Retail partners for the clinic were Duane Reade, H-E-B, Wal-Mart, and Walgreens. A unit of Stephen M. Caes Revolution Health Care Group, the group's expansion plans include having 1,000 clinics by the end of 2007.
- **TelaDoc:** A membership physician-based service with whom patients can talk to licensed primary care doctors 24/7/365. Offices are located in Florida, Idaho, South Carolina, and Tennessee.

- **OnSiteDoc:** Physician-based service offered 24/7/365. This group specializes in employee-based care for on-the-job injuries or illnesses.

- **Orthopedic Convenient Care:** Part of the Jewett Orthopedic Clinic P.A., in Winter Park, Florida, this care group has six local physician offices with 23 doctors. The group in May 2006 opened the Jewett Orthopedic Convenient Care Center, a specialty walk-in clinic that treats broken bones, sprains, strains, or lacerations, and also provides follow-up care and treats workers' compensation injuries. In addition to offering orthopedic care, it also has an in-house pharmacy and provides physical therapy, occupational therapy, and orthotic devices such as splints, MRI, and digital X-rays. It's now open on weekdays and Saturdays, but Jewett plans to offer evening hours by the end of 2006 (Lundine, 2006).

- Many independent, disease-management companies that are linked to health plans or are Medicaid or Medicare based are part of this movement. Most are nurse practitioner based.

Health care outside the physician's office in other settings is a significant trend, and it challenges independent and established medical groups. These groups have largely been excluded from this new market. If you doubt the potential power of this trend, keep in mind that Wal-Mart, the country's largest corporation, will establish 59 in-store clinics by the end of 2006. Similar in-store clinics are being established at Target, Cub Foods, Walgreens, Eckerds, Publix, and other grocery and pharmacy chains (Barbaro, 2006).

MinuteClinic

The most prominent and first to market of these new retail outlet clinics was MinuteClinic, which opened its first clinic in Minneapolis in 2000. MinuteClinic now has more than 80 clinics in metropolitan areas in Minneapolis, Atlanta, Seattle, Baltimore, Nashville, Indianapolis, Raleigh-Durham, Charlotte, Orlando, and Columbus (MinuteClinic.com). Major health plans, including Aetna and Cigna, are now promoting these clinics as convenient places to receive care for their members. Health care professionals—usually nurses, nurse practitioners, or physician assistants—in these clinics (which are concentrated at or near pharmacies) treat such nonemergency illnesses as strept throat, ear infections, sinus infections, mononucleosis, cold sores, seasonal allergies, deer tick bites, pinkeye, bronchitis, and female bladder infections. These clinics appeal to busy Americans, many of whom are families in which both mother and father work or who find it difficult to access care from doctors on weekends or off hours. Nurse practitioners treat common illnesses quickly (in about 15 minutes without need for an appointment), affordably ($39 to $110 and covered by most insurers), and conveniently (open 7 days a week).

Appeal and Credibility to Consumers

A *Wall Street Journal* Online/Harris Interactive Health-Care Poll in October of 2005 showed that although fewer than 7 percent of U.S. adults have ever used an onsite health clinic in a pharmacy or retail chain, many agreed retail-based clinics might be more convenient, accessible, and perhaps would offer some services at a lower cost than at doctors' offices. Among those who have never gone to an in-store clinic for health care services, 59 percent said they would be not or not at all likely to use such a clinic; 41 percent said they would be somewhat or very likely to use one for basic medical services. Many consumers expressed some concern about the quality of care they would receive at these clinics and from whom they would receive it (Harris Interactive, 2005).

The following are the results of that same online survey of 2,245 U.S. adults conducted by Harris Interactive between October 12 and 14, 2005, for the *Wall Street Journal* Online's Health Industry Edition. Among those who have used an onsite health clinic in a pharmacy or retail chain, most reported being somewhat or very satisfied with various aspects of their experience. Clinic users were most satisfied with its convenience (92 percent said they were somewhat/very satisfied), followed by the quality of care (89 percent), having qualified staff to provide the care (88 percent), and the cost (80 percent).

Despite the current low incidence of onsite clinic use at retail chains or pharmacies, large majorities of all adults see the convenience and affordability benefits these sites offer.

- More than four in five (83 percent) adults strongly or somewhat agreed onsite health clinics at retail stores could provide basic medical services to people at times when doctors' offices are closed, like evenings and weekends.
- Seventy-eight percent strongly or somewhat agree that onsite health clinics could provide busy people with a fast and easy way to get basic medical services.
- Three quarters of adults strongly or somewhat agree that onsite health clinics could provide low-cost basic services to people who otherwise might not be able to afford care.

However, many have concerns about these clinics and do not see them as purely helpful to consumers.

- Three in four adults strongly or somewhat agreed they would be worried serious medical problems might not be accurately diagnosed by someone working in an onsite health clinic in a retail store or pharmacy.
- Seventy-one percent strongly or somewhat agree they would be worried about the qualifications of the staff providing care in a health clinic not run by medical doctors.
- About two thirds strongly or somewhat agree onsite health clinics might be merely another way for big companies to make more money. (Harris Interactive, 2005)

Innovation Talking and Action Points

From the data just listed, it is clear retail outlets for routine medical care are still an idea in progress. The concept has yet to persuade the majority of consumers that these clinics are the places to go for routine care. At the same time, retail outlets are clearly a major innovation, filling demographic needs for quicker, more convenient, and less-costly care. However, the phenomenon of convenient retail outlets has caught the attention of the public and the media (Spencer, 2006).

Some physicians regard these outlets as competition; others look at them as an opportunity. Jack Reed, executive director of ProHealth Physicians, Inc., head-quartered in Farmington, Connecticut, says his group is opening two of these retail clinics in grocery chains in Connecticut by the end of 2006, and six to eight in the first half of 2007. "Our philosophy," says Reed, "is to go with the market flow, rather than resisting it. We are just beginning to learn how to work in the retail marketplace, and we do not yet know what other services we can offer in this retail space." In a consumer-driven, market-based health care economy, ProHealth's philosophy may soon be shared by other physicians who see opportunities outside their offices.

Retail clinics as a source of convenient affordable care for minor illness is a classic example of an innovation created by converging need or gaps in the current health system:

- The need for convenient affordable care delivered 24/7 by certified health professionals; nurse practitioners qualified to write prescriptions for minor illnesses
- The need for a credible alternative to expensive emergency room care for non-emergent ailments
- The need to offer a supplement to primary care physicians, who are declining in numbers and who are overwhelmed in many ways
- The need for affordable care for patients covered by high-deductible plans with HSAs, who want to spend their money sensibly and to have money left to roll over to the following year
- The need for affordable care for uninsured patients, who can afford to spend $50 or so for care, but who either cannot afford to pay health care premiums or choose not to
- The need for convenient care for time-strapped baby boomers, often with both spouses working

As Uwe E. Reinhardt, professor of economics and public affairs at Princeton University notes, "Primary care is a neglected field in the United States, lagging other economically advanced countries. The clinics can teach the rest of our health system how primary care could be done and brought to the public. That is very important" (Freudneheim, 2006a).

Case Study

MinuteClinic–Meeting the Need for Quick, Convenient Health Care

By Brent Burkhart, TBC, a public relations firm representing MinuteClinic

Since this study was written, MinuteClinic has been acquired by CVS Corporation. As of this writing, MinuteClinic has 114 locations in 17 states.

The need for convenient, walk-in health care is something most people face. When Rick Krieger experienced that need first-hand, it got him thinking about the retail health care center that eventually became MinuteClinic. On a wintry weekend in 1999, Krieger took his sick son to an urgent care center in Minneapolis. The boy needed a strep throat test and, after a 2-hour wait, finally got one. With that, Krieger knew there had to be a quicker, more convenient way.

A year later, Krieger and partners Dr. Douglas Smith and Steve Pontius founded a series of retail health care centers that ultimately became MinuteClinic, recognized nationally today as the pioneer and largest provider of retail-based health care in the United States.

Those first health care centers opened in the Minneapolis–St. Paul area Cub Foods grocery stores, focusing on seven common medical conditions: strep throat, mono, flu, female bladder infections, ear infections, sinus infections, and pregnancy testing. Patients paid much less than at urgent care, emergency, or other health care centers.

Walk-in Convenience Leads to Aggressive Expansion

The demand for walk-in convenience led to quick growth for the privately held Minneapolis-based management company, and by August 2004, the company expanded its operations to the Baltimore area. Less than a year later, MinuteClinic opened its first health care centers in CVS pharmacy stores in Minneapolis–St. Paul and Baltimore.

This led to a national expansion in CVS pharmacy locations in 10 markets nationwide and ultimately in July 2006, the CVS Corporation announced it had struck a definitive agreement to purchase MinuteClinic. The acquisition was scheduled to be completed by the fourth quarter of 2006 and MinuteClinic will operate as a wholly owned subsidiary of the CVS Corporation (the acquisition occurred on July 13, 2006).

In July of 2006, there were a total of 83 MinuteClinic health care centers located in Atlanta, Baltimore, Charlotte, Columbus, Indianapolis, the Maryland Capital area, Minneapolis–St. Paul, Nashville, Orlando, Providence-Woonsocket, Raleigh-Durham, and Seattle (as noted earlier by November 2006 there were 114 locations in 17 states).

While most MinuteClinics are found in CVS pharmacy stores, MinuteClinics will remain in select Bartell Drugs, Cub Foods, and QFC stores and additional retail hosts will continue to be sought. MinuteClinic health care centers are also located in corporate and government office buildings, corporate and college campuses, and shopping centers.

Six years after that first patient walked through the doors, more than 500,000 patients have visited MinuteClinics; surveys reveal greater than 97 percent of customers rate their experience as excellent. Since its launch, MinuteClinic has helped individuals, self-insured employers, and health insurance companies substantially reduce the costs of health care. In addition to saving millions of dollars, the walk-in health care clinics have saved countless hours of wasted time.

Treatment for a Variety of Common Illnesses

MinuteClinic offers quick, convenient, and affordable treatment for many common illnesses. MinuteClinic also offers common vaccinations, such as flu shots, tetanus, pneumonia, MMR, hepatitis A and B, meningitis, and tetanus-diphtheria. Additional treatments include chlamydia, flu, mono, swimmer's ear, pregnancy testing, and skin conditions, including athlete's foot, cold sores, deer tick bites, impetigo, minor burns and rashes, minor skin infections, minor sunburn, poison ivy, ringworm, swimmer's itch, and wart removal.

Combining Quality Medical Care with an Understanding of Today's Demanding Lifestyles

MinuteClinics are open 7 days a week, require no advance appointment, and visits typically take 10 to 15 minutes. For most customers, MinuteClinic will accept the office visit copay indicated on their health insurance card as payment. Customers paying by cash or credit card will find treatment prices posted outside each health care center. Most treatments at MinuteClinic cost between $49 and $59.

MinuteClinics serve as a high-quality adjunct to emergency rooms, urgent care centers, and physician offices. The result is a convenient care system that saves patients, employers, and insurers time and money.

Staffed by Certified Family Nurse Practitioners and Physician Assistants

MinuteClinics are staffed by certified family nurse practitioners and physician assistants who are trained to diagnose, treat, and write prescriptions (when clinically appropriate) for common family illnesses—and, because most clinics are located within a retail pharmacy, patients can choose to fill their prescriptions right then and there.

Every MinuteClinic patient assessment and treatment follows nationally established clinical practice guidelines from the American Academy of Family Physicians and the American Academy of Pediatrics that are embedded in MinuteClinic's electronic medical records system.

MinuteClinic nurse practitioners use a software program that guides diagnosis, treatment, and billing. At the conclusion of each visit, the software generates educational material, an invoice, and a prescription for the patient (when clinically appropriate), as well as a diagnostic record that is sent to the patient's primary care provider's office. A supervising physician is on call during all hours of operation.

Individuals with illnesses outside MinuteClinic's scope of services—or who exhibit signs of a chronic condition—are referred to their physician or, if critical, the nearest urgent care center or emergency room. Patients who can't be treated are not charged for their visit. MinuteClinic only serves patients over the age of 18 months.

MinuteClinic services are a complement to primary care providers. MinuteClinic nurse practitioners and physician assistants stress the importance of a regular medical exam with every patient they see. If the individual doesn't have a medical home, a list of physicians in the area is provided.

An Experienced Executive Team

MinuteClinic's seasoned, creative management team is one of the factors responsible for the company's success in delivering top-quality care of common illnesses.

Dr. Glen Nelson, chairman of the board, is a former surgeon who holds a B.A. from Harvard University and doctor of medicine degree from the University of Minnesota. He has a strong interest in emerging medical technologies and exploring other avenues for improving health care. Dr. Nelson served as vice chairman of Medtronic from 1988 until 2002.

Michael C. Howe was appointed CEO of MinuteClinic in June 2005 after serving as president and CEO of Arby's, Inc. Highly regarded for his *Fortune* 100 experience with companies such as Procter & Gamble and KFC (PepsiCo), as well as entrepreneurial organizations, Howe's determination and drive have generated turnaround and high-growth opportunities for nationally known consumer brands. Howe graduated magna cum laude from the University of Minnesota–Duluth earning two degrees, a bachelor of business administration and a bachelor of accounting.

Dr. James Woodburn, chief medical officer, has 22 years experience as a physician: administrative, emergency, and occupational medicine. He is responsible for the clinical integrity and quality of medical care provided by all MinuteClinics. For 12 years, he was corporate medical director for Blue Cross Blue Shield of Minnesota where he developed innovative employer-based health programs to improve the lives of employees nationwide. Dr. Woodburn attended the University of Wisconsin–Madison Medical School and also has degrees in electrical and biomedical engineering.

In addition to the management team, MinuteClinic's National Clinical Quality Advisory Council is a panel that brings together nationally recognized health care leaders from a variety of specialties and backgrounds to contribute strategic creativity, clinical guidance, and quality improvement ideas to MinuteClinic services.

The advisory council discusses new clinical and health improvement programs, evaluates current clinical performance, and reviews the nationally established guidelines for the services provided by MinuteClinic at existing and new health care centers. There are eight members on the advisory council including a permanent representative from the American Academy of Family Physicians.

You're Sick. We're Quick

The result—in just a few years, a new category of health care delivery/retail-based health care centers—has taken hold, and with MinuteClinic as its recognized innovator and leader. The insurance industry, medical community, and employers have each embraced the retail-based health care centers as a viable and proven complement to traditional health care delivery.

The rapid growth to date of MinuteClinic and its aggressive plans for the future speaks directly to the value and importance that consumers attach to these centers, which is what the founders set out to provide following that wintry weekend experience in 1999.

Chapter 32

Self-Care, Self-Service, and Self-Empowering Consumer Care

Prelude: Care for yourself, serve yourself, empower yourself, but when you're really sick, the doctor knows best.

An ATM (Automatic or Automated Teller Machine) is a computerized machine designed to dispense cash to bank customers without need of human interaction. The ATM can also take deposits, transfer money between bank accounts, and provide other basic financial services. Most banks feature one or more "on premises" ATMs so that customers have access to services 24 hours a day, seven days a week. During banking hours the ATM can reduce long lines inside the bank by providing an alternative to a human teller. Even better, the ATM continues to be available long after the bank is closed. If you need cash in the evening, on a holiday or Sunday, the ATM is there to serve.

WiseGEEK, 2006

Twenty-four hours a day, consumers are entering data freely, conveniently, and voluntarily into ATM machines, gas pump dispensers, electronic airport check-in machines, and supermarket check-out machines. Consumers are Googling, Yahooing, and Microsofting the Internet any time of the day or night to search for health care information for themselves, relatives, or friends—so why not health care, too?

Why? Because it's already happening. Health plans market their products on the Internet through transparent Web sites. These sites can be defined as sites allowing consumers to compare prices, outcomes, and quality of drugs, doctors, and hospitals. Consumers can go to Healthgrade.com and, for $7.95, compare prices and outcomes for 50 procedures or so for hospitals and doctors in their zip code or region. They can also go to Medicarecompare.gov and compare hospital outcomes and Medicare prescription drug plans. About every hospital has a Web site, and more and more doctor practices have Web sites, too—so, too, do health plans. These sites allow consumers to compare hospitals and doctor prices.

Today's health care consumers are part of the consumer-driven self-care, self-service, and self-empowering health industry revolution. They are smart, knowledgeable about what ails them, computer savvy, assertive, and, on occasion, disrespectful of authority. However, beyond all of this, as Dr. James F. Fries, professor of medicine at Stanford University, and his colleagues have proven, health professionals can use electronic and printed matter to activate consumers to pursue self-care (Fries, Harrington, Edwards, Kent, & Richardson, 1994).

Healthtrac Self-Care Programs

Through self-care programs at their place of employment called Healthtrac, Fries and colleagues have taught people how to cope with the "five Ds": death, disability, discomfort, drug toxicity, and dollar cost. The overall goal of Fries and his associates is to reduce need and demand for medical services by focusing on the following:

- Improving personal self-efficacy and autonomous consumer behavior
- Increasing self-management skills
- Increasing chronic disease self-management skills
- Decreasing behavioral health risks related to smoking, lack of exercise, and high-fat diets
- Increasing the intensity of interventions for high-risk interventions compared to low-risk ones
- Decreasing the number of very low birth-weight babies
- Decreasing the frequency of inhumane and undignified care at the end of life

If these activities can succeed in the workplace, they can succeed in the wider consumer health marketplace.

Prophet of Consumer-Driven Care

Dr. Tom Ferguson pioneered and articulated the concept of health care consumers using the Internet to educate themselves. Dr. Ferguson studied and wrote about the empowered medical consumer starting in 1975 and about online health resources for consumers beginning in 1987. In 1993, he organized the world's first conference devoted to computer systems for medical consumers. After attending Reed College, earning a master's degree in creative writing from San Francisco State University and a medical degree from Yale University School of Medicine, he launched a prolific career in consumer-focused medical writing as founder of *Medical Self-Care Magazine.*

From 1980 to 1996, he authored or co-authored over a dozen books and was section editor for health, medicine, and self-care for the *Whole Earth Catalogue.*

Dr. Ferguson led the movement to advocate informed self-care as the starting point for good health. He promoted a new kind of relationship between knowledgeable medical consumers and medical professionals. His goal was to encourage medical professionals to treat clients as equal partners in achieving better outcomes. With the advent of broad Internet access, he was positioned to become a leading proponent of online health information resources.

Using the Internet is no longer an option; it is a necessity. According to Harris Interactive surveys, 98 percent of graduating medical students and 80 percent of practicing doctors have Internet access (Peck, 2002). Today more than 85 percent of practicing doctors have broadband Internet access, but only 16.6 percent communicate with patients by e-mail for a variety of reasons, medical, legal, fear of being inundated with e-mails, lack of reimbursement (Brooks & Menachiemi, 2006). Doctors now live in a wireless world; so too do consumers who commonly search the Net for health care information. Increasingly, these consumers wirelessly visit their doctor via e-mail, refilling prescriptions and scheduling appointments.

Ferguson foresaw all of this. He predicted the Internet's potential for disseminating medical information long before its time. He coined such terms as "e-patients" and "disease tribes" for patients who searched the Net and who gathered together in Internet chat rooms.

Ferguson established a journal called *Medical Self-Care,* serving as its editor from 1975 to 1989. In 1998, he became editor and publisher of a newsletter *The Ferguson Report: The Newsletter of Consumer Informatics and Online Health.* In addition, he was senior associate at the Center for Clinical Computing, a Harvard Medical School–based research institution, an associate faculty member at the Texas Health Science Center and the University of Arkansas Medical Sciences Center, and as a senior research fellow at the Pew Internet and American Life Project, where he specialized in reports on how people use the Internet to obtain health information. Ferguson laid much of the groundwork for consumer-driven health care. Regina Herzlinger, a Harvard Business School professor, deserves credit for officially christening the movement, but it was Ferguson who almost single-handedly got the ball rolling.

Consumers Are Extremely Smart People

Like Herzlinger, Ferguson recognized health care consumers as extremely smart people, perfectly capable of fending for themselves, doing their own research, and, in concert with doctors, figuring out how to wend their way through the medical maze.

In an interview, Ferguson observed:

> *Online technology has made it possible for people to gain access to disease support groups and to research information about their diseases. It provides an environment in which some patients can play a role that's different from the role they've played traditionally. The online revolution is changing the roles of both physicians and patients. Patients spend a good portion of their time away from the physician's office, caring for themselves. When patients are motivated they are willing to put almost endless time and energy into being a resource for their own care.*
>
> *Patient knowledge is different from physician knowledge. Depending on their specialty, a specialist might have to stay current on 30, 200, or 400 medical conditions. A general practitioner might have to keep up with 600. Patients only have to know about one disease—their own.* (Reece, 1999)

And for Physicians...

For physicians, online patient self-education means that those who live in high-tech urban areas and want to treat well-educated young adults will have to be proficient on the Internet or they won't have any patients left. Most educated people now have Internet access, can use search engines to gather data on their condition, and expect their physician to have the same level of expertise.

EHRs and Physician Web Sites Serve Different Purposes

There is much talk these days of personal health records (PHRs) and electronic health records (EHRs). PHRs are for patients who want a running record of their health and who wish to present it to physicians before office visits, so patients do not have to re-answer the same questions again and again. By and large, EHRs are for physicians' internal practice efficiency, documentation, coding, claims processing, patient safety, and avoiding test duplication.

These EHR features are important, indeed essential functions, but they may be largely invisible to consumers seeking convenient, time-saving, money-saving, and self-serving access to routine physician services. What are needed are consumer add-on services to existing physician EHRs or through physician Web sites, even without EHRs.

Medfusion, Inc.

A company in Raleigh, North Carolina, called Medfusion has pioneered development of physician Web sites that offer such consumer-friendly services as office location and hours, physician credentials, prescription refills, scheduling an appointment, and patient education information. On these physician Web sites, the company seeks to satisfy those consumer who are either irritated by the inconvenience of being "on-hold" or seeking conveniences offered by being online. Medfusion characterizes its services as "secure patient and physician communication portals" (Medfusion.com). Consumer self-service capabilities reduce phone calls, improve efficiency, reduce costs, and improve revenue. Workflow enhancements include patient preregistration, appointment requests and reminders, outbound messaging, lab results delivery, prescription renewals, patient online bill payment, personal health records, and virtual office visits.

Consumer-Friendly Online Services

Through their Web sites, physicians can cater to time-bankrupt consumers. They seek no-nonsense, quick-hitting, relevant information and services. The information includes practice location, maps, physician backgrounds, and practice expertise. Through this portal, consumers can schedule appointments; refill prescriptions; arrange for a virtual e-mail visit with their doctors; obtain laboratory, X-ray, and imaging results; and even create their own medical histories before seeing their doctors. These kinds of services save not only the patients but the physicians time and are convenient.

Innovation Talking and Action Points

Given the size of the self-care movement, the electronic data entry self-services already common in U.S. retail establishments, and widespread use of Internet search engines, innovations in self-care, self-service, and self-empowerment are powerful and inevitable. An additional benefit of this consumer-driven revolution may be a decrease in the demand, need, and cost of medical services.

Case Study

Self-Care, Self-Service, and Self-Empowerment in Action

By Richard L. Reece, MD

A number of the doctors and practice managers involved with the Web sites of Medfusion clients were contacted. They included a solo concierge physician in Atlanta; a large primary care group in Mississippi; two solo family physicians, one in Washington, D.C., and the other in Oregon; a 37-person group of cardiovascular specialists in Oklahoma; and a 12-person orthopedic group in California. All said their Web sites automated and facilitated interactions of patients and clients and saved them time and staff time in explaining what the practice offered. The Web site helped bypass many time-consuming interactions between patients and staff and doctors. These interactions include time required for phone calls and telephone "tag"—and by so doing, free up time for "real" patient care. In addition, to problems such as overburdened phone lines and patient no-shows, there are other benefits: less staff is required to run the practice (online patients substitute for staff time), reduced expenses for yellow page listings (the Web sites are a form of advertising); and being able to charge for virtual online office visits. In the past, unlike their lawyer counterparts, doctors had a way to charge for phone calls to discuss minor problems. But now most doctors can charge for e-mail visits, which are tailored for minor problems, formerly discussed on the phone.

Furthermore, patient-empowering Web sites are adaptable and affordable for almost any type of practice in any part of the country. Perhaps, more important, tech-savvy health consumers enjoy this new brand of medicine too. No more waiting on hold to schedule an appointment, no more waiting to get the doctor to comment on the phone about some minor ailment, no more doctor visits to get a routine prescription refill, no more phone calls to get lab results, and in some cases, no more searching elsewhere to be educated about a disease (many Web sites contain educational videos).

Finally, through a software program on the physician Web site, patients can choose to be interviewed by a computer before their visit. That way, when the patient enters the exam room, the person's history has been laid out from his or her point of view before the doctor. For the doctor and the patient, this computer interview saves time and confusion and facilitates a faster route to a proper diagnosis.

Chapter 33

Malpractice Innovations

Prelude: This chapter suggests innovations that will help manage malpractice, not eliminate it. Malpractice will be with us as long as adverse outcomes occur, doctors make mistakes, patient expectations are not met, and our present legal system prevails.

A major medical malpractice crisis is unfolding in the United States today. The American Medical Association has identified 18 states in which doctors and institutional health care providers are having grave difficulties obtaining affordable professional liability insurance. In the past two years, insurance premiums in these states have increased dramatically for doctors in high-risk specialties such as obstetrics, emergency medicine, general surgery, surgical subspecialties, and radiology.

Another 26 states are on "orange alert," with indicators suggesting a serious and worsening situation. Doctors in West Virginia, New Jersey, Florida, Pennsylvania, Mississippi, Illinois, Texas, and Missouri have held or threatened work stoppages to draw attention to their plight, and several hospitals in the states that have been hit the hardest have temporarily closed or threatened to close emergency room, obstetrical, or other services.

Michelle M. Mellor et al., 2003

Many physicians want someone to do something, anything, to manage persistent malpractice problems. However, most of them know it will take alert, coordinated actions at all levels to manage the problem—which will never go completely away in a litigious United States with its high expectations of miraculous medical results. Physicians cannot depend on malpractice lawyers, state legislatures, or Congress to help. Given human nature and the stakes involved, "solving" all malpractice problems will be impossible. But pragmatic innovations to lessen malpractice are possible.

Managing the problem is probably the closest to a solution that the industry will come. As long as trial attorneys believe they can hit the malpractice jackpot, earning one third to one half of the settlement in contingency fees, nothing is likely to happen nationally. As long as patients have expectations of perfect outcomes, are confused about what the doctor said, think all complications result from something the doctor did wrong, and continue to wait in overcrowded emergency rooms, prospects for malpractice cure will remain grim. As long as doctors continue to write illegible prescriptions or prescribe powerful drugs with dangerous side effects, perform high-risk operations on fragile patients, communicate poorly with patients and family members, fail to clearly document patient histories, and do not work closely with hospitals to systematically follow risk-avoidance protocols, they will have malpractice settlements. As long as there is a reliance on Congress—45 percent of whom are lawyers—to set national malpractice caps, no single piece of legislature will resolve the problems (Time to change, n.d.).

Without corrective measures, a few things are certain.

- The costs of "defensive medicine," all those tests doctors order and things they do to avoid future malpractice suits, will continue to cost in the neighborhood of $60 billion to $108 billion (Carroll, 2005).
- Specialists with exorbitant malpractice rates (i.e., $100,000 to $250,000 per annum) will either retire, stop performing high-risk procedures, move to other states with lower rates, or pass on those malpractice costs to patients (Bean, 2005).
- Specialists will stop seeing nonpaying high-risk patients in emergency departments (Glabman, 2005).
- Doctors will approach hospitals to become full-time employees anticipating that the institution will take care of their malpractice expenses (Mays et al., 2005).
- Doctor shortages with limited access to care will develop (CBS News, 2006).
- Young doctors will avoid specialties with high malpractice rates (Fletcher, 2003).

What Young Doctors Think

According to an AMA survey, almost half of medical students in their third and fourth years say the malpractice environment is a factor when they choose a specialty. Though the AMA survey did not indicate how malpractice concerns influenced the students' choice of specialty, lawsuit data shows the highest malpractice risks are in OB/GYN, neurosurgery, emergency medicine, radiology, and orthopedic surgery. The AMA says its division for market research and analysis survey received responses from nearly 4,000 medical students in 45 states and the District of Columbia.

The survey found among students:

- 86 percent indicated medical liability is a "crisis" or a "major problem."
- 39 percent said the malpractice environment was a factor in their decision about a state in which they would like to complete residency training.
- 69 percent whose professors discussed malpractice said those professors also discussed defensive medicine, including increasing unnecessary or excessive care.
- 61 percent of students say they are extremely concerned that the current malpractice environment is decreasing physicians' ability to provide quality care.

"We watched, horrified, as the crisis was forcing our most experienced mentors to stop performing high-risk procedures or providing care in crisis states," says AMA medical student trustee David Rosman. "It is frightening to realize that because this crisis is affecting specialty choice, there may not be anyone to take their place" (American Medical Association Press Release). Depending on the specialty, young doctors often take into account those states with the highest premiums. Table 33-1 offers some sample states.

Minimizing Malpractice Risks and Worries

Young doctors will learn malpractice risks can be minimized using these techniques:

- Document patient encounters using electronic history taking and macro keys to record findings and treatment plan.
- Give patients a record of details of their visit before they leave the office.
- Communicate, communicate, and communicate, both through language and paper documentation.
- Make absolutely certain patients understand what they're being told. Have them repeat what was said.

Table 33-1 *High Annual Premium States in 2002 by Specialty (K stands for 1000s of dollars)*

State	OB-GYNs	Surgeons	Internists
Florida	$211K	$124K	$56K
Nevada	$142K	$85K	$17K
Michigan	$141K	$107K	$46K
New York	$115K	$66K	$17K
Illinois	$102K	$70K	$26K
Texas	$98K	$71K	$26K

Source: US Department of Health and Human Services, Special Update on Medical Liability Crisis, September 25, 2003.

Patients Viewed as Enemies

According to a survey of 736 doctors by the Doctors' Company, a physician-owned insurance company, more than 72 percent of doctors view their patients as potential malpractice adversaries. Nearly 40 percent of surveyed doctors said they limited services to minimize liability risk (Thedoctors.com). A survey in 2000 by Merritt, Hawkins & Associates of doctors aged 50 to 65 found more than half plan to quit practice in the next 3 years. Their greatest source of frustration was malpractice worries (28 percent), followed by managed care (16 percent), Medicare/ Medicaid regulations (13 percent), and long hours and pressure of running a business (10 percent each).

Doctor Avoidance Actions

Doctors are taking actions. Many have dropped malpractice insurance altogether. Others are abandoning high-risk procedures, moving to more physician-friendly states, or asking patients to sign forms of waivers promising not to sue for frivolous reasons. When people speak of "frivolous" lawsuits, they are generally referring to lawsuits without merit that cost doctors money and tarnish their reputation.

Yet another approach is that of Dr. Neil Baum, an advisory board member of *Physician Practice Options,* a monthly newsletter for physicians addressing their practice business options. Baum advises considering these questions to spot those 15 percent of patients who create 90 percent of the malpractice lawsuits:

- **Does the patient have chronic medical or psychological problems?** These patients often arrive with a briefcase of downloaded Internet material for you to review.
- **Does the patient understand what you're saying?** Patients who don't understand a course of treatment or a procedure account for most malpractice litigation.
- **Does the patient complain about former physicians?** If the patient criticizes another doctor, take meticulous notes on his or her chart as a precaution. Avoid criticizing another physician.
- **Does the patient require complex care?** Physicians are frequently involved in cases involving complex patient management and difficult communication with family members, either because of multiple physicians working on the case or a confusing care regimen.
- **Has the patient given informed consent?** For physicians in surgical specialties, a lack of informed consent causes many lawsuits, especially for patients with a complication or unfavorable result. Give the patient sufficient information about all known potential complications so he or she can make an informed decision about a treatment. (Baum, 2004b)

Dr. Steven H. Farber, a cardiologist in Houston, agrees with Dr. Baum, but he adds these three simple pieces of advice.

1. Communicate, communicate, communicate!
2. Document, document, document!
3. Write legibly!

The Malpractice Climate

Malpractice threats erode quality of health services. Respondents in a 2002 Harris Interactive survey, which included doctors, nurses, and hospital administrators, said malpractice litigation harmed their ability to provide quality care. Among other findings, the Harris survey showed:

- 79 percent of doctor respondents said they ordered unnecessary tests because they feared litigation.
- 74 percent said they made unnecessary referrals.
- 51 percent said they suggested unnecessary biopsies.
- 45 percent said they prescribed antibiotics unnecessarily. (Taylor, 2002)

Twenty states are currently experiencing a medical liability crisis: Arkansas, Connecticut, Florida, Georgia, Illinois, Kentucky, Massachusetts, Mississippi, Missouri, Nevada, New Jersey, New York, North Carolina, Ohio, Oregon, Pennsylvania, Texas, Washington, West Virginia, and Wyoming. Of the remaining states, 24 have the potential to be deemed "in crisis." Only six—California, Colorado, Indiana, Louisiana, New Mexico, and Wisconsin—are considered stable; all six have longstanding state laws placing caps on noneconomic damage awards.

Despite continuing rises of medical liability premiums, in 2004, the U.S. Senate announced it will not pass comprehensive medical liability reform. According to the Medical Group Management Association (MGMA), medical groups faced average premium increases of 37 percent between 2003 and 2004, on top of 40 percent between 2002 and 2003. In 2003, primary care premiums rose 51 percent while specialty care premiums climbed 40 percent.

According to an MGMA Online Survey, average increases by specialties from 2002 to 2003 included:

- general surgery, 49 percent
- cardiology, 49 percent
- gastroenterology, 45 percent
- ophthalmology, 41 percent
- neurosurgery, 39 percent
- obstetrics and gynecology, 35 percent

- orthopedic surgery, 34 percent
- internal medicine, 33 percent
- urology, 32 percent
- anesthesiology, 31 percent

Highest increases by state were:

- Indiana, 85 percent
- Missouri, 64 percent
- Pennsylvania, 63 percent
- Arizona, 56 percent
- Ohio, 49 percent
- North Carolina, 44 percent
- Florida, 40 percent
- Georgia, 36 percent
- Oregon, 36 percent

No Single Solution

Much of the current debate about who is at fault for soaring malpractice rates (avaricious lawyers versus careless hospitals and dangerous doctors) may be at a standoff. Most of this debate focuses on tort reform. Adversarial positions taken by lawyers and doctors are understandable, but it may be more practical, realistic, and productive to reduce malpractice suits by promoting safety and educating patients about what to expect from medical care.

Reducing Malpractice Rates by Promoting Safety

In a June 21, 2005, *Wall Street Journal* article, the reporter described how anesthesiologists have developed a model to lower premiums by improving safety. The rising cost of medical malpractice insurance has hit many doctors, especially surgeons and obstetricians, but one specialty has largely escaped escalating premiums—the 30,000 anesthesiologists of the American Society of Anesthesiology (Hallinan, 2005).

Twenty years ago, the society decided that, rather than lobbying for laws to protect themselves against lawsuits, they would focus on patient safety. They concentrated on devices to alert anesthesiologists to potentially fatal problems and to correct those problems. The anesthesiologists built high-tech mannequins to practice responses to overwhelming allergic reactions and to life-threatening airway obstructions. With a mannequin, anesthesiologists could slit open an obstructed airway, something they couldn't practice on patients.

Anesthesiologists also began to use pulse oximetry devices clipped on patient fingers to instantly detect dropping oxygen levels signaling airway obstruction. Another device was a capnographic instrument measuring carbon dioxide in a patient's expelled breath. Rising carbon dioxide levels help anesthesiologists determine at a glance if a patient is breathing properly.

By 1990, virtually every American hospital had pulse oximeters and capnographs. Malpractice suits dropped from 7.9 percent of all claims in 1972 to 3.8 percent of all claims from 1985 to 2001. Malpractice premiums dropped too; in 2005 dollars, from $33,000 in 1985 to $21,000 in 2005, roughly one tenth of what some high-risk specialties like obstetricians and neurosurgeons pay in high-risk states (Hallinan, 2005).

Six Keys to Reducing Hospital Deaths

In a 2005 *Newsweek* article, Dr. Donald Berwick, president and CEO of the Institute for Health Care Improvement and clinical professor of pediatrics and health care policy at Harvard Medical School, made another step toward improving hospital safety. Berwick offered six pragmatic safety suggestions, developed by the Institute for Health Improvement during their 100,000 Lives Campaign. This campaign, inspired by an Institute of Medicine study, showed that as many as 100,000 Americans were dying needlessly in hospitals every year.

On June 14, 2006, Berwick announced that the campaign to reduce lethal errors and unnecessary deaths in the nation's hospitals had saved an estimated 122,300 lives in the previous 18 months. Berwick said, "I think this campaign signals no less than a new standard of health care in America" (Associated Press, 2006). About 3,100 hospitals participated in the project, sharing mortality data and carrying out study-tested procedures that prevent infections and mistakes. Experts say the cooperative effort was unusual for a competitive industry that does not like to focus publicly on patient deaths.

The safety keys to saving lives were:

1. Preventing ventilator-associated pneumonia (VAP): Simple maneuvers, like elevating the head of the hospital bed and frequently cleaning the patient's mouth, can eliminate VAP.

2. Preventing IV-catheter infections: Make it easy for doctors and nurses to wash their hands between patients, adopt simple procedures for changing bandages around catheters, and make sure no catheter remains in a vein even 1 hour longer than needed.

3. Stopping surgical-site infections: Surgical-site infections are a major cause of complications and deaths after operations. Give the right antibiotics at the right time during surgery, enforce hand-washing, and avoid shaving the surgery site before the operation (clipping hair avoids nicking the skin and is safer).

4. Responding rapidly to early warning: A nurse or visitor is often the first to notice a patient is in trouble. By setting up special rapid-response teams, hospitals can ensure these critical warnings are never missed or

ignored. Take family members and nurses' concerns seriously. Respond within minutes.

5. Making heart attack care reliable: Correct treatments for heart attacks could save far more lives. The 100,000 Lives Campaign simply asked hospitals to ensure every patient gets every medication and treatment recommended by the American College of Cardiology and other expert bodies. These measures include aspirin and a beta blocker on arrival and a stent or clot buster promptly after administration.

6. Stopping medication errors: Medication errors are easily prevented. One secret is to "reconcile" medications whenever patients move from one care setting to another—from hospital to home, or even from one place to another within a hospital. (Berwick, 2005)

Managing Patient Expectations

Most malpractice claims aren't about medical negligence; they're about miscommunication. Doctors may fail to impart to patients the risk and real outcomes of procedures. People sue when expectations don't match reality. Patients don't understand their procedure and aren't prepared for how they might feel after surgery. Most patients don't read consent forms, and they aren't aware of the risks involved with their procedure. Studies show patients may forget 85 percent of what doctors tell them within 10 minutes after leaving a doctor's office.

One answer to this failure to communicate or understand may be interactive videos, now provided free by hundreds of hospitals, clinics, and doctors, to about 85,000 patients around the country. These video programs are called Expectation Management and Medical Information (EMMIs) and feature computer animation. They were developed by Rightfield Solutions in Chicago to walk patients through more than 60 surgical procedures (Landro, 2005).

Hospitals can obtain EMMIs for $1,200 per surgeon or for $75,000 for hospitals under 100 beds and for $300,000 for hospitals of 400 beds or more. These videos, actually a sophisticated form of informed consent, not only educate patients but in a lawsuit provide documentation of what the patient heard and saw.

A rival system, the Iowa City–based Patient Education Institute, provides interactive systems for 1,000 hospitals and countless doctors' waiting rooms (Landro, 2005). Both systems offer evidence for hospitals and doctors to defend themselves against patients who claim they weren't fully informed about risks.

Alternative Risk Organizations

What can hospitals or doctors do when commercial insurers, beset by losses, abandon a market? One increasingly attractive option is to self-insure through so-called risk retention groups, captive insurers, or purchasing groups. According to the Wilmington Trust, alternative risk organizations, when structured and run properly, can effectively manage risk and control insurance costs. The advantages of alternative risk organizations, including those run by joint hospital–physician ventures, or hospitals and physicians separately, are direct involvement in risk and loss control, along with reduced premiums for health care practitioners. These organizations can provide a viable alternative to waiting out the medical malpractice storm.

These groups are allowed in certain states (Vermont and Hawaii), but often must be set up offshore in Bermuda, the Cayman Islands, or Barbados. The Boston-based law firm McDermott, Will, and Emery is doing a brisk business setting up 20 or so of these entities each year. Organizing these new organizations is easiest for single-specialty groups like orthopedic surgeons or cardiovascular groups, because single specialties speak common languages and perform limited numbers of procedures. Increasingly hospitals and medical groups together are participating. Setting up these organizations is complicated and requires knowledge of international law, state jurisdictional laws, and Stark, Office of the Inspector General, and IRS regulations.

Estimates of the alternative market size vary. Conning Research & Consulting Inc., a unit of Swiss Reinsurance Co., pegs it at $18 billion in annual premiums, compared to $12 billion estimated for conventional insurance companies. Actuarial firm Milliman, Inc., estimates the alternative-market premium at $9 billion, or about 40 percent of a $21 billion market. These estimates suggest 4 in 10 medical professionals have turned to alternative sources for coverage (Anand, 2005).

For alternative risk organizations to work, doctors must feel they have a stake and must receive incentives—lower premiums, acquisition of desired equipment, and a financial share of premium savings. Alternative risk organizations, like any form of insurance, have upsides (premium reductions and a closer relationship between hospitals and doctors) and downsides (failure to control risks, financial losses, and clashes with medical staff over enforcement of rules).

Hospital Risk-Management Programs

Conducting hospital risk-management programs isn't easy. Risk management basically consists of systematic activities to minimize financial loss for hospitals and doctors who work within those institutions. The mainstays of risk management are credentialing of medical staff, incidence monitoring and tracking, patient complaint monitoring and tracking, infection control, and documentation of medical record, including patient education about expectations and risks. Risk management requires close coordination and communication between patients, nurses, doctors, and hospital staff.

The physician culture may be a particular problem. Through their training and acculturation, physicians develop a mindset that they must be right in everything they do. They are reluctant to be open about mistakes or to set up organizations to reduce errors that may lead to high malpractice rates. Furthermore, some physicians are not accustomed to teamwork and may become disruptive when confronted. In addition, the role of the hospital medical director is complicated by the problems of misdiagnosis, mismanagement, investigating patient complaints, helping to settle claims, and frequent meetings with attorneys to reach agreement.

Obviously, there is more to the malpractice crisis than tort reform. A complementary and potentially more productive approach may be for doctors to initiate safety improvement programs on their own, to identify those clinical procedural errors that cause the most problems, to manage patient expectations through interactive videos, to investigate alternative risk entities, and to systematically pursue hospital-based risk-management programs.

Case Study 1

Lawyer Says Lawyer Colleagues Are Wrecking Health Care

By Henry Kopel, Assistant U.S. Attorney, Connecticut

Here is an account by Henry Kopel, an assistant U.S. attorney in Connecticut, in the April 4, 2004, *Hartford Courant* entitled "My Colleagues Are Wrecking Health Care." His story is poignant on two counts: (1) he is a lawyer, and (2) he is married to a doctor suddenly confronted with high malpractice premiums.

• •

"My wife is an obstetrician-gynecologist. As is true of most Connecticut obstetricians, her medical malpractice insurance premiums for one year are more than $80,000. This premium is expected to increase by several thousand dollars every year. If she seeks to change jobs or retire, she will need more than $150,000 to maintain lawsuit protection against all past patients—who retain the right to sue for at least 20 years. Those who bring such frivolous lawsuits suffer no penalty for the financial and emotional havoc they cause."

Case Study 2

Using an Electronic Medical History as a Defense

By Allen Wenner, MD

Dr. Allen Wenner is a family practitioner in Columbia, South Carolina. Over the last 15 years, he has developed the Instant Medical History, a software program that allows patients to tell their own history based on their chief complaint, age, and sex (see Chapter 3).

Wenner maintains that with universal patient-generated medical histories clearly stating the patient's view of their clinical problem, frivolous lawsuits in doctors' offices would virtually disappear. There would be no more "he said–she said" in court, because it would be clear precisely what the patient said.

● ●

To my knowledge, the Instant Medical History is the first medical software program to be used by a physician to successfully defend against medical malpractice in the United States. The final judgment was rendered April 15, 2001, in Circuit Court for the Fifth Judicial Circuit of South Carolina, the *Estate of William Stroud v. Allen Wenner, M.D., and Doctors Care, Inc.* and was decided in my favor after a short 20-minute deliberation.

The dispute involved the deceased patient's symptoms when he initially presented in my office for clinical examination. The jury verdict ruled in my favor. The case involved a difficult-to-diagnose proximal aortic dissection in a 47-year-old male who died during surgery several days after being seen by me. The patient did not complain of pain or other symptoms of dissecting aneurysm in his electronic medical history.

Failure to diagnose is a growing cause of tort actions against physicians and a leading cause of malpractice suits. A recent illustration of this is John Ritter, the actor who died of a dissecting aortic aneurysm. His family sued for malpractice and won. Typical in this type action is disagreement between the family and the doctor over the presenting condition of the patient.

Before my clinical exam, the patient completed a structured interview using Instant Medical History software. The software is an expert decision-support knowledge base that branches to new questions depending on the patient's answers. Patients document in detail their exact symptoms and complaints. Every interview is unique to each patient visit. The jury found that patient-entered data was "testimony from the grave" that could not be disputed.

Aortic dissection is a frequent diagnosis in tort actions because of its catastrophic nature, unexpected occurrence, and difficulty in diagnosis. Aortic dissections are initially not diagnosed in 40 percent of the cases. Of the total 1,000 cases per year in United States, 300 cases per year are involved in court actions. Aortic dissection is statistically the most difficult diagnosis for a physician to encounter, partly because of physician ignorance but often because of lack of clear presenting symptoms, which was the case with my patients. Indeed, Kevin Helliker and Thomas Burton won a Pulitzer Prize for explaining the medical and legal difficulties surrounding diagnosis and death from dissecting aortic aneurysms (Helliker & Burton, 2003).

Health care information systems have long been on the rise as a way for physicians to remove ambiguity from paper-based medical record keeping. This case became the first test for software in a medical liability action put before a jury. Instant Medical History is a product of Primetime Medical Software.

Chapter 34

An Innovator's Personal Experience and Vision

Prelude: The author shares his experiences with innovation and his vision of the future of innovation.

Courage rather than analysis dictates the truly important rules for identifying priorities:

- *Pick the future as against the past;*
- *Focus on opportunity rather than on problem;*
- *Choose your own direction—rather than climb on the bandwagon; and*
- *Aim high, aim for something that will make a difference rather than for something that is "safe" and easy to do.*

Peter F. Drucker, 1966

Making a Difference

What will make a difference in raising quality, improving outcomes, and lowering costs in the U.S. health system? The answer lies in the hearts, minds, and actions of health consumers and physicians, not with business or government activism. Consumers' choices and physicians' pens, with which they write orders, have always generated, in one way or another, the majority of health costs. Physicians prescribe drugs, perform procedures, hospitalize, transfer patients to other health care institutions, and order most of the myriad of procedures that go into caring for patients. Most of these things are done as the result of physicians' written orders.

Hospitals consume 31 percent of the health care dollar compared to 22 percent for doctors, 11 percent for prescription drugs, and 36 percent for all other costs. But doctors issue the orders (U.S. Department of Justice, 2004). Hospitals recognize physicians' ordering powers. In 2002, Dr. Charles A. Peck, an internist and an Arthur Andersen Partner in Atlanta, wrote:

> *Physicians and hospitals collectively suffer from "mural dyslexia," characterized by an inability to read the handwriting on the wall. The handwriting is indeed clear. To survive, hospitals must collaborate with doctors because the most expensive piece of medical technology is the physician's pen. In turn, to survive, doctors must collaborate with someone, and the hospital remains the natural partner.* (Peck, 2002)

Patient Data

The physician's office is where data is collected that can be used to judge the patient's present health, predict future diseases, and create predictive models that will improve outcomes. Most doctors routinely collect four data sets in their offices:

1. Demographic data—age, sex, marital status, race, and occupation
2. Physical data—temperature, weight, blood pressure, height (which can be used to calculate body mass index and establish obesity status), and hip circumference (not usually measured but useful because ratio correlates with coronary risk)
3. Clinical data—medications, allergies, past and present medical history, recent surgeries, chief complaint, and symptoms
4. Laboratory, cardiac, and X-ray data—routine electrocardiograms, stress test results, chemistry profiles, lipid profiles, hematology profiles, chest X-rays, and increasingly, CT, MRI, and echo images

In recent years, unknown to most doctors, another piece of data has been routinely collected in doctors' offices—their prescribing habits. This has proved controversial for two reasons:

1. Selling data on doctors' prescribing habits is lucrative for information companies, such as IMS Health of Fairfield, Connecticut
2. Doctors, who may be confronted by drug company representatives bearing this data, regard exposing their prescription habits as invading their privacy. (Steinbrook, 2006a)

The Power of Mundane Data

Data sets collected in physicians' offices may seem mundane to the average consumer, but they are not. The data includes demographic information, date of death, results of laboratory and ex-ray tests, and hospitalizations. These data sets have predictive power in judging patients' future health and the effectiveness of health interventions and behavioral changes influencing health.

The very routineness of these data is what is important. In constructing any predictive model of what lies ahead, it is essential to have data nearly universally available. This fundamental data should be included in personal health records, which is why those records will be so essential to the efficiency and effectiveness of any future health system. Cutting costs to reduce spending is not enough. Developing a center to compare data showing the relative cost and outcome effectiveness is a much sounder and fairer approach (Wilensky, 2006).

As the co-owner of a large Minneapolis-based clinical laboratory, Lufkin Medical Laboratories, with the aid of University of Minnesota physics professor, Russell Hobbie and I, using an early version of the Internet, wrote a software program based on disease patterns of 700 abnormal tests performed at our clinical laboratory. This is useful to clinicians because at a glance of the laboratory report, the clinician can consider the various diagnostic possibilities.

Using this program, we constructed and attached the report, Unified Presentation of Relevant Tests (UNIPORT), based on that information with every set of abnormal test results that emanated from the laboratory. Six million of these reports, which included the top 10 diagnostic possibilities, were generated over a 5-year span, without complaints from laboratory clients (indeed, the business grew at about 20 percent a year) and without any medical legal suits based on the physicians' failure to follow-up on diagnostic suggestions.

When multiple abnormal tests were present, the top 10 list of diagnostic possibilities contained the precise diagnosis 80 percent of the time. The software program was shut down when Smith Kline and French acquired the laboratory in 1985. Presumably, Smith Kline stopped the program because of its expense and because listing possibilities that were not acted on raised medical legal issues.

The Health Quotient

In the early 1980s, again working with Doctor Hobbie, I used software to develop an algorithm for health using the health quotient (HQ) as the physical health analogy of the IQ, the instrument for measuring intelligence. We realized estimates of future health often rest on physical measurements—blood pressure, pulse, body mass index (a function of height and body weight), waist and hip circumferences, blood chemistries, and a past personal or family history of heart attacks or strokes.

The program classified patients as being in superb health (HQ of 120 or more), average health (HQ of 80 to 120), subpar health (HQ of 50 to 70), and poor health (HQ of 50 or less).

With these HQ reports, a personal letter was sent to each patient explaining what the HQ meant and what to do about it, including seeing a doctor if HQ values were subpar or poor.

Among the values requiring immediate medical attention was a total cholesterol/HDL of 9.0 or more as a strong indicator of a possible future heart attack and a total cholesterol/HDL of 13.5 or more as an indicator of an impending heart attack. This information is of value because, given the knowledge of an impending heart attack, patients and their doctors can quickly take steps to avoid an attack.

Clinical Observations

Six years ago, in 2000, Doctors Allen Wenner, Donald Copeland, and I founded the High Performance Physician Institute. Its mission was to give conferences for practicing doctors to persuade and to teach them how to introduce electronic health records into their clinical practices. The institute's founders believed the electronic health record, in conjunction with an electronic medical history, generated by patients, would increase office efficiency, enhance patient and doctor satisfaction, and improve care.

One of the obstacles of introducing these records, however, outside of costs and practice disruption, is the high price of clinical history data entry. To introduce such data, either a nurse or data assistant is hired or someone takes the time to handwrite (approximately 30 words a minute) or dictate (about 150 words a minute) the data. The slowness and expense of any of these approaches are why clinical histories in medical offices tend to be sketchy and incomplete.

The institute, however, suggested that this data could be entered virtually for free. How? By the patients themselves. Patients could enter their own data using a software program such as Instant Medical History. This particular software program uses yes-or-no algorithms based on age, sex, and chief complaint, and requires less than 10 minutes to complete. Nobody, after all, knows more about why they are at the doctor's office than the patient, and no one is more accurate in entering their own personal data.

Patient data entry represents a missing piece in constructing a predictive model. It is:

- inexpensive (each doctor pays about $50 a month to hook it into an existing electronic record)
- uniform
- complete
- digitized

Google and Similar Data-Entry Models

Think for just a moment about the power of Google, the Internet's largest and fastest-growing search engine. Type in any combination of search terms into its search box. Immediately a list of prioritized possibilities will appear. This action gives new meaning to the word "instantaneity." Although the Google logic may be awesomely complicated, its use is amazingly simple. Google is the quintessential "disruptive technology" (Christensen, 2000) as exemplified in this letter to the editor in the *New England Journal of Medicine:*

...And a Diagnostic Test Was Performed

To the Editor: At a recent case conference with a distinguished visiting professor, a fellow in allergy and immunology presented the case of an infant with diarrhea; an unusual rash ("alligator skin"); multiple immunologic abnormalities, including low T-cell function; tissue eosinophilia (of the gastric mucosa) as well as peripheral eosinophilia; and an apparent X-linked genetic pattern (several male relatives died in infancy). The attending physicians and house staff discussed several diagnostic possibilities, but no consensus was reached.

Finally, the visiting professor asked the fellow if she had made a diagnosis, and she reported that she had indeed and mentioned a rare syndrome known as IPEX (immunodeficiency, polyendocrinopathy, enteropathy, X-linked). It appeared to fit the case, and everyone seemed satisfied. (Several weeks later, genetic testing on the baby revealed a mutation in the FOXP3 gene, confirming the diagnosis.)

"How did you make that diagnosis?" asked the professor. Came the reply, "Well, I had the skin-biopsy report, and I had a chart of the immunologic tests. So I entered the salient features into Google, and it popped right up."

"William Osler," I offered, "must be turning over in his grave. You Googled the diagnosis?"

Where does this lead us? Are we physicians no longer needed? Is an observer who can accurately select the findings to be entered in a Google search all we need for a diagnosis to appear, as if by magic?

The cases presented at clinicopathological conferences can be solved easily; no longer must the discussant talk at length about the differential diagnosis of fever with bradycardia.

Even worse, the Google diagnostician might be linked to an evidence-based medicine database, so a computer could e-mail the prescription to the e-druggist with no human involvement needed. The education of house staff is morphing into computer-search techniques. Surely this is a trend to watch.

> **Robert Greenwald, M.D.**
> **NorthShore–Long Island Jewish Health System**
> **Lake Success, New York (Greenwald, 2005)**

Innovation Talking and Action Points

Combine what you have just read with the descriptive information about the Archimedes and MedAI Models in Chapter 9,and you will see: The future is here. Focus on this opportunity.

Don't talk about it, do it.

Case Study

Data Mining and Innovation: Keys to U.S. Health Reform

By Richard L. Reece, MD

This is an edited version of an article that appeared on June 27, 2006, on Healthleadersmedia.com

. . . .

HealthLeaders contributor Preston Gee asserts that a political divide exists between market-driven and single-payer advocates who seek to resolve cost, coverage, and quality problems. Either solution, the title implies, harbors profound consequences for health care stakeholders.

It's possible that a powerful force embedded in American culture—our genius for innovation—will bridge the divide.

A New Solution

Experts point to four basic reform solutions that exist for the United States:

1. A national universal system of coverage
2. A consumer-driven, market-based system covering those able to pay
3. State-by-state universal coverage, Massachusetts-style
4. A national consumer-driven, market-based model with universal coverage through federal employee health benefits plan or the universal health voucher plan, as proposed by the Mayo Clinic

I propose another approach incorporating all these solutions—systematic innovation by government and market-based organizations. This solution will take time. It overlaps government and private sectors, and it is not without doubters.

Major Innovations

Six major innovations—sometimes inspired by government, sometimes undertaken independently or in concert with the private sector—are driving health reform:

1. data-mining reform
2. consumer-driven care
3. pay-for-performance initiatives

4. national electronic infrastructure building
5. state-by-state reform experimentation
6. "disruptive simplification" innovations at the practice-management level

Data mining may be the most important and sweeping innovation, because it gives the tools to restructure and rebuild the existing system based on irrefutable and impersonal data. According to Webopedia, the computer technology dictionary, data mining may be defined as:

> The class of database applications that look for hidden patterns in a group of data that can be used to predict future behavior. For example, data mining software can help retail companies find customers with common interests.

> The term "data mining" is commonly misused to describe software that presents data in new ways. True data mining software doesn't just change the presentation, but actually discovers previously unknown relationships among the data.

Four areas of data mining are transforming health care:

1. **Medicare Data Mining** This form of data mining is not new, but it remains an inexhaustible innovation source because of its size. John Wennberg and Alan Gettlesohn first explored the Medicare "mine" in 1973 when they published their classic findings on how medical care varied from one region of the country to the other.

   Ever since, Medicare data has been considered the sine qua non for studying and judging health costs and outcomes. Wennberg considers medical service variation across regions and academic centers as "unwarranted." The variation data, he concludes, does not correlate with better outcomes data (Wennberg, 2006).

   Fisher, Wennberg, and their colleagues at Dartmouth have proven beyond statistical doubt that "more is not better" (Fisher, 2003). Employers and health plans are aware Medicare data is a treasure trove for data miners wishing to improve quality and outcomes and to pay hospitals and doctors for performance, which is why the Business Roundtable, an association of chief executive officers representing 10 million employees and providing coverage for 34 million Americans, is pressuring the Bush administration to release all Medicare claims data (Business Roundtable, 2006).

2. **Pharmaceutical Data Mining** It isn't generally recognized that 75 percent of UnitedHealth Group profits come from outside the traditional HMO business. In 2005, Dr. Brian Gould, a former senior executive for UnitedHealth, remarked:

   > In early 1990, I moved to Minneapolis. I was in charge of United's Specialty Operations Division—all the non-HMO businesses. These included a pioneering pharmaceutical benefit company, Diversified Pharmaceutical Services. In 1993, we sold DPM to Smith Kline Beecham for an astonishing price of $2.3 billion.

   Under the terms of agreement, UnitedHealth Group agreed to provide Smith Kline Beecham "with access to medical data and outcomes analysis." This meant access to United's pharmaceutical data mining operation data. For example, if United had pharmaceutical claims data indicating who was taking insulin, Smith Kline could use that data to study a huge population of diabetics.

   United has not abandoned pharmaceutical data mining. Its Ingenix division provides clinic research services, medical education services, and therapeutic outcomes and epidemiology research data to pharmaceutical companies, biotechnology companies, and medical device manufacturers.

3. **Printed Word Data Mining** Google is so powerful that it has become a verb. One no longer looks up information in medical libraries, one "googles" medical information. Google is turning the medical world upside-down. Medical journals, for example, are struggling to survive because of drops in advertising and readership.

4. **Clinical Practice Management and Practice Pattern Data Mining** The real potential of practice management clinical data mining lies in two areas:

   1. practice pattern grouping using existing data to define costs and consequences
   2. predictive modeling using broad clinical and financial databases to define the effect of current patient behavior, diagnoses, and interventions on future outcomes and costs

Practice pattern grouping often goes by the name of episode grouping. As government and private health care organizations seek to deliver top-quality care more cost effectively, episode grouping has come into vogue. By clustering costs around a clinical episode—everything from doctors involved, to diagnoses, to medications, to interventions, to hospitalization, to rehabilitations, to nursing home care, to outcomes—you can more precisely analyze total outcomes and costs.

You can also more accurately—and fairly—assess physician performance. Much of the total cost, for example, of hospitalizations resides in the hospital's costs. Hospital charges make up about 80 percent of physician costs in the hospital setting. The hospital charges may be beyond the doctor's control.

On the other hand, drugs doctors prescribe or interventions they choose are not. It has been found that total episode costs may vary by factors of as much as 20 to 1. In these instances, and even with smaller variations, systematic or structural reforms are in order. True reform lies in rationalizing, not rationing, care.

Predictive modeling requires a more sophisticated mathematical approach and artificial intelligence deployment. One of the pioneers in this field is Dr. David Eddy, who, over the last 10 years at Kaiser Permanente, has developed a predictive model called the Archimedes model. This model provides a mathematically based lever that moves and manipulates vast amounts of data in a way that simulates reality.

Many proponents of consumer-driven care, pay-for-performance, electronic health and personal health records, and a national electronic information infrastructure believe electronic handling and application of data will change health care for the better. Certainly electronic data is one element for positive change. Not whether one can use data alone to identify and segregate the top performance is questionable. The broad consensus of the consumer community and other health professionals has an equally important role. That is why publications like the annual *U.S. News and World Report* of America's best hospitals and Castle and Connolly Medical Ltd.'s books on America's top doctors have been so widely read.

Role of Medical Schools

Innovation and entrepreneurship are not subjects medical schools teach. For the most part, the academic medical educational establishment completely ignores both subjects in their curricula. This may not hold true in MD-MBA programs, but it is the case for those acquiring an MD. It's possible the whole process is considered too commercial. Besides, innovation and entrepreneurial behavior are not something reputable doctors talk about. Openly science and professionalism are what count.

One does not talk about money: its making, investing, or spending. That will come if you are a good doctor. Unfortunately, as almost any "good" primary care doctor will tell you, being a "good doctor" does not correlate with income. One is not paid for intellect—or performance. One is paid for procedures.

Peter F. Drucker, the 20th century's leading management philosopher, would have regarded the medical establishment's monetary attitudes as vacuous and shortsighted.

Indeed, in *Innovation and Entrepreneurship: Practice and Principles,* Drucker said this:

> Innovation is the specific tool of entrepreneurs, the means by which they exploit change as an opportunity for a different business or a different service. It is capable of being presented as a discipline, capable of being learned, capable of being practiced. Entrepreneurs need to search purposefully for the sources of innovation, the changes and symptoms that indicate opportunities for successful innovation. And they need to know and to apply the principles of successful innovation. (Drucker, 1986)

Many health care professionals learn about innovation the hard way—through personal experimentation and failure. One thing they don't teach you in medical school is how to fail or to react to failure. For good reason, as a doctor, you are expected to succeed.

Until recent years, as a business, medicine has been relatively secure and risk free. That is too bad, because with accelerating technological and competitive changes, too many doctors are risk adverse, just when they need to be trying new approaches. What doctors need to accept is that failure is OK. It is alright to fail—as a businessperson. That is how you learn to innovate—and to succeed the next time around.

Conclusions—What to Expect

Key innovations will continue to transform U.S. health care. These innovations include information technology tools to better manage care and its costs, consumer-driven and -centered care, intensive management of chronic illnesses outside traditional settings, private-public partnerships to manage Medicare and Medicaid patients, and proliferating, customized ambulatory care and retail clinics to provide convenient and less costly care.

Innovations from the private sector will be insufficient to solve all cost, access, and quality problems. The problems are simply too big, too pervasive, and too intertwined with government payment. Government will have to play more decisive roles in oversight and payment. These roles may grow with the November 7, 2006, elections, which turned over control of the House and Senate to Democrats. Expect government to pay more concentrated attention to covering the 47 million uninsured, to government negotiation with pharmaceutical companies for Medicare coverage, congressional action to close the Medicare Drug "donut hole," more federal funding of stem cell research, more talk and action at the state level toward a single payer system, and to demands for more cost and quality transparency.

Abelson, R. (2005, September 22). Possible conflicts for doctors are seen on medical devices. *New York Times*, p. 1.

Academy of Medicine of Cleveland and Northern Ohio. (2006, July 13). CVS purchases Minute-Clinic for reported $170 million. Available: http://www.amcnoma.org/.

Agency for Health Care Research Quality (AHRQ). Press release. (2005, Sept.14). Available: http://www.ahrq.gov/news/press/pr2005/lowehrpr.htm.

Altman, S. H., & Doonan, M. (2006). Can Massachusetts lead the way in health care reform? *New England Journal of Medicine, 354*, 2093–2095.

American Academy of Family Physicians. (2006, June 22). America's family physicians urge retail health clinics put patients' health first. Available: http://www.aafp.com.

American Medical Association. (2003a, November). AMA survey: Medical students' opinion of the current medical liability environment. Chicago, IL: American Medical Association Division of Market Research and Analysis.

American Medical Association. (2003b, December 8). Medical students not immune to nation's medical liability crisis [press release]. Available: http://goliath.ecnext.com/coms2/gi_0199-1181610/Medical-Students-Not-Immune-to.html.

Anand, S. (2005, August 17). Doctors' creed: Insure thyself. *Wall Street Journal*, p. 1.

Anders, G. (2006, April 18). As patients, doctors feel pinch, insurer's CEO makes a billion. *Wall Street Journal*, p. 1.

Armstrong, D. (2005, May 3). Referral arrangements between doctors and medical imaging centers. *Wall Street Journal*, p. 1.

Asch, S. M., Kerr, E. A., Keesey, J., Adams, J. L., Setodji, C. M., Malik, S., & McGlynn E. (2006). Who is at greatest risk for receiving poor quality care? *New England Journal of Medicine, 354*, 1147–1154.

Assistant Secretary for Planning and Evaluation (ASPE). (2005, May). Long-term growth of medical expenditures—public and private [issue brief]. Available: http://aspe.hhs.gov/health/MedicalExpenditures/index.shtml.

Associated Press. (2006, June 15). Hospital initiative to cut errors, finds almost 122,000 lives saved. *New York Times*.

Average hospital margins by bed, size, 1997–2004. (2006, April 1). *Managed Healthcare Executive.* Available: http://www.managedhealthcareexecutive.com/mhe/article/articleDetail. jsp?id= 315075.

Axelrod, R., & Vogel, D. (2003). Predictive modeling in health plans. *Disease Management and Health Outcomes, 11*(12), 779–787.

Bachman, J. (2004). The patient-computer interview. *Mayo Clinic Proceedings*, *78*, 67–78.

Baldwin, F. D. (2004, August). Managing customer relationships. *Health Care Informatics*.

Barbaro, M. (2006, February 24). Wal-Mart to expand health plans. *New York Times*, p. 1.

Barry, P. (2006, July–August). Coverage for all. *AARP Bulletin Online*. Available: http://www.aarp.org.

Bartlett, J. (1992). *Familiar Quotations* (16th ed.). Boston: Little, Brown.

Baum, M. (1996). Quack cancer cures or scientific remedies? *Journal of the Royal Society of Medicine*, *84*, 543–547.

Baum, N. (2004a, October). Clinicians can learn from alternative practitioners. *Physician Practice Options*.

Baum, N. (2004b, May). Physicians become wary of litigious patients. *Physician Practice Options*.

Baum, N., with Zablocki, E. (1996). *Take Charge of Your Practice Before Someone Else Does*. Baltimore, MD: Aspen Publishers.

Bean, J. (2005, February 10). Statement of the Alliance of Specialty Physicians before House Energy and Commerce Subcommittee. *Current Issues Related to Medical Practice Reform*.

Beinfeld, M., Gazeel, G. S. (2005). Diagnostic imaging costs: Are they driving up costs of hospital care? *Radiology*, *235*, 934–939.

Belasco, J. A. (1990). *Teaching the Elephant to Dance: Empowering Change in Your Organization*. New York: Crown Publishers.

Belluck, P. (2006, April 4). Massachusetts sets health plan for nearly all. *New York Times*, p. 1.

Bent, S., Kane, C., Sheno, K., Neuhaus, J., Hudes, E. S., Goldberg, H., & Avias, A. (2006, February 9). Saw palmetto for benign prostatic hyperplasia. *New England Journal of Medicine*, *354*, 557–566.

Berk, M., & Monheirt, A. (2001, March/April). The concentration of health expenditures revisited. *Health Affairs*, *20*, 9–18.

Berry, L., & Bendapudi, N. (2003, February 1). Clueing in customers. *Harvard Business Review*, *81*, 100–106.

Berwick, D. (2005, December 12). Six keys to safer hospitals: A set of simple principles could prevent 100,000 needless deaths each year. *Newsweek*.

Betbeze, P. (2005, December 30). The employers' last stand. *HealthLeaders Magazine*. Available: http://www.healthleadersmedia.com/view_feature.cfm?content_id=75917.

Betbeze, P. (2006, April 19). Attention healthcare shoppers. *HealthLeaders Magazine*. Available: http://www.healthleadersmedia.com/view_feature.cfm?content_id=79112.

Blackwell, B. (1973). Drug therapy: Patient compliance. *New England Journal of Medicine*, *289*, 249–252.

Blair, R. (2006, February). RHIO nation. *Health Management Technology*.

BlueCross BlueShield Association. (2006, December 5). Blue Healthcare Services: Blue brings it all together. Available: http://www.bcbs.com/innovations/healthcare/.

Blumenthal, D. (2006, July 6). Employer-sponsored health insurance in the United States: Origins and implications. *New England Journal of Medicine*, *355*, 82–88.

Bogdanich, W. (2006, July 17). Hospital chiefs get paid for advice on selling to hospitals. *New York Times*, p. 1.

Bogdanich, W., Meier, B., & Walsh, M. (2002, March 4). Medicine's middlemen: Questions of conflicts at 2 hospital buying groups. *New York Times*, p. 1.

Brennan, T. (2002). Luxury primary care—market innovation or threat to access? *New England Journal of Medicine*, *346*, 1165–1168.

Brody, J. E. (2005, February 8). A new set of knees comes at a price—a whole lot of pain. *New York Times.*

Brooks, R., & Menachiemi, N. (2006). Physicians' use of email with patients: Factors influencing electronic communication and adherence to best practices. *Journal of Medical Internet Research, 8,* 2.

Business Roundtable. (2006, August 22). Business Roundtable applauds signing of executive order to increase health care quality and transparency [press release]. Available: http://www.businessroundtable.org/taskForces/taskforce/document.aspx?qs=7015BF159FC49514481138A74EA1851159169FEB56A36B2AC.

Butcher, L. (2005, September 16). St. Luke's helps consumers determine costs upfront. *Kansas City Business Journal,* p. 1.

Cain, B. (2006, June). Physician P4P pioneer. *HealthLeaders Magazine.*

Califano, J. (1977). Remarks before the American Medical Association. *Minnesota Medicine, 60,* 601–605.

Cannon, D., & Appleby, J. (2006, January 3). Hospital building boom in "burbs." *USA Today,* p. 1.

Carey, B. (2006, February 3). When trust in doctors erodes, other treatments fill the void. *New York Times,* p. 1.

Carey, W. P. (2006, April 6). Transforming U.S. health care: Supply-chain makeover rejuvenates health center. *Knowledge@W.P. Carey.* Available: http://knowledge.wpcarey.asu.edu/index.cfm?fa=viewArticle&id=1223&specialId=42.

Carroll, J. (2005, March). Going on the offensive against defensive medicine. *Managed Care Magazine.*

CBS News. (2006, June 17). A future doctor shortage? A growing lack of new doctors could be American's next health crisis. Los Angeles.

Cherney, E. (2006, April 18). New ways to monitor patients at home. *Wall Street Journal,* p. 1.

Chin, T. (2005, June 6). Medem launches personal health record service. *American Medical News,* p. 1.

Christensen, C. M. (2000). *The Innovator's Dilemma.* New York: HarperBusiness.

Cilingerian, J. A. (2004). Who has star quality? In Herzlinger, R. (ed.), *Consumer-Driven Health Care: Implications for Providers, Payers, and Policymakers.* San Francisco: Jossey-Bass.

Citizen's Health Care Working Group. (2006, June). *Preliminary Report.* Washington, D.C.: Author.

Clancy, C. (2006, March 27). Pay for performance: The train has left the station, but where is it taking us? [editorial]. Medscape General Medicine. Available: http://www.medscape.com.

Claxton, G., Gabel, J., Gill, I., Pickreign, J., Whitemore, H., Finder, B., Rouhani, S., Hawkins, S., Rowland, D. (2005, September 14). What high-deductible plans look like: Findings from a national survey of employers, 2005. A Web exclusive. *Health Affairs, 10,* 1377.

CNNMoney.com. (2006, July 26). The senator from Starbucks: Howard Schultz's mission: Get CEOs to step-up health-care reform. Available: http://www.cnn.com.

Coburn, T., & Herzlinger, R. (2006, May 18). They'd sooner fix Medicaid [editorial]. *Wall Street Journal.*

Cogan, J. F., Hubbard, R. G., & Kessler, D. P. (2005). *Healthy, Wealthy, and Wise: Five Steps to a Better Health System.* Washington, DC: AIE Press and the Hoover Institute.

Commonwealth Fund. (2006, April). Gaps in health insurance: An all American problem. *Commonwealth Fund Digest.* Available: http://www.cmwf.org.

Consortium for Southeastern Hypertension Control. (2006, June 1). Home page. Available: http://www.cosehc.com.

Cortese, D. A., & Smoldt, R. K. (2006). Healing America's ailing health system. *Mayo Clinic Proceedings, 81*, 492–496.

Council of Supply Chain Management Professionals. (2004). Home page. Available: http://www.supply-chain.org.

Cumming, R., Knutson, A., Cameron, B., & Derrick, B. (2002, May 24). Comparative analysis of claims-based methods of health risk assessment for commercial populations [research study]. Schaumburg, IL: Society of Actuaries.

Cutler, C. (2006, May 30). Aetna to offer secure, reimbursed online communications between members and doctors [press release].

CVS Corporation. (2006, July 13). CVS Corporation to acquire MinuteClinic, largest provider of retail-based health clinics in U.S. [press release].

Dalzell, M. (1999, October). California physicians struggling: Problems ahead for other states? *Managed Care Magazine.*

Daniels, S. (2005). *Leader's Guide to Hospital Case Management.* Sudbury, MA: Jones and Bartlett.

Dash, E. (2006, January 27). Health savings accounts attract Wall St. *New York Times*, p. 1.

Dash, E., & Freudenheim, M. (2006, October 16). Chief executive at health insurer is forced out in options inquiry. *New York Times*, p. 1.

De Kruif, P. (1943). *Kaiser Wakes the Doctors.* New York: Harcourt, Brace and Company.

Dell. (2006, April 10). Dell to enhance personal health records for U.S. employees with capability to import claims information: Initiative with WebMD provides online tool for managing personal health information. Available: http://www.dell.com/content/topics/global.aspx/corp/pressoffice/en/2006/2006_04_10_nv_000?c=us&l=en&s=corp.

Dionne, E. J. (2006, June 9). Lessons for Liberals in California. *Washington Post.*

Dingel says Bush ignores U.S. automakers. (2006, January 27). ConsumerAffairs.com. Available: http://www.consumeraffairs.com/news04/2006/01/auto_sales_dingel.html.

Drucker, P. F. (1960). *Managing in Turbulent Times.* New York: Harper & Row.

Drucker, P. F. (1968). *The Age of Discontinuity: Guidelines to Our Changing Society.* New York: Harper & Row.

Drucker, P. F. (1985). *Innovation and Entrepreneurship.* New York: Harper & Row.

Drucker, P. F. (2004). *The Daily Drucker.* New York: HarperBusiness.

Emanuel, E., & Fuchs, V. (2005, March 24). Health care vouchers—a proposal for universal coverage. *New England Journal of Medicine, 352*, 1255–1260.

Emergency room visits reach record high. (2005, May 26). MSNBC. Available: http://www.msnbc.msn.com/id/7995137/.

Executive Health Resources. (2006, November 17). Home page. Available: http://www.ehrdocs.com/.

Farber, S. (2001). *Beyond the White Coat: Intimate Reflections on Being a Doctor in Today's World,* The Woodlands, TX. Available: http://www.booklocker.com.

Federated Ambulatory Surgery Association. (2006). Physician ownership of ambulatory surgery centers. Available: http://www.fasa.org/docs/PhysicianOwnershipFactSheet.pdf.

Fisher, E. (2003, October 23). Medical care—is more always better? *New England Journal of Medicine, 349*, 1665–1667.

Fitzgerald, C. L. (2005, October). Highmark reins in diagnostic imaging. *Physician News Digest.*

Fletcher, A. (2003, December 12). Some states' laws scare off doctors in "high risk" specialties. *Denver Business Journal.*

Fletcher, A. (2006, February 20). New study sheds light on just who are the uninsured. *Denver Post.*

Florida, Pfizer urging state to restart drug rebate program. (2004, December 19). *Disease Management News*. Available: http://www.pfizerhealthsolutions.com/pdf/PHSNews/121004_disease_mgmt_news.pdf.

Ford, E. S., Giles, W. H., & Mokhad, D. (2004, October 27). Increasing prevalence of metabolic syndrome in U.S. *Diabetes Care, 10*, 2444–2449.

Fox, M. (2006, January 3). Primary care about to collapse. Reuters. Available: http://www.nonprofithealthcare.org/documentView.asp?docID=320.

Fox, W., & Pickering, J. (2006, May 20). Payment level comparison between public programs and commercial health plans in Washington State hospitals and physicians. Premera Blue Cross. Available: https://www.premera.com/stellent/groups/public/documents/pdfs/dynwat%3B5724_13206660_3636.pdf.

Freudenheim, M. (2006a, May 14). Attention shoppers: Low prices on shots in the clinic off aisle 7. *New York Times*, p. 1, Business Section.

Freudenheim, M. (2006b, May 25). The check is not in the mail. *New York Times*, p. 1, Business Section.

Freudenheim, M. (2006c, September 26). Health care costs rise twice as fast as inflation. *New York Times*, p. 1, Business Section.

Freudenheim, M. (2006d, June 25). Market forces pushing doctors to be more available. *New York Times*, p. 1, Business Section.

Friedman, T. L. (2005). *The World Is Flat: A Brief History of the Twenty-First Century*. New York: Farrar, Straus, and Giroux.

Fries, J. F., Harrington, H., Edwards, R., Kent, L. A., & Richardson, N. (1994). Randomized controlled trial of cost reductions from a health education program: The California Public Employees Retirement System (PERS) Study. *American Journal of Health Promotion, 8*, 216–223.

Fuchs, V. (1982). The battle for control of health care. *Health Affairs, 1*, 5–13.

Fuchs, V., & Emaneul, E. (2005). Health care reform: Why? What? When? *Health Affairs, 24*, 1399–1414.

Fuchs, V., & Sox, H. (2001). Physicians' views of the relative importance of thirty medical innovations. *Health Affairs, 20*, 30–42.

Fuhrman, V. (2005, August 18). Aetna reveals what doctors really charge to help people compare fees, a potential bargaining tool. *Wall Street Journal*, p. 1.

Fuhrman, V. (2006, April 11). An insurer tries a new strategy: Listen to patients. *Wall Street Journal*, p. 1, Personal Section.

Galewitz, P. (2005, October 17). Healthcare builds up. *HealthLeaders Magazine*.

Gerber, M. (2004). *The E-Myth Physician: Why Most Medical Practices Don't Work and What to Do About It*. New York: HarperBusiness Edition.

Glabman, M. (2005, May–June). Specialists shortage shakes emergency room: More hospitals forced to pay for specialist care. *Physician Executive*, pp. 1–10.

Gladwell, M. (2002). *The Tipping Point: How Little Things Make a Difference*. Boston: Back Bay Books.

Goldfield, N., Kelly, W., Averill, R., McCullough, E., and Vertexes, J. (2005, January–March). Pay for performance: An excellent idea that simply needs implementation. Quality Management in *Health Care. 14*(1), 31–44.

Goodman, D. C., Stukel, T. A., Chang, C., & Wennberg, J. E. (2006, March/April). End-of-life care at academic medical centers: Implications for future workforce requirements. *Health Affairs, 25*, 521–531.

Goodman, J. C., Musgrave, G., & Herrick, D. (2004). *Lives at Risk: Single-Payer Insurance Around the World.* Lanham, MD: Rowan & Littlefield.

Gore, L., & Hughes, C. (2004, September 28). Two-thirds of emergency department directors report on-call specialty coverage problems [press release]. American College of Emergency Physicians. Available: http://www.acep.org/webportal/Newsroom/NR/general/2004/TwoThirdsofEmergencyDepartmentDirectorsReportOnCallSpecialtyCoverageProblems.htm.

Greenwald, R. (2005). And a diagnostic test was performed. *New England Journal of Medicine, 353,* 2089–2090.

Griggs, T. (2006, October). Imaging centers could take big hit from Deficit Reduction Act. *Acadiana Medical News,* p. 1.

Haines, E. (2006, March 14). In new health plan, patients pay their share—or else. *Wall Street Journal,* p. 1, Personal Section.

Hallinan, J. (2005, June 21). Once seen as risk, one group of doctors changes its ways: Anesthesiologists now offer model of how to improve safety, lower premiums. *Wall Street Journal,* p. 1.

Halvorson, G. C., & Isham, G. (2004). *Epidemic of Care.* San Francisco: Jossey-Bass.

Handler, J., & Forelle, C. (2006, May 12). UnitedHealth cites deficiency in options grants. *Wall Street Journal,* p. 1.

Harris Interactive. (2005, October 26). Many agree on potential benefits of onsite clinics in major retail stores that can provide basic medical services, yet large numbers are also skeptical. Available: http://www.harrisinteractive.com/news/allnewsbydate.asp?NewsID=983.

Hawkins, J. (2001, March). Doctor dearth. *Hospitals and Health Networks,* pp. 1–3.

The health care opportunity [editorial]. (2006, February 1). *Wall Street Journal.*

Helliker, K., & Burton, T. (2003, November 4). Medical ignorance contributes to toll from aortic illness. *Wall Street Journal,* p. 1.

Herrick, D. (June 15, 2006). Consumer-driven care spurs innovation in physician services. *National Center for Policy Analysis, 559,* 1.

Herzlinger, R. E. (2004). *Consumer-Driven Health Care: Implications for Providers, Payers and Policymakers.* San Francisco: Jossey-Bass.

Herzlinger, R. E. (2006a, May 18). They'd sooner fix Medicaid: Can market incentives save the system? *Wall Street Journal.*

Herzlinger, R. E. (2006b, May 1). Why innovation in health care is so hard. *Harvard Business Review, 84,* 58–66.

Herzlinger, R. E., & Nurney, T. (2005, August 2). Medicine for Medicaid. *Wall Street Journal.*

Hiatt, H. (1976, June 24). Too much medical technology? *Wall Street Journal.*

Himmelstein, D., Warren, E., Thorne, D., & Woolhandler, S. (2005). Illness and injury as contributors to bankruptcy. *Health Affairs, 24,* 63–72.

Hollmer, M. (2006, July 7). Costs drive primary care docs elsewhere. *Boston Business Journal.*

Hopkins, J. (2006, January 25). Boomers sore knees, bad hearts drive investments. *USA Today.*

Hospital shuts down CPOE system [news bulletin]. (2003, January 23). *Health Data Management.*

Hounsfield, G. N., Ambrose, J., Perry, B. J., & Bridges, C. (1973). Computerized transverse axial scanning (tomography). *British Journal of Radiology, 46,* 1016–1051.

Howland, D. (1999, January). When doctors go retail: Is it OK to sell products? *ACP-ASIM Observer.*

Hurley, R. (2006, May/June). A failure of politics—not policy: A conversation with Gordon Bunnyman. *Health Affairs, 25,* 212–225.

Iglehart, J. (2006, June 29). The new era of imaging—progress and pitfalls. *New England Journal of Medicine, 354,* 2822–2828.

Inlander, C. B. (2006, August). Medical care at your local retail store. *Bottomline Health*, p. 1.

Institute of Clinical Systems Improvement. (2006). Home page. Available: http://www.icsi.org.

Institute of Medicine. (2000). *To err is human: Building a safer hospital system.* Washington, DC: National Academies Press.

Institute of Medicine. (2001). *Crossing the quality chasm: A new health system for the 21st century.* Washington, DC: Committee on Quality of Health Care in America, National Academies Press.

Institute of Medicine. (2006). *Prevalence of drug errors in the United States.* Washington, DC: National Academies Press.

Japenga, A. (2000, October). Is a luxury hospital in your future? *USA Weekend.*

Jayashree, N. (2005). Clinical research outsourcing overview: Current scenarios and future outlook. International Biopharmaceutical Association Publication. Available: http://www.ibpassociation.org/IBPA_articles/Outsoursing.htm.

Jefferson University physicians selected Allscripts for electronic health record. (2006, February 21). *Healthcare II and Biotechnology News.* Available: http://www.allscripts.com/ahsNews.aspx?type=Press%20Release.

Johnson, C. (2006, May 19). Former president says health costs hurting U.S. competitiveness. *Chicago Tribune.*

Kaiser, L. (2001, September 18). *Proceedings* [transcript]. Commonwealth North Forum. Available: http://www.commonwealthnorth.org/transcripts/kaiser.html.

Kaisernetwork.org. American medical associate examines retail clinic, other issues at annual meeting. June 12, 2006.

Kesselheim, A. S., Ferris, T. J., & Studdert, D. M. (2005). Will physician-level measures of clinical performance be used in malpractice litigation? *Journal of the American Medical Association, 95,* 1831–1834.

Kirking, D. M., Le, J. A., Ellis, J. J., Breisdander, B., & McKerscher, P. L. (2006). Patient-reported underuse of prescription medicine. *Medical Care Research Review, 63,* 427–446.

Kirkpatrick, R. (2006). When ends don't meet. *Minnesota Medicine, 30,* 36–38, 48.

Kizer, K. (1996). Transforming the veterans health care system—the "new VA." *Journal of the American Medical Association, 275,* 1069.

Klepper, B. (2006, March 1). Health-care crisis for business: Business leaders push reform to rein in costs and protect coverage. *Charlotte Observer.*

Knauss, C. (2005, June 10). In blow to Canada's health system, Quebec's law is voided. *New York Times.*

Knauss, C. (2006, February 19). Canada's private clinics surge as public system falters. *New York Times.*

Kolata, G. (2006a, May 21). The health of nations: Here, if you've got a pulse, you're sick. *New York Times.*

Kolata, G. (2006b, August 28). Making health care the engine that drives the economy. *New York Times.*

Kolata, G. (2006c, October 22). Study sees gain on lung cancer. *New York Times.*

Kolata, G. (2006d, February 23). 2 top selling arthritis drugs found to be ineffective. *New York Times.*

Kopel, H. (2004, April 4). My colleagues are wrecking healthcare. *Hartford Courant.*

Kuhn, H. (2006, July 18). Payment for imaging services under the Medicare physician fee schedule. House Subcommittee on Health of the Committee for Energy and Commerce, Centers for Medicare and Medicaid.

Landro, L. (2005, December 14). Managing expectations of surgery. *Wall Street Journal.*

Lawlor, P., & McFadden, S. (2006, March 10–16). Area's fastest growing companies, and area's 100 largest private companies. *Boston Business Journal*, p. 26.

Lawrence, D. (2002). *From chaos to care: The promise of team-based medicine.* New York: Perseus Publishing.

Leavitt, M. (2006, March 14). Remarks as delivered by the Honorable Mike Leacitt, Secretary of Health and Human Services, Commonwealth Club of California.

Lohr, S. (2005, February 19). Health industry under pressure to computerize. *New York Times.*

The lopsided Bush health plan [editorial]. (2006, February 3). *New York Times.* Available: http://www.nytimes.com/2006/02/03/opinion/03fri1.html?ex=1296622800&en=94827fde05a3db38&ei=5090&partner=rssuserland&emc=rss.

Lueck, S. (2005, February 7). Surging costs for Medicaid ravage state, federal budgets. *Wall Street Journal.*

Lundine, S. (2006, May 12). Jewett Orthopaedic opens specialty walk-in clinic. *Orlando Business Journal.*

Lyall, S. (2006, May 7). In a dentist shortage, British (ouch!) do it themselves. *New York Times.*

Mann, D. (2006, March 24). Joint replacement surgery on the rise: Study: Sharp increase in artificial knees and hips. *WebMD Medical News.* Available: http://www.medicinenet.com/script/main/art.asp?articlekey=60714.

Market competition gives way to benefit of cooperation: Rival hospitals in Greater Cincinnati unite to share clinical information via an SSL VPN and to improve patient care. (2004, November 1). *Health Management Technology.* Available: http://www.healthmgttech.com/archives/1104/1104market_competition.htm.

Martin, D. P., Hunt, J. R., Hughes, M., & Conrad, D. A. (1990). The Planetree Hospital Project: An example of the patient as partner. *Hospital Health Services Administration, 35,* 591–601.

Mayo Clinic National Symposium on Health Care Reform, May 21–23, 2006. Mayo Clinic. Available: http://www.mayoclinic.org/healthpolicycenter/2006-symposium.html.

Mays, G., Bodenheimer, T. Felland, L. E., Gerland, A. M., Pham, H. H., Regopoulos, L. E. (2005, November). Growth fuels hospital competition and challenges Greenville safety net (Community Report No. 10). Center for Studying Health System Change. Available: http://www.hschange.com/CONTENT/797/.

McDonald, J. (2006, February 27). Natural remedy users loyal, studies or not. *Hartford Courant.*

McGee, M. (2004, January 19). $40 M booster shot: Insurers offer free PDAs and PCs hoping to speed adoption by doctors. *Information Week.*

Medem.com. (2003, February 3). Medem-Center agreement delivers online consultation and new patients to physician practices [press release].

Medicare Payment Advisory Commission (MedPac). (2005, March). *Report to the Congress: Physician-owned specialty hospitals.* Washington, DC: Author.

Meier, B. (2006, April 27). Doctors urge safety panels for devices. *New York Times.*

Merritt Hawkins and Associates. (n.d.). *2005 Review of Physician Recruiting Incentives.* Available: http://www.merritthawkins.com/pdf/2005_incentive_survey.pdf.

Meza, J. (1998, May). Waiting times in a physician office. *American Journal of Managed Care,* pp. 703–712.

MGMA. (2004). Malpractice Online survey of 770 group practices representing 12,357 physicians.

Miniter, B. (2006, April 12). Bad medicine: What's wrong with RomneyCare? *Opinion Journal.* Available: http://www.opinionjournal.com/columnists/bminiter/?id=110008218.

Molzen, G. (2003, September 3). New EMTALA regulation could increase shortage of on-call specialists in emergency department [press release]. American College of Emergency Physicians. Available: http://www.acep.org/webportal/Newsroom/NR/general/2003/New EMTALARegulationCouldIncreaseShortageofOnCallSpecialistsinEmergencyDepartments .htm.

Mongan, J., Mechanic, R., Lee, T. (2006, December). Transforming U.S. health care: Policy challenges affecting the integration and improvement of care. The Brookings Institution. Available: http://www.brookings.edu/views/papers/20061215_mongan.htm

Moore, Gordon (2006). Netting better results. Institute of Healthcare Improvement. Available: http://IHI. org.

Mullan, F. (2002). *Big doctoring in America: Profiles of primary care.* Berkeley: University of California Press.

Muneke, T. (2000, January 31). *Health and the Devil's Staircase, business enterprise solutions and the Devil's staircase, business enterprise solutions and technology.* Washington, DC: Veteran's Hospital Administration.

Naik, G. (2006, May 8). To reduce errors, hospitals prescribe innovative designs. *Wall Street Journal.*

Naisbitt, J. (1982). *Megatrends: Ten New Directions Transforming Our Lives.* New York: Warner Books.

National Center for Complementary and Alternative Medicine. (2002). Study shows St. John's wort ineffective for major depression of moderate severity [news release]. Bethesda, MD: National Institutes of Health.

National Center for Complementary and Alternative Medicine. (2006). What is complementary and alternative medicine. Bethesda, MD: National Institutes of Health. Available: http://nccam .nih.gov/health/whatiscom/.

National Committee for Quality Assurance. (2004). *State of health care quality: 2004.* Washington, DC: Author.

Neurath, P. (2005, October 28). Docs quit independent practices to join hospitals. *Puget Sound Business Journal.*

Newman, N. (2006, January 27). HSAs—a Wall Street bonanza. NathanNewman.org. Available: http://www.nathannewman.org/log/archives/003619.shtml.

Newton, J. (2006, June 23). High deductible: A dilemma. CNHI News Service. Available: http://www.cnhins.com/finance/cnhinsfinance_story_174110645.html.

Nolan, T., & Berwick, D. M. (2006). All-or-none measurement raises the bar in performance. *Journal of the American Medical Association, 295,* 1168–1170.

Nordernberg, T. (2000, January–February). The healing power of placebos. *FDA Consumer Magazine.*

Nowak, S. (2006, January 31). How consumerism is driving a fundamental shift in healthcare communication. *CRM Buyer.*

OBrien, J. (2006). *Alternative risk transfer solution.* Wilmington, DE: Wilmington Trust Corporation. Available: http://www.captive.com/service/WilmingtonTrust/images%20and%20pdf/medmalwhitepaper.pdf.

Ouchi, W. (1984). *The M-Form Society: How American Teamwork Can Recapture the Competitive Edge.* Reading, MA: Addison-Wesley.

Pack, T. (2006a, May 31). Healthways $307 M deal opens door to Medicaid market. *Nashville Tennessean.*

Pack, T. (2006b, May 1). Insurers to put patient files on Web. *Nashville Tennessean.*

Pack, T. (2006c, May 19). Saint Thomas Specialty Hospital maneuvers through cracks: Piggybacks on hospital campus, certificate of need. *Nashville Tennessean.*

Pallanto, K. (2006, February 28). Healing in the lap of luxury. *Forbes.*

Payer, L. (1989). *Medicine and culture: Varieties of treatment in the United States, England, West Germany, and France.* New York: Penguin Group.

Pear, R. (2003, September 3). Emergency rooms get new rules on patient care. *New York Times.*

Pear, R. (2006a, July 17). Bush administration plans Medicare changes. *New York Times.*

Pear, R. (2006b, April 11). Employers push White House to disclose Medicare data. *New York Times.*

Pear, R. (2006c, August 3). Scaling back changes to Medicare payments. *New York Times.*

Peck, C. A. (2002, January–February). The enterprise circle (partnerships between physicians and health care systems). *Physician Executive, 27,* 12–17.

Peitgen, H.-O., Jurgens, H., & Saupe, D. (1992). *Chaos and fractals: New frontiers of science.* Berlin, Germany: Springer-Verlag.

Pennington, B. (2006, April 16). Baby boomers remain active, and so do their doctors. *New York Times.*

Perry, D. (1997). Patient patients no more: Aging baby boomers and health care. In American College of Physician Executives (ed.), *Making Sense of Managed Care, Volume II: Strategic Positioning.* San Francisco: Jossey-Bass.

Peters, T. J., & Waterman, R. H., Jr. (1982). *In Search of Excellence: Lessons from America's Best-Run Companies.* New York: Harper & Row.

Pffeninger, J., & Fowler, G. (2003). *Pffeninger and Fowler's procedures for primary care* (2nd ed.). St. Louis, MO: CV Mosby.

Pfizer Health Solutions. (2004, November 9). Florida and Pfizer report innovative partnership has delivered on promise of better health at lower cost for thousands of Medicaid recipients [press release]. Available: http://www.prnewswire.com/cgi-bin/stories.pl?ACCT=104& STORY=/www/story/11-09-2004/0002399256&EDATE=.

Piette, J., Heisler, M., & Wagner, T. (2004). Cost-related medication use. *Archives of Internal Medicine, 164,* 1749–1755.

Planetree. (2006, November). Home page. Available: http://www.planetree.org/.

Porter, M., & Teisberg, E. (2005). *Redefining health care: Creating value-based competition on results.* Boston: Harvard University Press.

Portman, R., Vigilante, K., & Ecken, B. (2005, June 15). Can a national healthcare information system work? *Strategy and Business.* Available: http://www.strategy-business.com/ sbkwarticle/sbkw050615?tid=230&pg=all.

President Bush participates in panel on health savings accounts [press release]. (2006, April 5). Office of the Press Secretary, White House. Available: http://www.whitehouse.gov/news/ releases/2006/04/20060405-5.html.

Rauber, C. (2003, April 18). Quiet giant. *HealthLeaders Magazine.*

Reece, R. L. (1988a). *And Who Shall Care for the Sick? The Corporate Transformation of Medicine in Minnesota.* Minneapolis, MN: Media Medicus.

Reece, R. L. (1988b). Mayo diversifies into a national system: An interview with W. Eugene Mayberry, MD, Chairman of the Board of Directors, Mayo Clinic. In Reece, R. L. (ed.), *And Who Shall Care for the Sick: The Corporate Transformation of Medicine in Minnesota.* Minneapolis, MN: Media Medicus.

Reece, R. L. (1998, July 15). Mayo executive says federal fraud investigation is unfair, fragmented: Interview with Robert R. Waller, MD. *Physician Practice Options.*

Reece, R. L. (1999, December 15). Refusing to use the Internet will not be an option for physicians, expert says. *Physician Practice Options.*

Reece, R. L. (2003a, December 3). Realities and boundaries in revitalizing primary care: Part 1. HealthLeaders Media. Available: http://www.healthleadersmedia.com/view_feature.cfm?content_id=50658.

Reece, R. L. (2003b, December 12). Realities and boundaries in revitalizing primary care: Part 2. HealthLeaders Media. Available: http://www.healthleadersmedia.com/view_feature.cfm?content_id=50895.

Reece, R. L. (2004a, June 17). Payment obstacles to hospital, patient and physician telecommunication. HealthLeaders Media. Available: http://www.healthleadersmedia.com/view_feature.cfm?content_id=55632.

Reece, R. L. (2004b, January 16). Realities and boundaries in revitalizing primary care: Part 3. HealthLeaders Media. Available: http://www.healthleadersmedia.com/view_feature.cfm?content_id=51676.

Reece, R. L. (2005a). Disease management as means of reforming delivery of chronic care, interview with Victor Villagra, MD. Chapter in Reece, R. L., *Voices of Health Reform*. Independence, MO: Practice Support Resources.

Reece, R. L. (2005b, August). Physicians as retailers: Banking on convergence. HealthLeaders Media. Available: http://www.healthleadersmedia.com/view_feature.cfm?content_id=71229.

Reece, R. L. (2005c). *Voices of Health Reform*. Independence, MO: Practice Support Resources.

Reece, R. L. (2006a, April 6). Feeling the impact: Key operational trends in healthcare. HealthLeaders Media. Available: http://www.healthleadersmedia.com/view_feature.cfm?content_id=78736.

Reece, R. L. (2006b, January 20). Thoughts of being a doctor, Part 2: Seven tips for assessing trends and knowing your friends. HealthLeaders Media. Available: http://www.healthleadersmedia.com/view_feature.cfm?content_id=76237.

RelayHealth. (2006, April 19). Blue Cross and Blue Shield of Florida offers coverage for nonurgent care delivered online via RelayHealth Services [press release].

Review and outlook, Medicaid Rx [editorial]. (2005, February 2). *Wall Street Journal*. Available: http://ww2.aegis.org/news/wsj/2005/WJ050201.html.

Robinson, J. (2001, July/August). Physician organization in California: Crisis or opportunity? *Health Affairs*, *20*, 81–96.

Romney, M. (2006, April 11). Health care for everyone? We've found a way. *Wall Street Journal*.

Rosenblatt, R., Andrilla, H., Curtin, T., & Hart, L. G. (2006, March 1). Shortages of medical personnel at community health centers: Implications for planned expansion. *Journal of the American Medical Association*, *295*, 1047–1049.

Rosenthal, M., Landon, B., Sharon-Lise, N., Frank, R., & Epstein, A. (2006, November 2). Pay for performance in commercial HMOs. *New England Journal of Medicine*, *355*, 1895–1902.

Rowland, C. (2006a, April 14). Mass. health plan seems unlikely to be U.S. model: Demographics in state's favor. *Boston Globe*.

Rowland, C. (2006b, April 17). Medical records project has breakaway winner: 170 offices of 180 pick Westborough startup. *Boston Globe*.

Rowland, D. (2005, June 28). *Medicaid: Addressing the future*. Testimony before Senate Special Committee on Aging, Washington, DC.

Rubenstein, S. (2006, June 13). Patients get new tools to price health care. *Wall Street Journal*.

Ruff, L. (2006, November 2). *Medical technologies: Boomers embrace quality of life solutions*. Paper presented at Washington Biotechnology Conference, 19th Annual J. P. Morgan Healthcare Conference, Seattle, WA.

Sagan, L. (1987). *The health of nations: The cause of sickness and well-being.* New York: Basic Books.

Salisbury, H. (1959, March 3). Gasopolis. *New York Times.*

Salz, P. A. (2006, March 27). The key to sustainable success is unfettered innovation. *Wall Street Journal.*

Satcher, D., & Pamies, R. (2006). *Multicultural medicine and health differences.* Columbus, OH: McGraw-Hill.

Saul, S. (2006, May 16). Unease about industry's role in hypertension debate. *New York Times.*

Sharpe, A. (1998, August 12). Boutique medicine: For the right price, these doctors treat patients as precious. *Wall Street Journal.*

Shaywitz, D., & Ausiello, D. (2002, February 23). Enter the physician executive. *Boston Globe.*

Short, W. (2005, March 25). HSAs treat ills of health care payment system. *Kansas City Business Journal.*

Shortell, S. (2006, February 6). *Pay for performance: An overview of the California experiment.* Paper presented at the National Pay for Performance Preconference, Los Angeles, CA.

Society for Innovative Medical Practice Design (SIMPD). (2006, November). Survey. Available: http://www.simpd.org.

Spence, J. (2006, Spring–Summer). Centered. *Duke Medical Magazine, 6,* 1.

Steinberg, S. (2005, May 8). Chronic pain: The enemy within. *USA Today.*

Steinbrook, R. (2006a, June 29). For sale: Physician prescribing data. *New England Journal of Medicine, 274,* 2745–2747.

Steinbrook, R. (2006b). Health care reform in Massachusetts—a work in progress. *New England Journal of Medicine, 354,* 2095–2098.

Straube, B. (2006, November 16). The CMS quality roadmap: Quality plus efficiency. *Health Affairs, Web Exclusive.*

Sullivan, D. (2006, May). Retail health clinics are rolling your way. *Family Practice Management, 13*(5). Available: http://www.aafp.org/fpm/20060500/65reta.html.

Taylor, H. (2002, May 8). *Most doctors report fear of malpractice liability has harmed their ability to provide quality care: Caused them to order unnecessary tests, provide unnecessary treatment and make unnecessary referrals* [Harris Poll #22]. Available: http://www.harrisinteractive .com/harris_poll/index.asp?PID=300.

Time to change Congress? (n.d.). Scholastic.com. Available: http://content.scholastic.com/browse/article.jsp?id=4732.

U.S. Budget and Economic data, projected Medicare outlays, 2005 (Trustees Report). Washington, DC: U.S. Government Printing Office.

U.S. Department of Health and Human Services. (2003, September 25). *Special update on Medical liability crisis.* Washington, DC: Author. Available: http://aspe.hhs.gov/daltcp/reports/mlupd1.htm.

U.S. Department of Justice. (2004). Pie chart of health care spending. Available: http://www.usdoj .gov/publichealth_care.

U.S. Department of Labor, Bureau of Labor Statistics. (2006). Physician and surgeons. Available: http://www.bls.gov/oco/ocos074.htm.

Walsh, M., & Meier, B. (2002, April 30). Hospitals sometimes lose money by using a buying group. *New York Times.*

Walton, M. (1986). *The Deming management method.* New York: Perigree.

Wang, C. (2006, November 8). 12 most common questions about insurance and complementary/ alternative medicine. About: Alternative Medicine. Available: http://www.yorku.ca/ychs/ Compl_Altern_Health.pdf.

Weed, W. (2004, December 14). The way we live now: 12-14-2003, questions for Raymond Damadian, Scanscam? *New York Times.*

Wennberg, J. (2006, January 24). Duncan W. Clark Lecture, New York Academy of Medicine, New York, NY.

Wennberg, J., & Gittelson, A. (1973). Small area variations in health care delivery. *Science, 182,* 1102.

White, C., Fisher, C., Mendelson, D., & Schulman, D. (2006, March). *State Medicaid disease management: Lessons learned from Florida.* Paper prepared by Health Strategic Consultancy, Faqua School of Business, Duke University, Durham, NC.

White House, employers at odds over disclosure of cost, quality data from Medicare. (2006, April 13). *Medical News Today.* Available: http://www.medicalnewstoday.com/medicalnews .php?newsid=41463.

Wikipedia. (2006, July). Vilfredo Pareto. Available: http://en.wikipedia.org/wiki/Vilfredo_Pareto.

Wilensky, G. R. (2006, November 7). Developing a center for comparative effectiveness information. *Health Affairs,* Web Exclusive. Available: http://www.cmwf.org/usr_doc/Wilensky_ develctrcompareffect_967_itl.pdf.

Willemssen, J. (1997, May 16). *Medicare Transactions System: Serious managerial and technical weaknesses threaten modernization.* Testimony before U.S. Government Accounting Office, Washington, DC.

Winslow, R. (2006, May 16). Care varies widely at two medical centers. *Wall Street Journal.*

What is an ATM? (2007). WiseGEEK. Available: http://www.wisegeek.com/what-is-an-atm.htm.

World Health Organization. (2000). *Health system performance in all member states, WHO indexes, estimates for 1997.* Geneva, Switzerland. Available: http://www.who.int/whr/2000/en/annex10_ en.pdf.

Yang, C., with Cappel, K. (2005, April 11). Another case entirely. *BusinessWeek Online.* Available: http://www.businessweek.com/magazine/content/05_15/b3928093.htm.

Zimmerman, B., Lindberg, C., & Pisket, P. (1998). *Edgeware: Insights from complexity science for health care leaders.* Irving, TX: VHA, Inc.

Zismer, D. K. (2003a, December). Ambulatory strategies: Not your hospital department anymore. *Discovery Dorsey Health Strategies.*

Zismer, D. K. (2003b, October/November). New thinking for a new medical specialties marketplace: Ten recommendations for not-for-profit community hospital boards. *Discovery Dorsey Health Strategies.*

Zismer, D. (2003c, February). Physician relations: The Achilles heel of hospital CEOs. *Discovery Dorsey Health Strategies.*

Zismer, D. K., & Hamel, M. (2003, March). Health care faculties as strategy. *Discovery Dorsey Health Strategies.*

Zugar, A. (2005, October 30). For a retainer, lavish care by "boutique doctors." *New York Times.*

Index